Diagnosis and Management of Type 2 Diabetes

Twelfth Edition

Steven V. Edelman, MD
Professor of Medicine
Division of Endocrinology and Metabolism
University of California, San Diego

Robert R. Henry, MD
Professor of Medicine
Division of Endocrinology and Metabolism
University of California, San Diego

PROFESSIONAL
COMMUNICATIONS, INC.

S0-ARM-127

Professional Communications, Inc.

A Medical Publishing & Communications Company

400 Center Bay Drive
West Islip, NY 11795
(t) 631/661-2852
(f) 631/661-2167

PO Box 10
Caddo, OK 74729-0010
(t) 580/745-9838
(f) 580/745-9837

For orders only, please call
1-800-337-9838
or visit our website at
www.pcibooks.com

ISBN: 978-1-932610-89-5

Printed in the United States of America

DISCLAIMER

The opinions expressed in this publication reflect those of the authors. However, the authors make no warranty regarding the contents of the publication. The protocols described herein are general and may not apply to a specific patient. Any product mentioned in this publication should be taken in accordance with the prescribing information provided by the manufacturer.

This text is printed on recycled paper.

DEDICATION

To our families,
for their tolerance and patience during
the writing of this book.

ACKNOWLEDGMENT

The authors thank the many individuals who have been a major force in shaping the field of diabetes and influencing the authors' opinions.

We would like also to express our appreciation to Phyllis Freeny for her excellent editorial assistance and Nikki D. Merrill for her exceptional graphic design work. Our assistants, George Rivera and Sue Pryor, are invaluable sources of help. Last, we would like to thank Malcolm Beasley for his patience and unyielding support in the writing of this book.

TABLE OF CONTENTS

TABLES

FIGURES

x

1
Diabetes Statistics

The prevalence and incidence of type 2 diabetes are increasing, not only in the United States, but also around the world. Diabetes affects approximately 285 million people worldwide and is expected to affect 438 million by 2030. The prevalence of diabetes refers to the total number of people known to have the disease at a particular time. In 2010, approximately 25.8 million Americans (8.3% of the US population) had diabetes, with a higher rate of prevalence in certain geographic areas, and approximately one third of those individuals were estimated to have undiagnosed diabetes. The prevalence has increased from 4.9% in 1990 to approximately 8.3% documented in 2010. Possible reasons for the substantial increases in the prevalence of diabetes over time include:

- Advancing age of the US population
- Reduced diabetic mortality rates due to improved screening, detection, and health care
- An increase in risk factors, such as obesity and physical inactivity.

The prevalence of diabetes increases with advancing age, reaching nearly 26.9% for those in the age ≥65 years category (**Figure 1.1**). The prevalence is similar for men and women up to the age of 65; for those over 65, the prevalence rates are slightly higher for men.

The prevalence of individuals with type 2 diabetes is considerably different depending on the race, ethnicity, and gender in the US population. Diabetes is more prevalent in American Indians, Alaska natives, Hispanics and Latinos, and non-Hispanic blacks (**Figure 1.2**). The increasing number of ethnic minorities in the United States may also contribute to the increasing prevalence of type 2 diabetes.

The lowering of the clinical diagnostic criteria for diabetes from a fasting blood glucose (FBG) of 140 mg/dL to 126 mg/dL has also contributed to the higher

FIGURE 1.1 — Estimated Percentage of Diagnosed and Undiagnosed Diabetes in People Aged ≥20 Years by Age Group: United States, 2005-2008

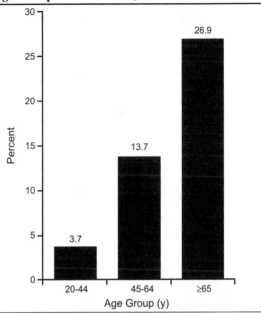

CDC National Diabetes Fact Sheet, 2011. CDC Web site. http://www.cdc.gov/diabetes/pubs/pdf/ndfs_2011.pdf. Accessed June 12, 2013.

prevalence of diabetes. Ethnic minorities not only have a higher prevalence of diabetes, but they also account for a greater number of individuals with undiagnosed diabetes as well as impaired fasting glucose (IFG), which is a risk factor for the development of type 2 diabetes.

The prevalence of undiagnosed diabetes also increases with age in both men and women. The rate of undiagnosed diabetes is estimated to be 7 million people in 2010. Undiagnosed type 2 diabetes is a serious problem. Insulin resistance and the associated macrovascular complications are well known to develop 10 to 15 years before the typical diagnosis of type 2 diabetes. In the United Kingdom Prospective Diabetes Study (UKPDS), 21% of newly diagnosed diabetics had diabetic retinopathy. Since diabetic retinopathy requires

FIGURE 1.2 — Estimated Age-Adjusted Total Prevalence of Diabetes in People Aged ≥20 Years by Race/Ethnicity: United States, 2005

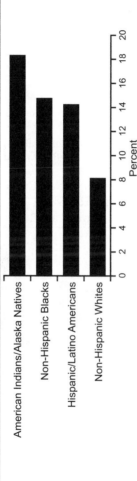

For American Indians/Alaska natives, the estimate of total prevalence was calculated using the estimate of diagnosed diabetes from the 2003 outpatient database of the Indian Health Service and the estimate of undiagnosed diabetes from the 1999-2002 National Health and Nutrition Examination Survey (NHANES). For the other groups, 1999-2002 NHANES estimates of total prevalence (both diagnosed and undiagnosed) were projected to year 2005.

CDC National Diabetes Fact Sheet. CDC Web site. http://www.cdc.gov/diabetes/pubs/estimates05.htm. Accessed June 12, 2013.

at least 4 to 7 years of hyperglycemia to develop, this indicates that diabetes went undiagnosed for this period of time. In addition, these newly diagnosed subjects also had a two to three times higher incidence of myocardial infarction (MI) and stroke compared with the general population.

The incidence of diabetes is the number of new cases diagnosed during a certain period of time, usually within the previous year. In 2010, about 1.9 million adults aged 20 years and older were newly diagnosed with diabetes. From 1998 through 2009, the number of new cases of diagnosed diabetes has increased sharply since the early 1990s (**Figure 1.3**). The estimated number of new cases of diagnosed diabetes by age in the United States in 2010 is shown in **Figure 1.4**.

From 1980 through 2009, the incidence of diagnosed diabetes was lower among adults aged 18 to 44 years

FIGURE 1.3 — Annual Number of New Cases of Diagnosed Diabetes Among Adults Aged 18 to 79 Years: United States, 2000-2009

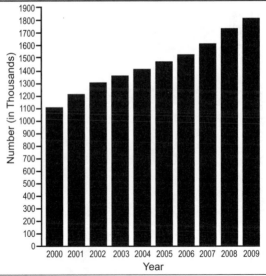

Adapted from CDC National Diabetes Fact Sheet: United States, 2011. CDC Web site. http://www.cdc.gov/diabetes/statistics/incidence /fig1.htm. Accessed June 12, 2013.

1

FIGURE 1.4 — Estimated Number of New Cases of Diagnosed Diabetes in People Aged ≥20 Years by Age Group: United States, 2010

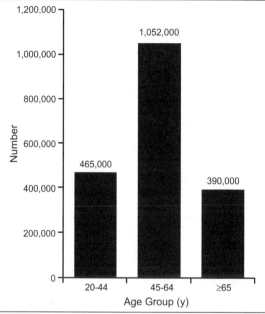

CDC National Diabetes Fact Sheet, 2011. CDC Web site. http://www.cdc.gov/diabetes/pubs/pdf/ndfs_2011.pdf. Accessed June 12, 2013.

compared with those older. During this period, the incidence of diagnosed diabetes increased among adults aged 18 to 44 years and 65 to 79 years. Among adults 45 to 64 years, the incidence of diagnosed diabetes showed little change during the 1980s but increased beginning in the 1990s through 2009 (**Figure 1.5**).

In a similar fashion to prevalence, the incidence rates for African Americans, Latinos, American Indians, Pacific Islanders, and Asian Indians are higher than for whites.

Some experts believe that the increasing incidence of diabetes is due to a genetic predisposition to diabetes commonly referred to as "the thrifty gene hypothesis," which theorizes that in the past, most individuals were hunters and gatherers doing physical labor for their daily existence. In times of famine, any individual

FIGURE 1.5 — Incidence of Diagnosed Diabetes per 1000 Population Aged 18 to 79 Years by Age: United States, 2000-2009

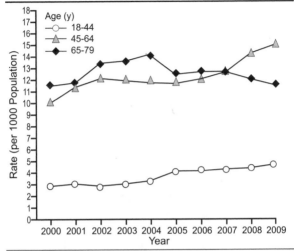

Adapted from CDC: National Diabetes Surveillance System. CDC Web site. http://www.cdc.gov/diabetes/statistics/incidence/fig3.htm. Accessed June 12, 2013.

who was not thin and had insulin resistance would be in a prime position to survive and not perish from starvation. In a relatively short period of time, individuals in our westernized societies are doing less physical labor, growing older, becoming much more obese, and consuming foods in greater amounts and with a much higher percentage of fat. What was a physiologic advantage in the past is now a physiologic disadvantage. All of these factors are thought to contribute to the increasing incidence of type 2 diabetes.

In conclusion, diabetes has achieved or is nearing epidemic proportions in many ethnic groups, not only in the United States, but also in other populations around the globe. Diabetes was the seventh leading cause of death in the United States in 2010. Much of the increase is due to our westernized society lifestyle that contributes significantly to the overall morbidity and mortality associated with type 2 diabetes. Overall, the risk of death for people with diabetes is about two times that of people without diabetes. In order to reduce the emotional and physical suffering of people with type 2 diabetes, a concerted effort should be undertaken toward the prevention, early detection, and aggressive management of this devastating condition.

SUGGESTED READING

Centers for Disease Control and Prevention. National diabetes fact sheet: national estimates and general information on diabetes and prediabetes in the United States, 2011. Atlanta, GA: U.S. Department of Health and Human Services, Centers for Disease Control and Prevention, 2011. CDC Web site. http://www.cdc.gov/diabetes/pubs/pdf/ndfs_2011.pdf. Accessed June 12, 2013.

International Diabetes Federation. *IDF Diabetes Atlas, 4th ed.* Brussels, Belgium: International Diabetes Federation, 2009. http://www.diabetesatlas.org. Accessed June 12, 2013.

World Diabetes Foundation Web site. http://www.worlddiabetesfoundation.org. Accessed June 12, 2013.

2 Pathophysiology and Natural History

Pathophysiology

Type 2 diabetes is known to have a strong genetic component with contributing environmental determinants. The genetic influence is readily apparent from data of twin and family studies. Identification of type 2 diabetes susceptibility genes has been elusive, and investigation of a number of candidate genes has been largely negative, yielding a very small population of patients (<5%) with genetic variation in any of the candidate genes studied to date.

It is likely that no single genetic defect will emerge to explain type 2 diabetes; thus the disease is heterogeneous, probably multigenic, and likely has a complex etiology. Even though the disease is genetically heterogeneous, there appears to be a fairly consistent phenotype once the disease is fully manifest. Most patients with type 2 diabetes and fasting hyperglycemia are characterized by:

- Insulin resistance
- Impaired insulin secretion
- Increased hepatic glucose production.

Although these three metabolic abnormalities have been well studied and characterized, the etiologic sequence has now come into focus.

It is probable that the increased hepatic glucose production of type 2 diabetes is secondary and can be fully reversed with a variety of forms of antidiabetic therapy. In addition, increased hepatic glucose production rates do not occur in the state of impaired glucose tolerance (IGT). This leaves insulin resistance, impaired insulin secretion, or both, as initiating abnormalities.

Accumulated evidence strongly supports the idea that both insulin resistance and impaired insulin secretion precede the onset of hyperglycemia and the type 2 diabetes phenotype. However, insulin resistance is quantitatively more severe in the prediabetic phenotype. In fact, studies have also shown that insulin secretion, including first-phase insulin responses to intravenous (IV) glucose, are either normal or increased in the prediabetic or IGT state. Thus substantial evidence from the literature indicates that those individuals who evolve from IGT to type 2 diabetes begin with insulin resistance.

Although genetic factors underlie the etiology of type 2 diabetes in most patients, acquired factors may also be contributory, such as:

- Obesity, particularly central or visceral obesity
- Sedentary lifestyle
- High-fat diet.

The aging process also contributes to the expression of type 2 diabetes in genetically susceptible individuals. When the β-cell function is able to compensate for insulin resistance, hyperinsulinemia develops, which maintains relatively normal glucose tolerance. Therefore, in the compensated insulin-resistant, hyperinsulinemic state, one has either normal glucose tolerance or IGT, but not diabetes. A subpopulation of individuals with compensated insulin resistance eventually go on to develop type 2 diabetes. The magnitude of this subpopulation depends on the methods used to detect glucose intolerance, the particular ethnic groups studied, and several other acquired and metabolic abnormalities that may be present. In addition, during the transition from the compensated state to frank type 2 diabetes, at least three pathophysiologic changes can be observed:

- First, basal hepatic glucose production rates increase, which is a characteristic feature of essentially all type 2 diabetes patients with fasting hyperglycemia.
- Second, the insulin resistance usually becomes more severe, which may be due to the degree of genetic load and/or acquired conditions, such as obesity, sedentary lifestyle, and aging. Antidiabetic treatment can completely normalize the elevated hepatic glucose production rates and partially ameliorate the insulin resistance so that the degree of insulin resistance returns approximately to the level present in the IGT state. Thus increased

hepatic output and the worsening of insulin resistance are likely to be secondary phenomena.

- The third and most marked change is a decrease in β-cell function and decline in insulin secretory ability. Whether this decline in insulin secretion is because of preprogrammed genetic abnormalities in β-cell function or acquired defects, such as glucose toxicity or β-cell exhaustion, or both, remains to be elucidated. Nevertheless, a marked decrease in β-cell function accompanies this transition and is thought to be a major contributor to the transition from IGT to type 2 diabetes.

In summary, the proposed etiologic sequence is that insulin resistance (probably genetic in origin) and abnormalities of pancreatic insulin secretion are manifest initially. The pancreas tries to compensate for insulin resistance, which leads to increased insulin secretion to maintain the prediabetic state. In time, the compensation fails and β-cell function declines, leading to hyperglycemia. Note, however, that most type 2 diabetic patients, particularly the majority who are obese at the time of initial diagnosis, are still hyperinsulinemic. In addition, the conversion of IGT to type 2 diabetes can also be influenced by:

- Ethnicity
- Degree of obesity
- Distribution of body fat
- Sedentary lifestyle
- Aging
- Other concomitant medical conditions.

The heterogeneous nature of type 2 diabetes and its natural history result in a varied response to the different antidiabetic agents over time.

The Natural History of Diabetes

Type 2 diabetes is at one end of the continuum represented by the fully compensated insulin-resistant state to IGT to frank type 2 diabetes. A triad of metabolic defects characterize type 2 diabetes: insulin resistance, nonautoimmune β-cell dysfunction, and inappropriately increased hepatic glucose production (**Figure 2.1**). The natural history of type 2 diabetes directly reflects the interrelationships between these three defects. The primary and earliest pathogenic lesion is insulin resistance, and the β-cell is able to compensate for a variable length of time by secreting supraphysiologic amounts of insulin. Insulin resistance, compensatory hyperinsulinemia, and mild postprandial hyperglycemia characterize IGT. Over time, however, the β-cell begins to fail and as relative insulin deficiency occurs, fasting hyperglycemia and full-blown type 2 diabetes develops. In addition, as insulin levels fall, the inhibitory effect of insulin on hepatic glucose production decreases and significant fasting hyperglycemia develops. Further progression of the disease is marked by an absolute insulin deficiency. Obesity, aging, weight gain in adulthood, and physical inactivity are some of the environmental factors that impact the

FIGURE 2.1 — The Natural History of Type 2 Diabetes

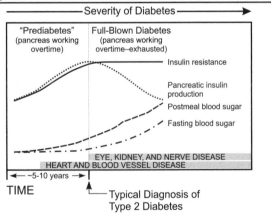

Insulin resistance can be present for many years before the diagnosis of diabetes. Blood glucose levels are not markedly elevated in the early stages of diabetes. Once the pancreas becomes exhausted, blood glucose values increase dramatically. As the pancreas becomes exhausted, the chance of achieving good glucose control with diet and exercise alone or with one oral agent is reduced.

natural history of diabetes, affecting its progression at all points in the continuum.

Screening patients for IGT is probably the best way for early identification of high-risk individuals since postprandial hyperglycemia occurs typically before the onset of fasting hyperglycemia in the natural history of type 2 diabetes. However, the diagnosis of IGT has required that an oral glucose tolerance test (OGTT) be performed. This procedure is cumbersome and has largely been replaced by fasting plasma glucose testing in general clinical practice because of convenience and greater reproducibility. This change in practice patterns underscores the importance of the new IFG criterion (ie, glucose between 110 and 125 mg/dL) in the clinical setting to detect people with glucose intolerance at an earlier stage in the natural history of the disease. The presence of IFG and IGT both indicate an increased risk for other syndromes associated with insulin resistance, such as hypertension and dyslipidemia, that also require an aggressive diagnostic and therapeutic plan.

Understanding the natural history of type 2 diabetes aids the clinician in identifying those patients most at risk for developing diabetes and aids in devising an effective treatment plan for those who already have the disease. Each of the available classes of oral antidiabetic agents has a different mechanism of action and is, therefore, potentially most effective at different stages in the continuum from IGT and IFG to frank diabetes. Given that insulin resistance is the major pathogenic factor in the prediabetic state of IGT and continues to persist in frank diabetes, efforts to enhance insulin sensitivity primarily in peripheral tissues using thiazolidinedione (TZD) therapy or in the liver using the biguanide metformin (MET) as first-line agents may be extremely useful in the prevention and early treatment of diabetes.

The potential benefits of intervention before the onset of diabetes and aggressive treatment once the disease becomes manifest are tremendous. Identifying and treating the individual with IGT will most likely reduce the incidence of macrovascular disease and type 2 diabetes. Early intervention in type 2 diabetes certainly reduces the incidence of microvascular disease and will most likely slow the progression of the disease itself. The primary care provider is uniquely positioned to promote and provide early prevention and to have a substantial impact on lessening the burden placed on individuals and society by type 2 diabetes.

SUGGESTED READING

DeFronzo RA, Ferrannini E. Insulin resistance. A multi-faceted syndrome responsible for NIDDM, obesity, hypertension, dyslipidemia and atherosclerotic cardiovascular disease. *Diabetes Care*. 1991;14:173-194.

Granner DK, O'Brien RM. Molecular physiology and genetics of NIDDM. Importance of metabolic staging. *Diabetes Care*. 1992;15:369-395.

Hamman RF. Genetic and environmental determinations of non–insulin-dependent diabetes mellitus (NIDDM). *Diabetes Metab Rev.* 1992;8:287-338.

Kobberling J, Tillil H. Genetic and nutritional factors in the etiology and pathogenesis of diabetes mellitus. *World Rev Nutr Diet*. 1990;63:102-115.

Olefsky JM. Etiology and pathogenesis of non–insulin-dependent diabetes (type II). In: *DeGroot: Endocrinology.* 2nd ed. New York, NY: Grune and Stratton, Inc; 1989:1369-1388.

Ramlo-Halsted BA, Edelman SV. The natural history of type 2 diabetes. *Primary Care Clin North Am.* 1998;26:771-789.

Rich SS. Mapping genes in diabetes: genetic epidemiological perspective. *Diabetes*. 1990;39:1315-1319.

Seely BL, Olefsky JM. Potential cellular and genetic mechanisms for insulin resistance in common disorders of obesity and diabetes. In: Moller D, ed. *Insulin Resistance and Its Clinical Disorders.* London, England: John Wiley and Sons, Ltd; 1993:187-252.

Tominaga M, Eguchi H, Manaka H, Igarashi K, Kato T, Sekikawa A. Impaired glucose tolerance is a risk factor for cardiovascular disease, but not impaired fasting glucose. The Funagata Diabetes Study. *Diabetes Care.* 1999;22:920-924.

Tuomilehto J, Lindstrom J, Eriksson JG, et al. Prevention of type 2 diabetes mellitus by changes in lifestyle among subjects with impaired glucose tolerance. *N Engl J Med.* 2001;344:1343-1350.

United Kingdom Prospective Diabetes Study Group. Overview of 6 years' therapy of type 2 diabetes: a progressive disease (UKPDS 16). *Diabetes.* 1995;44:1249-1258.

Weyer C, Bogardus C, Moss DM, Pratley RE. The natural history of insulin secretory dysfunction and insulin resistance in the pathogenesis of type 2 diabetes mellitus. *J Clin Invest.* 1999;104:787-794.

3 Classification

Diabetes mellitus and other categories of glucose intolerance can be divided into three main clinical categories:

- Diabetes mellitus (with four clinical subclasses)
- IGT
- Gestational diabetes mellitus (GDM).

The common denominator of a group of disorders that constitute the syndrome of diabetes mellitus is fasting or postprandial (random) hyperglycemia with plasma glucose levels above the limits established by the American Diabetes Association (ADA) Clinical Practice Recommendations. The four clinical classes of diabetes mellitus are:

- Type 1 diabetes mellitus (insulin-dependent)
- Type 2 diabetes mellitus (non–insulin-dependent)
- GDM
- Other specific types of diabetes associated with certain conditions.

Each of these subclasses has distinctive characteristics (**Table 3.1**).

Type 1 Diabetes Mellitus

Type 1 diabetes is defined by the presence of ketosis caused by complete or almost complete lack of insulin. Immunologic destruction of the β-cells is the etiologic basis of type 1 diabetes. An autoimmune cause is suggested by evidence of circulating antibodies to islet cells, to endogenous insulin, and/or to other antigenic components of islet cells at the time of diagnosis. Patients commonly are lean and may have experienced considerable weight loss prior to diagnosis. Most are diagnosed before age 20, although type 1 diabetes can develop at any age. Approximately 5% to 10% of all individuals who have been diagnosed with diabetes have type 1 diabetes. Daily

TABLE 3.1 — Distinguishing Characteristics of Diabetes Mellitus and Other Disorders of Glucose Intolerance

Category	Distinguishing Characteristics
Type 1 diabetes (insulin-dependent)	Any age, usually not obese, often abrupt onset, signs/symptoms usually before age 20, positive urine ketone test with hyperglycemia, insulin therapy necessary to sustain life and prevent ketoacidosis
Type 2 diabetes (non–insulin-dependent)	Usually over age 30 at diagnosis, obese, few classic symptoms, not prone to ketoacidosis unless under severe physical stress (eg, infection), exogenous insulin usually not needed to control hyperglycemia for many years
Gestational diabetes mellitus	Onset or discovery of glucose intolerance during pregnancy
Malnutrition-related diabetes mellitus	Young age (10 to 40), usually symptomatic, not prone to ketoacidosis, most require insulin therapy

Other Types of Diabetes Mellitus Associated With Certain Conditions

Secondary to:
- Pancreatic disease — Pancreatectomy, hemochromatosis, cystic fibrosis, chronic pancreatitis
- Endocrinopathies — Cushing's syndrome, acromegaly, pheochromocytoma, primary aldosteronism, glucagonoma
- Drugs and chemical agents — Certain antihypertensive drugs (thiazides, diuretics, or β-blockers), glucocorticoids, estrogen-containing preparations, nicotinic acid, phenytoin, catecholamines

Associated with:
- Insulin receptor abnormalities — Acanthosis nigricans
- Genetic syndromes — Lipodystrophic syndromes, muscular dystrophies, Huntington's chorea

- Miscellaneous conditions

Polycystic ovary disease

Impaired glucose tolerance

Plasma glucose levels are higher after a glucose load than normal but not diagnostic of diabetes mellitus

Adapted from American Diabetes Association. *Diabetes Care*. 2013;36(suppl 1):S11-S66.

3

therapy with exogenous insulin is required throughout the patient's life to prevent metabolic decompensation, ketoacidosis, and death.

Type 2 Diabetes Mellitus

Type 2 diabetes is the most common type of diabetes, accounting for 90% to 95% of all diagnosed cases in the United States, and is more prevalent among various non-Caucasian ethnic/racial populations, such as American Indians, African Americans, Pacific Islanders, and Hispanics. A strong genetic basis exists for type 2 diabetes (approximately 90% of patients with type 2 diabetes have a positive family history of this disorder). In addition, identical-twin studies have revealed a 60% to 90% concordance for diabetes. An absence of ketosis is one of the primary features that distinguish type 2 diabetes from type 1 diabetes, although it is possible to have ketonemia with type 2 diabetes.

Patients with type 2 diabetes can vary considerably in their ability to secrete insulin. Insulin secretion, however, is inadequate to overcome the insulin resistance associated with this type of diabetes. Defects of insulin action (insulin resistance) are typical of type 2 diabetes.

Obesity is frequently present in type 2 diabetes. Approximately 90% of people with type 2 diabetes are obese (20% over ideal body weight), and the chances of developing type 2 diabetes double for every 20% increase in body weight in susceptible individuals. However, type 2 diabetes also can develop in nonobese individuals; this is more commonly observed in older patients. The incidence of type 2 diabetes increases with age and obesity in part because people tend to gain weight and especially develop central abdominal obesity as they age.

Type 2 diabetes usually is diagnosed after the age of 30, although it is being diagnosed more frequently at a younger age (eg, at age 20) in certain ethnic groups prone to developing diabetes. The age at onset for type 2 diabetes is progressively decreasing and now develops in adolescents as well as in young adults. Initially, patients are often asymptomatic and only occasionally display the classic symptoms of hyperglycemia (polydipsia, polyuria, polyphagia, weight loss). Because type 2 diabetes can go unrecognized for many years, the early stages of microvascular disease and frank macrovascular complications may be present by the time a diagnosis is made.

Other Specific Types of Diabetes Mellitus

This category of diabetes mellitus is the least common and includes diabetes related to certain other diseases, conditions, or drugs. Hyperglycemia is present at a level that is diagnostic of diabetes. Patients are placed in this category if their diabetes has a known or probable cause or is part of a specific condition or syndrome (**Table 3**.1). Treatment of the underlying disorder may ameliorate the diabetes; more frequently, however, it is necessary to treat the diabetes with lifestyle modifications, such as diet and exercise, and medication.

Impaired Glucose Tolerance

Individuals who have postprandial plasma glucose levels that are higher than normal but lower than established diagnostic values for diabetes mellitus are classified as having IGT (diagnostic criteria in **Table 3**.2). This condition is common (occurring in approximately 5% to

TABLE 3.2 — Diagnostic Criteria for Impaired Fasting Glucose and Impaired Glucose Tolerance Using the Oral Glucose Tolerance Test[a]

World Health Organization/American Diabetes Association Criteria	
IFG	FPG ≥100 – <125 mg/dL
IGT	
Fasting	<126 mg/dL
and 2 hour	140 – 199 mg/dL
Diabetes	
Fasting	≥126 mg/dL
and 2 hour	≥200 mg/dL

[a] 75-g glucose load.

American Diabetes Association. *Diabetes Care*. 2013;36(suppl 1):S11-S66.

7% of the US population) and is considered a precursor of type 2 diabetes. Although individuals with IGT are more likely to eventually develop diabetes mellitus, only approximately 25% do develop type 2 diabetes, and a similar percentage subsequently have normal glucose levels. The rate of progression is approximately 5% to 10% per year and can be influenced by:

- Ethnic origin
- Degree of obesity
- Distribution of body fat
- Sedentary lifestyle
- Aging
- Concomitant medical conditions.

Individuals with IGT are more susceptible to macrovascular disease (coronary artery, peripheral vascular, cerebrovascular), which often is present at the time of diagnosis. Pharmacologic therapies and nonpharmacologic interventions, such as weight reduction, improved diet, and increased physical activity through lifestyle modifications, have been shown to prevent the progression of IGT to type 2 diabetes.

Impaired Fasting Glucose

The ADA introduced a new diagnostic category called IFG, which is defined as a fasting glucose value of between 100 and 125 mg/dL. This new IFG classification has major clinical implications because it allows for the earlier identification and eventual treatment of people who have undiagnosed diabetes and IGT. Individuals with IFG need to be investigated further for the cardiovascular (CV) risk factors associated with diabetes and followed closely. In addition, nonpharmacologic therapies should be instituted early, such as diet, exercise, and lifestyle modification.

Gestational Diabetes Mellitus

Glucose intolerance that is first detected during pregnancy is classified as GDM. Excluded from this group are women who had diabetes before conception. GDM occurs in about 2% to 4% of pregnant women, usually during the second or third trimester, and is more common in women who are older, obese, of high-risk ethnic groups, or have a family history of diabetes. This condition is important to identify because of the increased risk of fetal morbidity and mortality with GDM.

Pregnant women at average risk should be screened with a 75-g OGTT, with plasma glucose measurement fasting and at 1 and 2 hours, during the 24th to 28th weeks of pregnancy. Women at high risk for GDM should undergo glucose testing as soon as possible. Approximately 81% to 94% of women with GDM return to normal glucose tolerance after delivery. However, women who have had GDM are at increased risk for developing type 2 diabetes, with approximately 30% to 40% developing type 2 diabetes or IGT within 10 to 20 years.

Problems With Classification

Sometimes it is difficult to distinguish between type 1 and type 2 diabetes. For example, younger type 2 patients who are thin and taking insulin may resemble type 1 patients. In addition, some patients display the characteristics of type 2 diabetes and are not susceptible to ketoacidosis, yet they are taking insulin. These patients should not be classified as type 1 based solely on their insulin regimen, because they are taking insulin for glycemic control rather than as a life-sustaining therapy to prevent ketoacidosis and death.

Type 2 diabetes sometimes is found in children or adolescents who usually are above their ideal body weight and a member of a high-risk ethnic group susceptible to type 2 diabetes. A unique type of diabetes found in the pediatric and young-adult population is called maturity-onset diabetes of the young and is an example of an autosomal-dominant form of inheritance of diabetes. Age alone should not be considered the diagnostic variable in these patients; they should be classified as having type 2 and not type 1 diabetes.

Another classification problem that can occur involves older patients who develop ketosis-prone type 1 diabetes. The onset of this form of diabetes is slower in older adults and may resemble type 2 diabetes for a considerable length of time. These individuals tend to be at or slightly below their ideal weight and respond poorly to oral antidiabetic agents. The appearance of ketones in their urine may indicate a true lack of insulin. The insulin requirements thus become obvious and insulin therapy must be started to avoid severe ketoacidosis, coma, and death. These patients tend to be more insulin sensitive than their obese counterparts with type 2 diabetes and require less insulin to control their diabetes. A positive blood test for glutamic acid decarboxylase (GAD) antibodies is indicative of type 1 diabetes.

SUGGESTED READING

American Diabetes Association. Standards of medical care in diabetes–2013. *Diabetes Care*. 2013;36(suppl 1):S11-S66.

American Diabetes Association. *Diabetes 2002 Vital Statistics*. Alexandria, VA: American Diabetes Association; 2002.

Porte D, Sherwin RS. *Ellenberg and Rifkin's Diabetes Mellitus*. 5th ed. Stamford, CT: Appleton and Lange; 1997.

4
Diagnosis of Diabetes and the Metabolic Syndrome

A diagnosis of diabetes can be suspected in the presence of the following signs and symptoms of hyperglycemia:

- Polydipsia (increased thirst)
- Polyuria (increased urinary frequency with increased volume)
- Fatigue
- Polyphagia (increased appetite)
- Weight loss
- Abnormal healing
- Blurred vision
- Increased occurrence of infections, particularly those caused by yeast.

Only a minority of adults who are diagnosed with diabetes are symptomatic initially. Consequently, the onset of type 2 diabetes may occur years before a diagnosis is made. Individuals who are asymptomatic tend to be diagnosed during a routine physical examination, during treatment for another condition, or through specific diabetes screening. The risk of diabetes is increased in asymptomatic individuals if any of the following risk factors are present:

- A strong family history of diabetes (first-degree relatives)
- Obesity (body mass index [BMI] ≥ 25 kg/m^2), particularly central adiposity
- Certain races (American Indian, Hispanic, African, Asian, or Pacific Islander ancestry)
- Women with previous GDM or a history of newborns ≥ 9 pounds at birth
- Previously identified IFG or IGT
- High-density lipoprotein (HDL) cholesterol ≤ 35 mg/dL and/or triglycerides ≥ 250 mg/dL
- Hypertension (blood pressure $\geq 140/90$ mm Hg)
- Polycystic ovary syndrome
- History of vascular disease

- Physically inactive
- Age $\geq$45 years.

Measuring plasma glucose concentrations is currently the only way to confirm a diagnosis of diabetes. Normal plasma glucose values are presented in **Table 4.1**, and the criteria for diagnosing diabetes in nonpregnant adults are shown in **Table 4.2**.

Three approaches to glucose testing can be used to diagnose diabetes:
- Fasting plasma glucose measurements
- Random plasma glucose measurements
- OGTT.

TABLE 4.1 — Normal Plasma Glucose Values for Nonpregnant Adults

Fasting	Time zero	<100 mg/dL
After 75-g oral glucose load	120 min	<140 mg/dL

American Diabetes Association. *Diabetes Care.* 2006;29(suppl 1):S43-S48.

TABLE 4.2 — Criteria for the Diagnosis of Diabetes Mellitus

- A1C $\geq$6.5%. Test should be performed in a laboratory using a method that is NGSP certified and standardized to the DCCT assay[a]
  OR
- FPG $\geq$126 mg/dL (7.0 mmol/L). Fasting is defined as no caloric intake for at least 8 hours
  OR
- 2-Hour plasma glucose $\geq$200 mg/dL (11.1 mmol/L) during an OGTT. The test should be performed as described by the World Health Organization, using a glucose load containing the equivalent of 75-g anhydrous glucose dissolved in water
  OR
- In a patient with classic symptoms of hyperglycemia or hyperglycemic crisis, a random plasma glucose $\geq$200 mg/dL (11.1 mmol/L)

[a] In the absence of unequivocal hyperglycemia, results should be confirmed by repeat testing.

Adapted from American Diabetes Association. *Diabetes Care.* 2013;36 (suppl 1):S11-S66.

The fasting plasma glucose test is the diagnostic test of choice and is used to diagnose approximately 90% of all individuals with type 2 diabetes. Plasma glucose testing also may be performed in individuals who have had food or beverages shortly before the test. This type of testing is referred to as random plasma glucose testing. An OGTT measuring only the fasting and 2-hour blood glucose can give excellent diagnostic data and is fairly easy to perform. Because the glycosylated hemoglobin (A1C) test has not been standardized, it is not currently used for diagnosing diabetes.

Regardless of the type of test used, all abnormal laboratory values should be documented at least twice to avoid a misdiagnosis caused by laboratory errors, unless all values are extremely high or classic symptoms are present. An OGTT generally is not necessary for diagnosing diabetes. However, an OGTT can be useful for evaluating high-risk individuals so that preventive measures can be started (diet modification, exercise, weight loss) at an early stage. The ADA and the World Health Organization have prepared criteria for diagnosing diabetes mellitus and IGT based on the OGTT (**Table 4.2**).

In the absence of an elevated fasting glucose ($\geq$126 mg/dL) or a casual plasma glucose >200 mg/dL (confirmed on a subsequent day), pregnant women should undergo risk assessment for GDM at the first prenatal visit. Women at low risk for developing glucose intolerance during pregnancy need not be tested for GDM. Women at high risk (marked obesity, previous history of GDM, glycosuria, high-risk racial/ethnic groups, or strong family history of diabetes) should undergo glucose testing as soon as possible. Testing involves a 50-g glucose load without regard to the time of the last meal or the time of day. If not found to have GDM at initial screening, retesting should be conducted during the 24th to 28th weeks of gestation. This test is only recommended in individuals at risk for diabetes. A 1-hour plasma glucose concentration >130 mg/dL is considered a positive reading that calls for a formal OGTT with a 100-g glucose load and sampling at fasting and 1, 2, and 3 hours after glucose challenge. The diagnosis of GDM is made when two or more of these samples meet or exceed the following values: fasting, 95 mg/dL; 1 hour, 180 mg/dL; 2 hour, 155 mg/dL; and 3 hour, 140 mg/dL.

A complete medical evaluation is indicated following a positive diagnostic blood test for diabetes. Patients should not be diagnosed on the basis of age alone. The purpose of this evaluation is to:

- Appropriately classify the patient
- Detect any underlying diseases that may require further evaluation
- Determine whether any of the complications of diabetes are present.

Figure 4.1 shows a Diabetes Warranty Program developed as a reference for patients, outlining evaluations at every visit and annually. Getting patients involved in their own care is an important tool for improving compliance and motivation.

Diabetes and Cardiovascular Disease Risk Assessment

Diabetes is now recognized as a CV disease equivalent. That is, an individual with diabetes but without evidence of overt heart disease has the same risk of an MI as a nondiabetic individual who has had a previous CV event. Diabetes is an independent risk factor for CV disease in both men and women. Women lose the protective effect against CV disease when they develop diabetes. Of every three people with diabetes, two die of CV disease. Once a person with diabetes develops clinical evidence of CV disease, their likelihood of survival is worse than that of nondiabetics with CV disease.

Most patients with type 2 diabetes have tissue resistance to insulin. The presence of insulin resistance is associated with and predisposes to both CV disease and type 2 diabetes. Like type 2 diabetes, insulin resistance is influenced by genetic susceptibility, obesity, physical inactivity, and advancing age. Patients with insulin resistance tend to develop the metabolic or dysmetabolic syndrome. This is associated with:

- Abdominal obesity
- Atherogenic dyslipidemia

- Hypertension
- Glucose intolerance
- A procoagulant state
- Evidence of vascular inflammation.

The National Cholesterol Education Program (NCEP) published guidelines on detection, evaluation, and treatment of high blood cholesterol in adults (Adult Treatment Panel III). These guidelines are based on clinical trial data and other scientific rationale.

The NCEP guidelines emphasize multiple risk factors (two or more) in its primary-prevention strategy. The primary target of therapy and a major cause of coronary heart disease (CHD) is elevated low-density lipoprotein (LDL) cholesterol. Numerous clinical trials clearly demonstrate that lowering LDL cholesterol reduces risk for CHD, even in individuals with type 2 diabetes. The NCEP advocates that the intensity of risk-reduction therapy or primary prevention of CHD be adjusted based on an individuals's absolute risk. Major risk factors include:

- High LDL cholesterol
- Cigarette smoking
- Hypertension ≥140/90 mm Hg or patient on antihypertensive therapy
- Low HDL cholesterol (<40 mg/dL)
- Family history of premature heart disease (at <55 years in male first-degree relative, at <65 years in female first-degree relative)
- Advancing age: ≥45 years of age in men, and ≥55 years of age in women.

Diabetes is considered a CHD risk equivalent and therefore a major risk factor. An HDL cholesterol level ≥60 mg/dL represents a negative risk factor and negates one positive risk factor from the total count.

The NCEP guidelines establish the goal of an LDL level <100 mg/dL when CHD or a risk equivalent such as diabetes is present. The ADA has established similar guidelines, including an order of priorities for the treatment of diabetic dyslipidemia in adults. After LDL cholesterol lowering, next in importance are HDL cholesterol

FIGURE 4.1 — Diabetes Warranty Program

What Should Be Done at *Every Visit* (3-6 months)

	Date	Result	Normal Range or Goal
Weight			
Blood pressure (sitting and standing)			
Foot examination[a]			
Glycosylated hemoglobin or fructosamine[b] (know the normal range)			

What Tests/Examinations Should Be Done at Least *Every Year*

	Date	Result (recommendations)	Normal Range
Cholesterol levels (fasting):			
• Total cholesterol			
• Triglycerides			
• High-density lipoprotein (HDL)			
• Low-density lipoprotein (LDL)			
Urine protein (microalbumin)			
Serum creatinine			
Thyroid function test (TSH)			

Eye examination (dilated) _____ _____

Dental examination _____ _____

Other tests/examinations (depending on
individual needs) by specialists:

• Cardiologist (for heart disease) _____ _____

• Podiatrist (for foot problems) _____ _____

• Gastroenterologist (for stomach problems) _____ _____

[a] Visual, tuning fork, 10-g monofilament, palpitation.

[b] Glycosylated hemoglobin and fructosamine are long-term diabetes control factors.

Edelman SV. Diabetes Warranty Program. VA Endocrinology Clinic, VA Hospital, UCSD, La Jolla, California.

4

raising, triglyceride lowering, and treatment of combined hyperlipidemia.

The Metabolic or Dysmetabolic Syndrome

The NCEP guidelines recognize the metabolic syndrome as a secondary target of risk-reduction therapy after LDL cholesterol lowering, which is the primary target. The constellation of abnormalities that constitute the metabolic syndrome enhance the risk for CHD at any given LDL level. By the NCEP criteria, the diagnosis of the metabolic syndrome requires three or more of the risk determinants shown in **Table 4.3**. Most individuals with type 2 diabetes have multiple risk determinants of the metabolic syndrome. First-line therapy for all components of the metabolic syndrome involves weight reduction/control and increased physical activity. Other components of the syndrome (high triglyceride levels, low HDL cholesterol levels, dyslipidemia, glucose intolerance, a procoagulant state, and hypertension) may require specific pharmacologic management to achieve adequate control.

Most individuals with type 2 diabetes and components of the metabolic syndrome usually receive:

- An angiotensin-converting enzyme (ACE) inhibitor and/or an angiotensin receptor blocker (ARB)

TABLE 4.3 — Clinical Criteria for the Metabolic Syndrome[a]

Risk Factor	Defining Level
Abdominal obesity (waist circumference)	Men >40 inches (102 cm) Women >35 inches (88 cm)
Triglycerides	≥150 mg/dL
HDL cholesterol	Men <40 mg/dL Women <50 mg/dL
Blood pressure	≥130/≥85 mm Hg
Fasting glucose	≥110 mg/dL

[a] The metabolic syndrome is synonymous to the dysmetabolic syndrome X or insulin-resistance syndrome.

Expert Panel on Detection, Evaluation, and Treatment of High Blood Cholesterol in Adults. *JAMA*. 2001;285:2486-2497.

as initial therapy for hypertension and/or microalbuminuria
- Enteric-coated aspirin at doses of 81 to 325 mg/day to reduce the prothrombotic or procoagulant state
- An HMG-CoA reductase inhibitor to reduce LDL cholesterol to <100 mg/dL, together with specific therapy for hyperglycemia and other possible risk determinants.

The Centers for Disease Control (CDC) recognize the metabolic or dysmetabolic syndrome X with a new ICD-9-CM code of 277.7. The CDC does not require that a given number of components be present to use this ICD-9 code, but instead relies on the professional opinion of the physician that the dysmetabolic syndrome X is present. The American Association of Clinical Endocrinologists (AACE) has suggested major and minor criteria to assist physicians in making the diagnosis. These are shown in **Table 4.4**. Many of the criteria advocated by AACE are similar to those of the NCEP guidelines.

TABLE 4.4 — Major and Minor Criteria for the Dysmetabolic Syndrome X[a]

Major Criteria
- Insulin resistance (denoted by hyperinsulinemia relative to glucose levels)
- Acanthosis nigricans
- Central obesity (waist circumference >102 cm for men and >88 cm for women)
- Dyslipidemia (HDL <45 mg/dL for women; <35 mg/dL for men, or triglycerides >150 mg/dL)
- Hypertension
- Impaired fasting glucose or type 2 diabetes
- Hyperuricemia

Minor Criteria
- Hypercoagulability
- Polycystic ovary syndrome
- Vascular endothelial dysfunction
- Microalbuminuria
- Coronary heart disease

[a] Criteria developed by the American Association of Clinical Endocrinologists.

SUGGESTED READING

American Diabetes Association. Standards of medical care in diabetes–2013. *Diabetes Care*. 2013;36(suppl 1):S11-S66.

American Diabetes Association. *Diabetes 2002 Vital Statistics*. Alexandria, VA: American Diabetes Association; 2002.

Porte D, Sherwin RS. *Ellenberg & Rifkin's Diabetes Mellitus*. 5th ed. Stamford, CT: Appleton & Lange; 1997.

Executive Summary of the Third Report of the National Cholesterol Education Program (NCEP) Expert Panel on Detection, Evaluation, and Treatment of High Blood Cholesterol in Adults (Adult Treatment Panel III). *JAMA*. 2001;285:2486-2497.

5 Nutrition

Nutrition Therapy

One of the more fundamental components of the diabetes treatment plan for all patients with type 2 diabetes is nutrition therapy. Specific goals of nutrition therapy in type 2 diabetes are to:

- Achieve and maintain as near-normal blood glucose levels as possible by balancing food intake with physical activity, supplemented by oral hypoglycemic agents and/or insulin as needed
- Normalize blood pressure
- Normalize serum lipid levels
- Help patients attain and maintain a reasonable body weight (defined as the weight an individual and health care provider acknowledge as possible to achieve and maintain on a short- and long-term basis)
- Promote overall health through optimal nutrition and lifestyle behaviors.

Because no single dietary approach is appropriate for all patients, and given the heterogeneous nature of type 2 diabetes, meal plans and diet modifications should be individualized to meet a patient's unique needs and lifestyle. Accordingly, any nutrition intervention should be based on a thorough assessment of a patient's typical food intake and eating habits and should include an evaluation of current nutritional status.

Some patients with mild-to-moderate diabetes can be effectively treated with an appropriate balance of diet modification and exercise as the sole therapeutic intervention, particularly if their FBG level is <140 mg/dL. The majority of patients, however, will require pharmacologic intervention in addition to diet and exercise prescriptions. It is important to note that pharmacologic treatment is often less successful when the patient is not on some type of dietary and exercise regimen.

Dietary changes do not have to be dramatic to produce clinically important results in terms of improving blood glucose, blood pressure, and lipid levels. Regular monitoring of blood glucose, glycated hemoglobin, lipid levels, blood pressure, and body weight serves as an ongoing assessment of the nutrition intervention.

Nutrition Consult

Because nutrition issues and meal planning are complex, a registered dietitian who is familiar with the current principles and recommendations for managing diabetes may be consulted after a patient is diagnosed with diabetes. This health care professional can be an essential member of the diabetes management team and perform a number of valuable functions:

- Conducts initial assessment of nutritional status:
  - Diet history
  - Lifestyle
  - Eating habits
- Provides patient education regarding:
  - The basic principles of diet therapy for diabetes
  - Meal planning
  - Problem-solving techniques for changing eating behaviors
- Develops an individualized meal plan:
  - Emphasizing one or two priorities
  - Minimizing changes from the patient's usual diet (to encourage compliance)
- Provides follow-up assessment of the meal plan to:
  - Determine effectiveness in terms of glucose and lipid control and weight loss
  - Make necessary changes based on weight loss, activity level, or changes in medication
- Provides ongoing patient education and support (particularly for those on weight-loss regimens), helping patients learn to adjust their meal plans for various situations.

Body Weight Considerations

Weight loss frequently is a primary goal of nutrition therapy because 80% to 90% of people with type 2 diabetes are obese. Caloric restriction and weight loss, even as small as 5 lb in body weight, can result in:

- Improved glucose control
- Increased sensitivity to insulin
- Improved lipid levels and blood pressure
- The need for a corresponding lowering of the dosage of pharmacologic agents (eg, oral antidiabetic medications and insulin).

Weight loss is associated with improved glucose uptake and insulin sensitivity as well as decreased hepatic glucose production. Consequently, the therapeutic regimen most useful for individuals with obesity and glucose intolerance is weight reduction via nutrition therapy and increased physical activity. If moderate weight loss does not improve metabolic parameters, however, pharmacologic therapy (oral antidiabetic agents or insulin) may need to be added to the regimen.

Weight loss and subsequent weight maintenance can be one of the more difficult and challenging aspects of managing diabetes. Therefore, emphasis should be placed on achieving and maintaining normal blood glucose control as the goal of nutrition therapy, using nutritionally balanced meal plans that promote gradual weight loss as a means of achieving this metabolic goal. A reasonable approach that provides a combination of the following strategies increases the chances of a successful outcome:

- Modest caloric restriction
- Restriction of saturated fat intake
- Spreading caloric intake throughout the day
- Increased physical activity
- Behavior modification techniques for changing eating habits and attitudes and promoting healthy, long-term lifestyle behaviors
- Psychosocial support.

Suggested weights for adults based on the United States Department of Agriculture (USDA) *Dietary*

Guidelines for Americans (1990) are shown in **Table 5.1**. The upper end of the ranges are considered appropriate weights for men, given their greater bone and muscle mass; the lower end of the ranges are for women, who have comparatively less bone and muscle mass.

TABLE 5.1 — Suggested Weight for Adults

Height (ft/in)	Weight (lb)	
	19-34 (y)	≥35 (y)
5′ 0″	97-128	108-138
5′ 1″	101-132	111-143
5′ 2″	104-137	115-148
5′ 3″	107-141	119-152
5′ 4″	111-146	122-157
5′ 5″	114-150	126-162
5′ 6″	118-155	130-167
5′ 7″	121-160	134-172
5′ 8″	125-164	138-178
5′ 9″	129-169	142-183
5′ 10″	132-174	146-188
5′ 11″	136-179	151-194
6′ 0″	140-184	155-199
6′ 1″	144-189	159-205
6′ 2″	148-195	164-210
6′ 3″	152-200	168-216
6′ 4″	156-205	173-222
6′ 5″	160-211	173-222
6′ 6″	164-216	182-234

US Department of Agriculture. US Department of Health and Human Services. *Nutrition and Your Health: Dietary Guidelines for Americans.* 3rd ed. Hyattsville, Md: USDA Human Nutrition Information Service; 1990.

Approximately 10% of patients with type 2 diabetes are of normal weight and do not need to restrict their caloric intake. For these individuals, nutrition therapy focuses on distributing caloric as well as nutrient intake and content throughout the day to achieve optimal glucose, lipid, and blood pressure control. The pattern of spreading out calories and carbohydrates between meals and snacks is individualized based on results of self-monitoring of blood glucose.

Caloric Intake

Adult caloric needs vary according to age, activity level, and desired weight change. The following formula can be used to determine adult caloric requirements. First calculate desired body weight:

- Women: 100 lb for the first 5 ft of height plus 5 lb for each additional inch over 5 ft
- Men: 106 lb for the first 5 ft of height plus 6 lb for each additional inch over 5 ft
- Add 10% for larger body builds; subtract 10% for smaller body builds.

5

Then, multiply the resulting weight by one of the following to compute caloric need based on desired weight:

- Men and physically active women: multiply by 15
- Most women, sedentary men, and adults over age 55: multiply by 13
- Sedentary women, obese adults, sedentary adults over age 55: multiply by 10.

If weight loss is indicated, daily caloric intake needs to be adjusted to produce the necessary deficit. Given that a 3500-calorie deficit per week is required to produce a 1-lb loss of fat, a decrease of approximately 500 to 1000 calories per day is needed to lose 1 to 2 lb of fat per week. Regular exercise is an excellent way to create a caloric deficit and has been associated with successful weight maintenance. Because caloric restriction alone can be difficult to maintain, some people have greater success by eliminating 250 to 500 calories from their daily diet and increasing daily activity by 250 to 500 calories.

Nutrient Composition of the Diet

A nutritionally balanced diet is as important for individuals with diabetes as for nondiabetics. Diet prescriptions for those with type 2 diabetes need to take into account the higher prevalence of dyslipidemia, atherosclerosis, and hypertension in this population. Practical dietary recommendations are outlined in **Table 5.2**.

TABLE 5.2 — Practical Dietary Recommendations

- Emphasize to the obese diabetic patient that even small amounts of weight loss can have substantial benefits for glucose, lipids, and blood pressure levels. Weight reduction should be constantly encouraged through lifestyle modification since the natural course with diabetes is to gain weight.
- Sugar (sucrose) and sugar-containing foods do not increase blood glucose levels to any greater extent than equivalent amounts of starch and do not need to be restricted. They can be substituted for other carbohydrate sources in the context of a healthy diet.
- When intensive insulin therapy is used, premeal insulin doses should be adjusted based on the carbohydrate content of the meal (carbohydrate counting). A rough guide is approximately 1 unit of insulin for every 15 g carbohydrate, but it should be individualized.
- When on a fixed daily insulin dose, day-to-day carbohydrate intake should be as consistent as possible.
- All fats are calorie dense and contribute to weight gain when consumed in excess. Not all fats are created equal. Monounsaturated fat (eg, olive oil) and polyunsaturated fats including fish oil (N-3 polyunsaturated fatty acids) have beneficial effects on lipid levels and may exert a cardioprotective benefit.
- Saturated (animal-derived) fats and transunsaturated fatty acids (processed hydrogenated vegetable oils) have detrimental effects on lipids and should be avoided as much as possible. This is best achieved by limiting intake of red meat, cheese, and whole milk.
- Exercise of any form is beneficial and more effective when regular and sustained. As little as 30 minutes five times per week is helpful in losing or maintaining weight, lowering glucose and blood pressure, and improving lipid profiles.
- Moderate alcohol intake can reduce cardiovascular risk, but should be limited to one drink for adult women and two drinks for adult men daily consumed with food. One drink is equivalent to 12 oz of beer, 5 oz of wine, or 1.5 oz of distilled spirits.
- High-salt intake contributes to hypertension (high blood pressure) and should be limited to that usually found in food. Patients should be encouraged not to eat processed meats, salty snacks, or add salt to food.
- Unless there is evidence of deficiency, vitamin, antioxidant, and mineral supplementation is generally not necessary. Folic acid supplements have benefit to prevent birth defects, and calcium, to prevent osteoporosis.

■ Protein Intake

The recommended dietary allowance for adults as advised by the USDA is used as the guideline for protein intake for patients with type 2 diabetes (0.8 g/kg body weight per day). This equates to a small-to-medium portion of protein once daily with either breakfast, lunch, or dinner. Protein allowance therefore amounts to 15% to 20% of daily calories and should be derived from both animal and vegetable sources. Vegetable protein may be less nephrotoxic than animal protein and thus restriction of vegetable protein may not be necessary. In following these recommendations, meat, fish, or poultry consumption would need to be limited to 3 to 5 oz daily.

The long-term consequences of high-protein (>30% of total daily calories) and low-carbohydrate diets are unknown, but may aggravate renal impairment in diabetic individuals. High-protein diets are often high in saturated fats, which have an adverse effect on LDL cholesterol.

Because excessive protein intake may aggravate renal insufficiency, type 2 patients with evidence of overt nephropathy should be encouraged to limit their protein intake to approximately 10% of daily calories or ≤ 0.8 g/kg body weight per day. In short-term studies, more severe restriction of protein (0.6 g/kg body weight per day) has been shown to be effective in slowing the progression of kidney disease in patients with diabetes who already have some renal insufficiency. However, severely restricted protein diets have also been reported to be associated with loss of muscle mass and strength. Evidence exists that a low-protein diet can reverse the rate of deterioration in renal function.

■ Fat Intake

The remaining 80% to 85% of daily calories are distributed between fat and carbohydrate intake, based on a patient's nutrition assessment and treatment goals (glucose, lipid, and weight outcomes). Several important benefits support the restriction of dietary fat in patients with type 2 diabetes:

- Excess consumption of dietary fat may contribute to obesity, which is common in the majority of patients with type 2 diabetes. Restricting dietary fat may limit the development or reduce the extent of obesity.

- Abnormal lipid levels often are associated with both obesity and diabetes and increase the risk of CV disease. Reduced intake of saturated fat can have beneficial effects by reducing triglyceride and LDL cholesterol and increasing HDL cholesterol.

Therefore, the following guidelines are recommended for fat intake to promote weight loss, achieve lipid goals, and reduce CV risk:
- Reduce dietary fat to <30% of total calories
- Limit saturated fat to <10% of total calories and to <7% of calories in patients with elevated LDL cholesterol
- Limit polyunsaturated fats to 10% of total calories
- Limit daily cholesterol consumption to 300 mg/day; limit to <200 mg/day if lipids are elevated
- Moderately increase intake of monounsaturated fats such as canola and olive oil (up to 20% of calories). A diet high in monounsaturated fats has been shown to improve glucose control, lower triglycerides, and raise HDL levels.

Effectiveness of dietary fat modification is determined by regular monitoring of glycemic control, triglyceride and cholesterol status, and body weight, with periodic adjustments based on metabolic response to the diet.

■ Carbohydrate Intake

The carbohydrate allowance is determined after protein and fat intake have been calculated and is individualized based on eating habits and glucose and lipid goals. Emphasis is placed on whole grains, starches, fruits, and vegetables to provide the necessary vitamins, minerals, and fiber in the diet. The recommended daily consumption of fiber is the same for people with diabetes as for nondiabetics (20 g to 35 g). Although dietary fiber can improve serum lipid levels, the effect on glycemic control is modest at best.

Traditionally, complex carbohydrates were thought to produce lower blood glucose responses than simple sugars because sugars are digested and absorbed more rapidly. This belief, which influenced previous recommendations of replacing simple sugars in the diet with complex carbohydrates, has been largely disproved by clinical research. For example, the glycemic response to fruits and milk has been found to be lower than the response to most starches, and sucrose has been found to produce a glycemic response similar to that with bread, rice, and potatoes. The rate of digestion of a given food seems to be more related to the presence of fat, degree of ripeness, cooking method, form, and preparation.

■ Sucrose

A modest amount of sugar is allowed in the daily diet of patients with type 2 diabetes. Sucrose and sucrose-containing foods may be substituted for other carbohydrates in the meal plan, but not simply added. Patients need to be taught how to make such substitutions using self-monitoring of blood glucose (SMBG) to evaluate the glycemic response. The total nutrient content of the sucrose-containing food should be considered, particularly because sugar and fat are the main ingredients in many sweets. Obese individuals usually are advised to avoid sweets because of the potential of a small portion triggering overconsumption.

■ Fructose

Fruits and vegetables are a natural source of dietary fructose. In addition, some sweeteners are derived from these sources. Moderate consumption is recommended, particularly concerning foods in which fructose is used as a sweetening agent. Although fructose has a lower glycemic effect than sucrose, it contains the same amount of calories and therefore should be limited in hypocaloric diets. People with dyslipidemia also are advised to limit their consumption of fructose because of the potential adverse effects on serum triglyceride and LDL cholesterol levels.

■ Other Nutritive/Nonnutritive Sweeteners and Fat Substitutes

Nutritive sweeteners such as corn syrup, fruit juice/concentrate, honey, molasses, dextrose, and maltose do not seem to have a greater advantage or disadvantage over sucrose in terms of impact on caloric content or glycemic response, but they need to be accounted for in the meal plan. Certain sugar alcohols (sorbitol, mannitol, xylitol) that are commonly used as sweeteners can produce a lower glycemic response than sucrose but seem to have no real advantage over sucrose or other nutritive sweeteners when consumed as part of mixed meals. Excessive consumption of sugar alcohols may cause laxative effects.

Nonnutritive sweeteners (saccharin, aspartame, acesulfame K, sucralose) have been approved by the Food and Drug Administration (FDA) for consumption by people with diabetes. These sweeteners are useful because they contribute minimal or no calories or carbohydrates to the diet when they are used as tabletop sweeteners or in soft drinks. However, when sweeteners are used in foods that contain other nutrients and calories (ice cream, cookies, puddings), the foods must be worked into the meal plan or consult with a nutritionist.

Because many of the fat substitutes, such as Olestra, currently being used are derived from carbohydrate or protein sources, the content of these compounds is increased above the usual amounts in such products. Patients need to be advised to review the carbohydrate and/or protein content when using products that contain fat substitutes.

■ Vitamins, Minerals, and Herbs

Supplementation generally is not recommended for people with diabetes when dietary intake is adequate and balanced. Patients who become chromium deficient as a result of long-term parenteral nutrition may require chromium supplementation. However, most people with diabetes are not chromium deficient and do not benefit from supplementation. Similarly, magnesium does not need to be added to the diets of most patients with diabetes unless routine evaluation of serum magnesium reveals a deficiency. Patients taking diuretics may need potassium supplementation. However, hyperkalemia may require potassium restriction in patients with renal insufficiency, or hyporeninemic hypoaldosteronism, or in those taking ACE inhibitors. One consideration may be the potential value of antioxidant supplements (vitamin C and β-carotene) in reducing atherosclerotic lesions and cataracts, both of which are common in type 2 diabetes. The value of such supplementation is yet to be confirmed.

There are many nonprescription herbal remedies being touted in health food stores as being beneficial for people with diabetes. While some of these herbs may have some rational scientific basis, most have not been well studied and the benefits are questionable. Some of these compounds have the potential to produce toxicity.

■ Alcohol Intake

The same recommendations used for the general population are appropriate for people with type 2 diabetes. Moderate consumption will not adversely affect blood glucose in patients whose diabetes is well controlled. Calories from alcohol should be included as part of the total caloric intake and reflected in the meal plan as a substitute for fat (one alcoholic beverage=two fat exchanges). For patients taking insulin, one or two alcoholic beverages per day are acceptable (one alcoholic beverage=12 oz beer, 5 oz wine, or 1½ oz distilled spirits; sweet drinks should be avoided) taken with or in addition to the meal plan. However, some special considerations exist regarding alcohol intake. Patients taking insulin or sulfonylureas (SFUs) are susceptible to hypoglycemia if alcohol is consumed on an empty stomach. Therefore, these individuals should be sure to take any desired alcohol with a meal and to perform frequent home glucose monitoring.

SUGGESTED READING

American Diabetes Association. Standards of medical care in diabetes–2013. *Diabetes Care*. 2013;36(suppl 1):S11-S66.

American Diabetes Association. *Medical Management of Non–insulin-dependent (Type II) Diabetes,* 3rd ed. Alexandria, VA: American Diabetes Association; 1994:22-39.

Henry RR. Protein content of the diabetic diet. *Diabetes Care*. 1994;17: 1502-1513.

Mudaliar SR, Henry RR. Role of glycemic control and protein restriction in clinical management of diabetic kidney disease. *Endocr Pract*. 1996;2:220-226.

Porte D, Sherwin RS. *Ellenburg and Rifkin's Diabetes Mellitus*. 5th ed. Stamford, CT: Appleton and Lange; 1997.

6   Exercise

Many adults with diabetes are sedentary and obese, which can contribute to the development of glucose intolerance. Therefore, physical activity should be included as an essential treatment component in the diabetes management plan unless contraindicated in a given individual. Current research suggests that even low-level regular exercise can prevent or delay the onset of type 2 diabetes in susceptible, high-risk individuals.

6

Benefits

The potential benefits of regular exercise include:
- Improved glucose tolerance because of enhanced insulin sensitivity
- Weight loss or maintenance of a desirable body weight because of increased energy expenditure
- Improved CV risk factors (lipids, blood pressure, etc)
- Improved response to pharmacologic therapy, with the potential of reducing the dosage or the need for insulin or OADs
- Improved energy level, muscular strength, flexibility, quality of life, and sense of well-being.

Precautions and Considerations

Because many people with diabetes have not been active and are deconditioned, exercise should be started cautiously at a low level and gradually increased to avoid adverse effects such as injury, hypoglycemia, or cardiac problems. Most adults with diabetes should have a physical examination, including a stress test, before beginning to exercise to rule out significant CV disease or silent ischemia and to determine the presence of any diabetic complications. Strenuous activity is not recommended for patients with poor metabolic control or for those with significant complications.

Patients being treated with insulin secretagogues or insulin alone or in combination are susceptible to hypoglycemia during exercise or for as much as 12 hours after. To prevent hypoglycemia, such patients should use SMBG both before and after exercising to determine their response to varying degrees of physical activity. Appropriate consumption of snacks and modification of pharmacotherapy, as needed, can help avoid most problems. More important, establishing and following a regular exercise program can reduce the likelihood of exercise-induced episodes of hypoglycemia.

Exercise Prescription

Any exercise prescription should be individualized to account for patient interests, physical status and capacity, and motivation. Although having a planned program of physical activity is ideal, exercise is so important and beneficial that just getting patients moving is a worthwhile initial goal. Patients should choose activities that are appropriate for their general physical condition and lifestyle, start slowly, and work up to the goal of performing an aerobic activity at 50% to 70% of maximum oxygen uptake at least three to four times per week, with a minimum duration of 20 minutes per session (ideally 30 to 40 minutes). Weight reduction is enhanced by exercising five to six times per week. Recommended aerobic activities include:

- Walking at a moderate pace (3 to 5 mph)
- Biking and stationary cycling
- Lap swimming and aerobic water exercises.

Muscle-strengthening exercises such as lifting light weights also should be included in an exercise program, as well as flexibility stretches during warm-ups and cool-downs.

Guidelines for safe exercise should be reviewed with patients (**Table 6.1**). Recommendations for a practical exercise prescription are outlined in **Table 6.2**.

TABLE 6.1 — General Exercise Guidelines

- An exercise stress test should be performed in most adults with diabetes to rule out significant cardiovascular disease or silent ischemia
- Start slowly at a low level; gradually increase intensity and frequency
- Carry identification including diabetes medical identification
- Monitor blood glucose preexercise and postexercise.
- Be alert for signs of hypoglycemia during and several hours after exercising; carry appropriate readily available carbohydrate source
- Closely monitor blood glucose when exercise intensity is increased
- Drink sufficient fluids before, during, and after exercise to maintain adequate hydration

TABLE 6.2 — Practical Exercise Prescription

- Most individuals with type 2 diabetes are overweight and in poor cardiovascular health prior to initiating an exercise program. Exercise should be part of an overall beneficial change in lifestyle (diet modification, reduced stress, etc)
- Exercise programs can be of low, moderate, or high intensity. The exercise prescription needs to be individualized and account for the presence of macrovascular and microvascular complications, weighing the benefits vs risks in a given patient. Most individuals with type 2 diabetes should focus on a low-to-moderate intensity program that is easy to initiate and maintain
- Low-to-moderate intensity exercise generally increases the heart rate up to approximately 60% of maximal heart rate. The maximal heart rate for an individual can be estimated by subtracting the age from 220 (maximal heart rate=220−age). Thus a 50-year-old individual exercising at a low-to-moderate intensity should keep the heart rate (220-50=170 × 60%) of no more than 100 beats per minute. Patients should be shown how to monitor their heart rate intermittently during exercise by palpation of the radial or brachial artery

SUGGESTED READING

American Diabetes Association. Standards of medical care in diabetes–2013. *Diabetes Care*. 2013;36(suppl 1):S11-S66.

American Diabetes Association. *Medical Management of Non–insulin-dependent (Type II) Diabetes.* 3rd ed. Alexandria, VA: American Diabetes Association; 1994:22-39.

7

Overview of Pharmacologic Therapy

The majority of patients with type 2 diabetes have less than ideal metabolic control despite our greater understanding of the underlying pathophysiologic mechanisms of hyperglycemia and the availability of a wide variety of new treatment options. Failure to achieve glycemic goals is related in part to a misconception by patients and caregivers that type 2 diabetes is a mild disease and not as serious as type 1 diabetes. In fact, in many respects, type 2 diabetes may have more severe consequences than type 1 diabetes because of the multiple CV risk factors and accelerated atherosclerosis associated with this form of diabetes.

Insulin resistance is an early and major cause of hyperglycemia and other metabolic abnormalities in type 2 diabetics (see *Chapter 2*). Hyperglycemia in type 2 diabetes often coexists with several other metabolic abnormalities, such as obesity, hypertension, dyslipidemia, and a procoagulant state, which themselves require prompt and aggressive diagnosis and treatment. Moreover, prolonged hyperglycemia leads to a worsening of the insulin resistance and endogenous insulin secretory inability (glucose toxicity), thus contributing to the primary and secondary oral-agent failure rate. Aggressive management to reduce the hyperglycemia, which in some cases may require temporary insulin therapy, is necessary to reverse the glucose toxic state.

Pharmacologic therapy with oral antidiabetic agents is required when dietary modification and exercise therapy do not result in normalization or near normalization of metabolic abnormalities. Pharmacologic therapy should always be considered as adjunctive therapy to diet and exercise, and not as a substitute. Although maintaining an optimal diet and exercise regimen is difficult, it is important to emphasize that no pharmacologic therapy can be expected to be successful if the patient is not following some type of dietary and exercise program. Effort should be made to diagnose type 2 diabetes early in the natural history of the disease when nonpharmacologic therapy tends to be most effective.

Pathophysiologic Basis of Pharmacologic Therapy

The treatment strategies selected for managing type 2 diabetes are based on understanding the pathophysiology of hyperglycemia and the unique clinical expression of the associated metabolic abnormalities in an individual. Type 2 diabetes is characterized by four basic abnormalities that contribute to the development of hyperglycemia:

- Peripheral insulin resistance, mainly in the skeletal muscle but also in the liver and adipose tissue
- Excessive glucose production by the liver
- Impaired insulin secretion by the pancreas
- Excessive glucagon secretion.

Fasting and postprandial hyperglycemia vary considerably among individuals, depending upon the extent, severity, and unique expression of each of these metabolic abnormalities, and these differences also play a role in the various responses to the different classes of OADs. Such differences are exemplified by the lean and obese varieties of type 2 diabetes, which exhibit the same underlying pathophysiology but differ in the extent to which each abnormality contributes to the development of the hyperglycemic state. In lean type 2 diabetic patients, impaired insulin secretion is usually the predominant defect, while insulin resistance tends to be less severe than in the obese variety. Insulin resistance and hyperinsulinemia are the classic abnormalities of obese individuals with type 2 diabetes. In obese type 2 diabetics, the oral antidiabetic agents that do not stimulate insulin secretion tend to be as effective as, but safer than, insulin secretagogues in terms of hypoglycemia when used early in the course of diabetes and when insulin deficiency is not the predominant abnormality. In addition, information is emerging regarding the importance of suppressing glucagon hypersecretion in the management of type 2 diabetes (see *Chapter 10*).

Importance of Controlling Postprandial Hyperglycemia

The evaluation of glycemic control and the response to antidiabetic therapy in type 2 diabetes has traditionally emphasized monitoring of fasting and preprandial glucose values. However, patients frequently demonstrate normal or near-normal preprandial glucose levels yet have distinctly abnormal postprandial glucose (PPG) values. Postprandial hyperglycemia is often the first clinical abnormality present in those individuals who eventually go on to develop type 2 diabetes. Although it is not well recognized, postprandial hyperglycemia contributes significantly to elevated A1C and has been implicated in development of CV and other diabetic complications. Abnormal PPG values in pregnant diabetic women have also been shown to contribute to perinatal morbidity and mortality and are more significantly correlated with adverse outcomes than fasting glucose levels. Many factors contribute to peak postprandial plasma glucose (eg, insulin resistance, impaired insulin secretion, excessive glucagon levels), but up to one third of the variance may be explained by differences in gastric emptying. Many type 2 diabetic patients demonstrate abnormally rapid gastric emptying after a high carbohydrate meal, which may contribute to excessive PPG excursions.

The importance of controlling PPG needs to be recognized and treated with modification of diet and use of antidiabetic medication as required. PPG levels are best evaluated 1 to 2 hours after meals by patients using home glucose monitoring devices. The AACE has published similar stringent guidelines for control of PPG with a 2-hour PPG goal of <140 mg/dL. The ADA has stated that the peak PPG level should be <180 mg/dL (**Table 7.1**).

Intensive Therapy in Type 2 Diabetes

Several long-term studies of intensive diabetes management in both type 1 and type 2 diabetes have provided clear-cut evidence that near normalization of glycemia can prevent and delay the development and

TABLE 7.1 — Targets for Glycemic Control

Biochemical Index	ADA Goal	AACE Goal
A1C	<7%	≤6.5%
Fasting/preprandial glucose	70-130 mg/dL	<110 mg/dL
Postprandial glucose	<180 mg/dL (peak)	<140 mg/dL (2 hours)

American Diabetes Association. *Diabetes Care*. 2013;36(suppl 1):S11-S66; American Association of Clinical Endocrinologists. *Endocr Pract*. 2007;13(suppl 1):S3-S68.

progression of retinopathy, nephropathy, and neuropathy in the disease. Patients with type 2 diabetes obtain benefits from improved glycemic control because the severity and duration of hyperglycemia have a critical role in the development and progression of microvascular complications, regardless of the etiology of the hyperglycemia. Studies demonstrate not only a reduction in microvascular disease in type 2 diabetes with improved glycemic control but also reductions in dyslipidemia and coronary artery disease.

The UKPDS demonstrated the benefits of glucose control in >5000 individuals with newly diagnosed type 2 diabetes. The subjects were randomized into a conventional-treatment group (nonpharmacologic diet treatment) with the goal to keep the FBG values <270 mg/dL and an intensive-treatment group (SFUs, insulin, or MET) with the goal to keep the FBG values <108 mg/dL. The average study duration of subjects was 11 years. Although the UKPDS was not ideally designed or conducted to achieve optimal glycemic control, several important messages have been derived from this study.

Most important, this study demonstrated a highly statistically significant reduction in microvascular disease in the intensive-treatment group on the same order of magnitude as occurred in the Diabetes Control and Complications Trial (DCCT) in type 1 diabetes (**Table 7.2**). In the UKPDS, the difference in A1C between the conventional- and intensive-treatment groups was only 0.9% compared with a 2% difference observed in the DCCT.

The natural history of type 2 diabetes was clearly demonstrated in both treatment groups, ie, that there

TABLE 7.2 — United Kingdom Prospective Diabetes Study: Intensive Blood Glucose Control

	Change in Risk (%)	P Value
Any diabetes-related end point	↓ 12	0.025
Myocardial infarctions	↓ 16	0.052
Microvascular disease	↓ 25	0.0099

Adapted from United Kingdom Prospective Diabetes Study (UKPDS) Group. *Lancet*. 1998;352:837-853.

was a definite secondary failure rate (~7% per year) in all subjects (**Figure 7.1**). Part of the explanation for the high secondary failure rate may be that subjects were diagnosed relatively late in the natural history of the disease, as they are in the United States: on average, >5 years after onset of hyperglycemia. In this situation, the disease process would be well established and therapeutic interventions less effective to prevent the natural progression of the disease. Another likely possibility is that the mechanism of action of the therapeutic agents utilized did not significantly impact one or more of the major pathophysiologic abnormalities of type 2 diabetes such as insulin resistance and β-cell dysfunction.

■ **Intensive Glucose Control and Cardiovascular Risk**

In the UKPDS, intensive glucose control with SFU/insulin therapy in patients with newly diagnosed type 2 diabetes was associated with a reduced risk of clinically evident microvascular complications as well as a nonsignificant ($P=0.052$) reduction of 16% in the relative risk of MI compared with patients receiving standard therapy (dietary restrictions). Patients whose body weight was >120% of their ideal weight primarily received MET. In these patients, there were reductions in the risk of MI of 39% ($P=0.01$) and of death from any cause of 36% ($P=0.01$). The results of long-term follow-up of the original UKPDS trial have been reported. After completion of the primary 5-year trial, 3277 patients of the 4209 initially randomized were followed for an additional 5 years. Within 1 year of the original study end, the between-group differences in A1C levels disappeared.

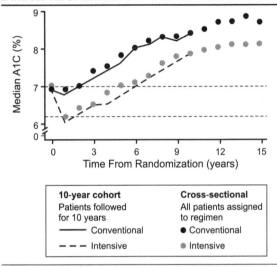

The trend toward loss of glycemic control was extended over the 10-year follow-up in the group of patients who received conventional treatment. Glycosylated hemoglobin (A1C) increased steadily over the 10 years. This can be seen in both the cross-sectional and 10-year cohort data. In patients who received intensive therapy, an initial decline in A1C was not sustained throughout the study. This result is similar to that seen in the conventional-treatment group, confirming that type 2 diabetes worsens over time. A comparable result was seen over the course of the study with regard to fasting plasma glucose levels—a gradual increase among patients who received conventional treatment and an initial reduction followed by deterioration among patients who received intensive treatment.

Adapted from United Kingdom Prospective Diabetes Study (UKPDS) Group. *Lancet*. 1998;352:837-853.

Nevertheless, the SFU/insulin group had a 15% ($P=0.01$) lower risk of MI and a 13% ($P=0.007$) lower risk of death from any cause compared with the diet group. The benefits were even greater among overweight patients who received MET, who had a 33% ($P=0.005$) lower risk of heart attack and a 27% ($P=0.002$) reduced risk of death. These results suggest that it may be very important to initiate early and aggressive treatment to maintain A1C at near-normal levels, possibly translating to long-term beneficial effects on CV disease and mortality.

The subsequent Steno-2 Trial looked at the cardiac event rate when multiple risk factors were aggressively treated in subjects with type 2 diabetes when compared with a control group. One hundred and sixty patients with type 2 diabetes with microalbuminuria (age ~55, BMI ~30, and duration of diabetes ~5.8 years) were randomized to aggressive treatment of their A1C, LDL, triglycerides, and blood pressure levels compared with a control group, and then followed for 7.8 years. Nonpharmacologic interventions in the intensive-therapy group included diet and increased exercise. Pharmacologic interventions included combinations of antihypertensives (ACE inhibitors or ARBs, with thiazides, calcium channel blockers [CCBs], and β-blockers added as needed), vitamin-mineral supplements (eg, vitamin C, D-α-tocopherol, folic acid, chrome picolinate), aspirin, oral hypoglycemic agents (MET, gliclazide), insulin (regular, NPH), and lipid-lowering agents (statins, fibrates). The composite end points were death from CV causes, nonfatal MI, coronary artery bypass grafting, percutaneous coronary intervention, nonfatal stroke, amputation, and surgery for peripheral atherosclerotic artery disease. The results were striking in that there was approximately a 50% reduction in the composite end points in <8 years (**Figure 7.2**).

However, the results of the Action to Control Cardiovascular Risk in Diabetes (ACCORD) and ADVANCE trials have raised questions as to whether CV events can be prevented in patients with type 2 diabetes by intensive metabolic control alone. In these large, prospective studies, intensive glycemic control resulted in a mean A1C of 6.4% (ACCORD) and 6.5% (ADVANCE) compared with standard control resulting in an A1C of 7.5% and 7.3%, respectively. In neither of these studies did the intensively treated group achieve a significantly reduced rate of CV events. In ACCORD, the study with the most ambitious goal (A1C <6%), all-cause mortality and CV mortality was greater in the intensive-treatment group. In the ADVANCE trial, mortality and

FIGURE 7.2 — STENO-2 Composite End Point: **Death From CV Causes**, **Nonfatal MI**, **CABG**, **PCI**, **Nonfatal Stroke**, **Amputation**, **Surgery for Peripheral Atherosclerotic Artery Disease**

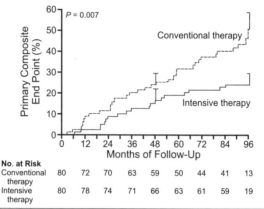

Gaede P, et al. *N Engl J Med*. 2003;348:383-393.

the incidence of CV events were not statistically different between the two treatment groups, whereas the risk of microvascular complications, especially nephropathy, was significantly decreased in the intensive-treatment group.

In addition, the Veterans Affairs Diabetes Trial (VADT) also showed that intensive glucose control had no significant benefit in terms of decreasing CV complications. Furthermore, any effect on CV risk disappeared with duration of the disease and that the risk of CV events increased in patients with severe hypoglycemic episodes. It is important to note that at baseline, the participants in VADT had an average A1C of 9.5%, 40% had previous CV events, >50% had abnormal lipids, 80% had hypertension, and most were obese. In these three studies, the hypoglycemic risk increased in the intensive-control group, which may have contributed to the reduced positive impact of better glucose control on CV complications.

These results from the ACCORD, ADVANCE, and VADT trials have raised questions about the benefits of intensive glycemic control on the risk of CV events. However, the ADVANCE study *did* show benefits of intensive glycemic control in terms of the reduced risk of the combined end point of major macrovascular and microvascular events, although not a significant reduction in the risk of macrovascular events considered separately. In the ACCORD trial, beginning at approximately 4 years, there was an increasingly favorable, although nonsignificant, separation in the curves for the primary composite end point of nonfatal MI, nonfatal stroke, or death from CV causes (**Figure 7.3**). One might speculate that this difference may have become significant if the study had gone to completion. It should also be noted there were differences in the patient populations in the ADVANCE and ACCORD trials. In ADVANCE, the percentages of patients treated with insulin at baseline were 1.5% (intensive group) and 1.4% (standard group), and by study end, the percentages were 40.5% and 24.1%, respectively. In ACCORD, the percentages of patients receiving insulin at baseline were 34.1% and 35.7% and 77% and 55%, respectively, at study end. Thus ACCORD probably included patients with more severe diabetes that required insulin at baseline, and that insulin was initiated more aggressively in ACCORD than in ADVANCE.

FIGURE 7.3 — Kaplan-Meier Curves for the Primary End Point[a] in the ACCORD Trial

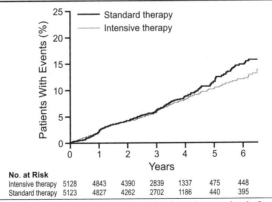

No. at Risk							
Intensive therapy	5128	4843	4390	2839	1337	475	448
Standard therapy	5123	4827	4262	2702	1186	440	395

[a] Combination of nonfatal MI, nonfatal stroke, or death from cardiovascular causes.

Adapted from The Action to Control Cardiovascular Risk in Diabetes Study Group. *N Engl J Med*. 2008;358:2545-2559.

Furthermore, the incidence of severe hypoglycemia was much higher in the intensive-treatment groups of ACCORD (10.5%) vs ADVANCE (2.7%) and it has been speculated that a high incidence of severe hypoglycemia may have contributed to the increased total and CV deaths in the intensive-treatment arm of ACCORD.

The results of the VADT clearly indicate that there was no benefit from intensive glycemic control, at least in that patient population. However, the VADT was probably underpowered to detect a significant difference among a patient population characterized by long-standing diabetes, poorly controlled hyperglycemia, previous CV events, and multiple coexisting CV risk factors. The observed lack of significant CV benefits in the ACCORD and VADT studies and the increased deaths associated with intensive glycemic treatment in ACCORD may not reflect the response of patients with a shorter duration of diabetes and without a strong history of CVD. It remains important to treat early with the goal of maintaining A1C at near normal levels without hypoglycemia.

In light of the above questions and concerns, the ADA currently recommends an A1C target of 7% for nonpregnant adults with the option of more stringent glycemic control in selected individuals where this can be achieved without significant hypoglycemia. Less stringent glycemic control is recommended for other groups, including those who have had severe hypoglycemia and those with a limited life expectancy. In addition, all CV risk factors should be addressed.

Secondary Failure of Oral Agents and the Importance of Early Glucose Control

Before the availability of the non–SFU antidiabetic agents in the United States, approximately 35% of type 2 patients were treated with insulin. In the United States, approximately two thirds of adults with type 2 diabetes use oral therapy during the first 5 years after diagnosis; this figure drops to about one third after a 20-year duration of diabetes. One of the explanations for this secondary failure rate of oral agents is that as the disease duration progresses, the endogenous insulin secretory ability of the pancreas diminishes, and the need for exogenous insulin increases. It is possible that by intensifying glycemic control early and by using non–insulin-secreting oral agents and "resting" the pancreas, one can possibly delay this consistently observed β-cell–exhaustion phenomenon.

SUGGESTED READING

Action to Control Cardiovascular Risk in Diabetes Study Group; Gerstein HC, Miller ME, Byington RP, et al. Effects of intensive glucose lowering in type 2 diabetes. *N Engl J Med.* 2008;358:2545-2559.

ADVANCE Collaborative Group; Patel A, MacMahon S, Chalmers J, et al. Intensive blood glucose control and vascular outcomes in patients with type 2 diabetes. *N Engl J Med.* 2008;358:2560-2572.

American Diabetes Association. *Medical Management of Type 2 Diabetes.* 6th ed. Alexandria, VA: American Diabetes Association; 2008.

Diabetes Control and Complications Trial Research Group. The effect of intensive treatment of diabetes on the development and progression of long-term complications in insulin-dependent diabetes mellitus. *N Engl J Med.* 1993;329:977-986.

Duckworth W, Abraira C, Moritz T, et al; VADT Investigators. Glucose control and vascular complications in veterans with type 2 diabetes. *N Engl J Med.* 2009;360:129-139.

Edelman SV. Importance of glucose control. *Med Clin North Am.* 1998; 82:665-687.

Festa A, D'Agostino R Jr, Howard G, Mykkanen L, Tracy RP, Haffner SM. Chronic subclinical inflammation as part of the insulin resistance syndrome: the Insulin Resistance Atherosclerosis Study (IRAS). *Circulation.* 2000;102:42-47.

Gaede P, Vedel P, Larsen N, Jensen G, Parving H, Pedersen O. Multifactorial intervention and cardiovascular disease in patients with type 2 diabetes. *N Engl J Med.* 2003;348:383-393.

Holman RR, Paul SK, Bethel A, Matthews DR, Neil HAW. 10-Year follow-up of intensive glucose control in type 2 diabetes. *N Engl J Med.* 2008;359:1577-1589.

Reichard P, Nilsson BY, Rosenqvist U. The effect of long-term intensified insulin treatment on the development of microvascular complications of diabetes mellitus. *N Engl J Med.* 1993;329:304-309.

United Kingdom Prospective Diabetes Study (UKPDS) Group. Intensive blood-glucose control with sulphonylureas or insulin compared with conventional treatment and risk complications in patients with type 2 diabetes (UKPDS 33). *Lancet.* 1998;352:837-853.

Weyer C, Funahashi T, Tanaka S, et al. Hypoadiponectinemia in obesity and type 2 diabetes: close association with insulin resistance and hyperinsulinemia. *J Clin Endocrinol Metab.* 2001;86:1930-1935.

8   Oral Agents

Current therapy for the treatment of hyperglycemia of type 2 diabetes includes the following oral antidiabetic agents:

- The biguanide metformin (MET)
- Dipeptidyl peptidase-4 (DPP-4) inhibitors sitagliptin, saxagliptin, linagliptin, and alogliptin
- The sodium-glucose transporter 2 (SGLT2) inhibitor canagliflozin
- The thiazolidinediones (TZDs) rosiglitazone and pioglitazone
- The alpha-glucosidase inhibitors (AGIs) acarbose and miglitol
- First- and second-generation sulfonylureas (SFUs)
- The D-phenylalanine derivative nateglinide
- The meglitinide repaglinide
- The bile acid sequestrant (BAS) colesevelam
- The dopamine receptor agonist bromocriptine mesylate.

According to the 2012 Position Statement from the ADA and the European Association for the Study of Diabetes (EASD), oral antidiabetic drug (OAD) therapy (specifically with MET) should be initiated concurrent with lifestyle intervention at diagnosis (see *Chapter 12*). MET is recommended as the initial pharmacologic therapy, in the absence of specific contraindications, for its effect on glycemia, absence of weight gain and hypoglycemia, generally low level of side effects, high level of acceptance, and relatively low cost. MET treatment should be titrated to its maximally effective dose over 1 to 2 months, as tolerated (see *MET* section, below).

OADs have different pharmacokinetics, potency, metabolism, and mechanisms of action that influence the choice of medication to use for initial and combination therapy (**Table 8.1**). Careful examination of the patient's metabolic profile, including weight, cholesterol levels, presence of glucose toxicity, duration of diabetes, and

TABLE 8.1 — Characteristics of Currently Available Oral Antidiabetic Agents

Generic Name	Trade Name	Recommended Starting Dose (mg)	Recommended Daily Maximum Dose (mg)	Dose Frequency
Alpha-Glucosidase Inhibitors[a]				
Acarbose	Precose	25 tid w/meals	100	bid-tid w/wo meals
Miglitol	Glyset	25 tid w/meals	50	bid-tid w/wo meals
Biguanide[a]				
Metformin	Glucophage	500 qd w/evening meal	2550	bid-tid
	Fortamet	500-1000 qd	2500	qd
	Glucophage XR	500 qd	2000	qd
	Glumetza	1000 qd	2000	qd
Bile Acid Sequestrant				
Colesevelam	Welchol	3750 mg[b]	3750 mg[b]	bid-qd
Dopamine Receptor Agonist				
Bromocriptine mesylate	Cycloset	0.8[c]	4.8	qd within 2 hours after awakening
DPP-4 Inhibitors				
Alogliptin	Nesina	25[d]	25[d]	qd w/wo meals
Linagliptin	Tradjenta	5[e]	5[e]	qd w/wo meals

74

Saxagliptin	Onglyza	2.5–5.0[d]	5.0[d]	qd w/wo meals
Sitagliptin	Januvia	100[d]	100[d]	qd w/wo meals
DPP-4 Inhibitor/Biguanide Combination Agents				
Alogliptin/metformin	Kazano	12.5/500	25/2000	bid w/meals
Linagliptin/metformin	Jentadueto	2.5/500	2.5/1000	bid w/meals
Saxagliptin/metformin XR	Kombiglyze XR	5/500 or 2.5/1000	5/2000	qd w/meal
Sitagliptin/metformin	Janumet	50/500	100/2000	bid w/meals
Sitagliptin/metformin XR	Janumet XR	50/500 or 50/1000	100/2000	qd w/meal
DPP-4 Inhibitor/Thiazolidinedione Combination Agent				
Alogliptin/pioglitazone	Oseni	25/15 or 25/30	25/45	qd w/wo meals
Glinides				
Nateglinide	Starlix	120 tid w/meals	360	bid-qid w/meals
Repaglinide[f]	Prandin	0.5 bid-qid w/meals	4	bid-qid w/meals
Glinide/Biguanide Combination Agent				
Repaglinide/metformin	Prandimet	1/500	10/2500	bid-qid w/meals
SGLT2 Agent				
Canagliflozin	Invokana	100	300	qd

Continued

TABLE 8.1 — *Continued*

Generic Name	Trade Name	Recommended Starting Dose (mg)	Recommended Daily Maximum Dose (mg)	Dose Frequency
Sulfonylureas[f,g]				
First Generation				
Acetohexamide	Dymelor	125 bid	1500	bid
Chlorpropamide	Diabinese	250 qd	500	qd
Tolazamide	Tolinase	100 qd	1000	bid
Tolbutamide	Orinase	250 bid	3000	tid
Second Generation				
Glimepiride	Amaryl	1-2 qd	8	qd
Glipizide	Glucotrol	5 qd	40	bid
Glipizide (extended release)	Glucotrol XL	5 qd	20	qd
Glyburide	DiaBeta, Micronase	2.5-5 qd	20	bid
	Glynase PresTab	1.5-3 qd	12	bid
Sulfonylurea/Biguanide Combination Agents				
Glipizide/metformin	Metaglip	2.5/250 qd w/meals	20/2000	bid w/meals
Glyburide/metformin	Glucovance	1.25/250 qd w/meals	10/2000	bid w/meals

Thiazolidinediones				
Pioglitazone	Actos	15-30 qd	45	qd
Rosiglitazone	Avandia	4 qd or 2 bid	8	bid-qd
Thiazolidinedione/Biguanide Combination Agents				
Pioglitazone/metformin	Actoplus Met	15/500 or 15/850 w/meals	45/2550	bid w/meals
Pioglitazone/metformin XR	Actoplus Met XR	15/1000 or 30/1000 w/meal	45/2000	qd
Rosiglitazone/metformin	Avandamet	2/500 bid w/meals	8/2000	bid w/meals
Thiazolidinedione/Sulfonylurea Combination Agents				
Pioglitazone/glimepiride	Duetact	30/2 or 30/4	45/8	qd
Rosiglitazone/glimepiride	Avandaryl	4/1 or 4/2	8/4	qd

[a] The dose of metformin, acarbose, and miglitol must be titrated slowly to limit GI side effects.

[b] Available either as a tablet or oral suspension formulation.

[c] Initial dose is 0.8 mg and increased by 1 tablet/week until a total maximum daily dose of 4.8 mg or until maximum tolerated daily dose.

[d] Dose adjustment required in patients with moderate or severe renal impairment or with ESRD.

[e] No dose adjustment is recommended for patients with type 2 diabetes who have renal or hepatic impairment.

[f] Selection of initial dose depends on the patient's glucose level.

[g] Starting dose for elderly and lean adults with diabetes may need to be reduced by up to 50%.

Modified from *Physicians' Desk Reference 2013*. 67th ed. Montvale, NJ: PDR Network, LLC; 2012.

8

concomitant use of other oral agents, will dictate the best OAD to use initially and in combination to achieve glycemic control. In general, OADs are contraindicated in patients who:

- Are pregnant or lactating
- Are seriously ill
- Have significant kidney or liver disease
- Have demonstrated allergic reactions.

In addition, patients with significant and prolonged hyperglycemia with marked symptoms, such as polyuria, polydipsia, or weight loss, should be considered for temporary insulin therapy before considering the institution of OADs. The rationale for insulin therapy is to acutely treat hyperglycemia to reduce glucotoxicity and enable the oral agents to be more effective.

Metformin

MET is a biguanide that works by:
- Mainly suppressing excessive hepatic glucose production
- Increasing glucose utilization in peripheral tissues to a lesser degree.

MET may also improve glucose levels by reducing intestinal glucose absorption. Because MET does not stimulate endogenous insulin secretion, hypoglycemia does not usually occur when this drug is used alone, although hypoglycemia may occur if MET is taken with insulin, an SFU, or an excessive amount of alcohol. MET is not metabolized and is excreted unchanged by the kidneys. MET is recommended as initial pharmacologic therapy in newly diagnosed patients concurrent with lifestyle intervention.

MET is effective as monotherapy or in combination with SFUs. MET can be added to the regimens of patients who have not responded initially to SFUs (primary treatment failure) or patients who responded initially to SFUs but who subsequently have deterioration of glycemic control (secondary treatment failure). SFUs can also be added to the regimens of patients in whom MET therapy has failed. The combination of MET and an SFU often achieves a better glycemic response than either agent given alone. When MET is added to an SFU, the dose of the SFU should be maintained.

The combination of MET with TZDs, AGIs, the glinides, DPP-4 inhibitors, GLP-1 analogs, colesevelam, or insulin has also been shown to be safe and effective. MET use with these agents is discussed further in this chapter and in *Chapter 10*.

Treatment with MET has beneficial effects on plasma lipids that are greater than expected from improved glucose control alone (it lowers triglyceride and LDL cholesterol levels while increasing HDL cholesterol). In addition, MET therapy has been associated with weight loss or less weight gain than other OADs. This may be particularly helpful in obese patients with type 2 diabetes.

■ Side Effects of Metformin

The major side effects of MET are:

- Gastrointestinal (GI) effects, consisting mainly of mild diarrhea or loose stools
- Anorexia
- Nausea
- Abdominal discomfort.

For most patients, these side effects:

- Are transient
- Are dose related
- Tend to decrease with chronic therapy.

They can be minimized by:

- Slow dosage titration
- Decreasing the dosage (sometimes only temporarily)
- Taking MET with meals.

Lactic acidosis is a rare complication of MET therapy but has a high mortality rate. Most of the cases of MET-associated lactic acidosis occurred in patients for whom the drug was contraindicated, ie, patients with renal dysfunction. MET should not be prescribed if the serum creatinine is >1.5 mg/dL in men or >1.4 mg/dL in women. In patients >80 years of age, it is recommended that a 24-hour urine collection be obtained to measure creatinine clearance (CrCl), which is a better indicator of kidney function. MET is also contraindicated in patients with significant hepatic disease, cardiac insufficiency, alcohol abuse, and any hypoxic condition or history of lactic acidosis. MET should not be used in any patient with CHF (compensated or uncompensated) who is currently on a loop diuretic and/or digoxin. MET should be temporarily discontinued at the time of or prior to any dye studies so that serum MET levels are low if the patient develops renal failure from the dye. MET should be withheld for 48 hours subsequent to dye studies and reinstated only after renal function has been evaluated and found to be normal. In any patient who is hospitalized with an acute severe illness, MET should be temporarily discontinued until the condition improves. During such circumstances, insulin is generally the preferred form of therapy.

■ Prescribing Metformin

The recommended starting dosage of MET is 500 mg twice a day or 850 mg once a day given with meals. However, we suggest an initial dosage of 500 mg/day with dinner for 1 week, then twice daily with breakfast and dinner to improve tolerability. The dosage should be titrated slowly, as needed, toward a maximum daily dose of 2550 mg. A third dose can be safely added at bedtime instead of at noon; compliance tends to be better. MET at bedtime works well to suppress hepatic glucose production overnight. Several weeks are required to observe the maximum effect of MET once a stable dosage is achieved.

■ Metformin/Glyburide Combination (Glucovance)

A combination pill (Glucovance) is available that consists of MET and glyburide (glyburide 1.25 mg combined with MET 250 mg and glyburide 2.5 mg or 5.0 mg combined with MET 500 mg) (Glucovance, **Table 8.1**). In the monotherapy pivotal trials, Glucovance was more effective at lowering the A1C and fasting and PPG values when compared with MET or glyburide alone. Even though Glucovance combines two medications that have been available for many years, early combination therapy with two different drugs that have different mechanisms of action have shown advantages.

MET is also available in an extended-release form (Glucophage XR, Fortamet, Glumetza). It can be taken once a day with equal efficacy compared with the short-acting form.

■ **Metformin/Glipizide Combination (Metaglip)**

A combination pill (Metaglip) is available that consists of MET and glipizide in various dosages (**Table 8.1**). Glipizide has a shorter duration of action and the metabolites have minimal hypoglycemic activity, leading to a lower rate of hypoglycemia compared with that which occurs with longer-acting SFUs.

DPP-4 Inhibitors

A potential role for intestinal peptides in the restoration of normal insulin secretion and regulation of PPG control was identified based on the observation that insulin responses to an oral glucose load exceeded those after IV glucose administration measured at the same blood glucose concentration. This so-called incretin effect is attributed to the insulinotropic action of gut hormones, particularly:

- Glucose-dependent insulinotropic polypeptide (GIP)
- Glucagonlike peptide 1 (GLP-1).

One approach to utilizing the therapeutic potential of GLP-1 has been the development of incretin mimetics (see *Chapter 10*).

Since incretin hormone actions are rapidly degraded through N-terminal cleavage by the enzyme DPP-4, the use of DPP-4 inhibitors offers another strategy for the treatment of patients with type 2 diabetes. Currently, four agents of this class of antihyperglycemic medications are approved in the United States. One of the advantages of these drugs is that they can be taken orally whereas the incretin mimetics are administered by subcutaneous injection.

■ **Sitagliptin (Januvia)**

Sitagliptin, a selective DPP-4 inhibitor, is indicated as an adjunct to diet and exercise to improve glycemic control in adults with type 2 diabetes mellitus. Specifically, it is approved:

- For initial therapy, either as monotherapy or in combination with MET or a TZD
- As add-on to MET, a TZD, or an SFU when the single agent alone does not provide adequate glycemic control
- In combination therapy with insulin
- As part of triple combination therapy with MET and a TZD when dual therapy does not provide adequate glycemic control.

Monotherapy Trials

The efficacy and tolerability of sitagliptin monotherapy in patients with type 2 diabetes were demonstrated in several randomized, double-blind, placebo-controlled trials. In an 18-week trial, 521 patients were randomized in a 1:2:2 ratio to receive placebo, sitagliptin 100 mg, or sitagliptin 200 mg qd after an appropriate washout and a diet/exercise or single-blind placebo run-in period. At the end of the treatment period, both sitagliptin 100 mg qd and 200 mg qd significantly decreased A1C compared with placebo (placebo-subtracted A1C: −0.60% and −0.48%, respectively). Patients with higher baseline A1C ($\geq$9%) experienced greater placebo-subtracted reductions with sitagliptin treatment (−1.20% for 100 mg and −1.04% for 200 mg) than those with a baseline A1C <8% (−0.44% and −0.33%, respectively) or 8% to 8.9% (−0.61% and −0.39%, respectively). After 18 weeks, both dosages of sitagliptin also significantly decreased FPG (placebo subtracted FPG: −12.6 mg/dL and −10.6 mg/dL, with 100 mg and 200 mg, respectively). Two-hour PPG also was significantly reduced with sitagliptin 100 mg and 200 mg compared with placebo (placebo subtracted PPG: −41.4 mg/dL and −48.6 mg/dL, respectively). The incidence of hypoglycemia or GI adverse events (AEs) was not significantly different with either dose of sitagliptin compared with placebo. There were similar reductions in mean body weight in the three treatment groups (sitagliptin 100 mg −0.6 kg; sitagliptin 200 mg −0.2 kg; and placebo −0.7 kg).

A 24-week study used a similar design and found similar results. After 24 weeks, both sitagliptin 100 mg and 200 mg produced significant placebo-subtracted reductions in A1C (−0.79% and −0.94%, respectively) and FPG (−17.1 mg/dL and −21.3 mg/dL, respectively). Both sitagliptin 100 mg and 200 mg significantly reduced 2-hour PPG from baseline (placebo-subtracted PPG: −46.7 and −54.1 mg/dL, respectively). There were no significant differences in the reductions in A1C, FPG, or PPG between the two sitagliptin doses. The incidence of hypoglycemia and GI AEs was not higher with either dose of sitagliptin compared with placebo. There were minimal reductions from baseline in body weight with sitagliptin 100 mg (−0.2 kg) and 200 mg (−0.1 kg); however, body weight was significantly reduced from baseline with placebo (−1.1 kg).

Sitagliptin was compared with MET as monotherapy in treatment-naïve patients with type 2 diabetes in a randomized, double-blind, noninferiority trial. Patients were treated either with sitagliptin 100 mg once daily ($n = 528$) or MET 1000 mg bid ($n = 522$) for 24 weeks. The criteria for noninferiority was if the upper boundary of the 95% CI for the between-group difference in A1C change from baseline was <0.40%. At week 24, A1C change from baseline was −0.43% with sitagliptin and −0.57% with MET. The between-group difference (95% CI) was 0.14%, thus confirming noninferiority.

Long-Term Efficacy of Sitagliptin Monotherapy

In order to look at the long-term efficacy of sitagliptin monotherapy, patients in the 24-week placebo-controlled trial entered an extension period lasting 54 weeks. Patients were given either 100 mg or 200 mg of sitagliptin once a day. The changes in A1C from baseline at week 54 were −0.6% (95% CI: −0.7, −0.4) with 100 mg and -0.6% (−0.8, −0.5) with 200 mg. Sitagliptin was well tolerated and there was no weight gain. The durability of sitagliptin efficacy was demonstrated over this 54-week study.

Combination or Add-On Therapy Trials

Sitagliptin was studied as combination or add-on treatment with MET, an SFU, or pioglitazone in randomized, parallel group, placebo-controlled studies of 18-weeks or 24-weeks duration. In these studies, patients were randomized after appropriate washout and placebo run-in periods.

The efficacy and tolerability of the initial combination of sitagliptin and MET in patients with type 2 diabetes inadequately controlled on diet and exercise were evaluated in a 24-week, study in which total of 1091 patients with A1C 7.5% to 11% were randomized to one of six daily treatments: sitagliptin 100 mg/MET 1000 mg (S100/M1000 group), sitagliptin 100 mg/MET 2000 mg (S100/M2000 group), MET 1000 mg (M1000 group), MET 2000 mg (M2000 group) (all as divided doses administered bid), sitagliptin 100 mg qd (S100 group), or placebo. The placebo-subtracted A1C changes from baseline were: −2.07% (S100/M2000), −1.57% (S100/M1000), −1.30% (M2000), −0.99% (M1000), and −0.83% (S100) ($P<0.001$ for comparisons vs placebo and for coadministration vs respective monotherapies). The proportion of patients achieving an A1C <7% and <6.5% was 66% and 44%, respectively, in the S100/M2000 group ($P<0.001$ vs S100 or M2000 monotherapies). The incidences of hypoglycemia ranged from 0.5% to 2.2% across active treatment groups and were significantly different from that in the placebo group (0.6%). There were significant reductions in body weight in treatment groups relative to baseline ranging from −0.6 kg to 1.3 kg, except in the sitagliptin monotherapy group in which there was no change from baseline.

A 24-week trial in 701 patients evaluated the efficacy and tolerability of sitagliptin in patients who had inadequate glycemic control on MET (≥1500 mg/day) monotherapy. Patients were randomized in a 1:2 ratio to receive adjunctive placebo or sitagliptin 100 mg qd for 24 weeks. Mean baseline A1C was 8.0% (**Figure 8.1**). After 24 weeks, sitagliptin/MET therapy resulted in a significant placebo-subtracted reduction in A1C (−0.65%) (**Figure 8.1-A**), FPG (−25.4 mg/dL), and 2-hour PPG (−50.6 mg/dL) (**Figure 8.1-B**). Overall, the incidences of hypoglycemia and GI AEs between the two groups were similar. Mean body weight changes from baseline were not significantly different between the sitagliptin group (−0.7 kg) and the placebo group (−0.6 kg).

Another 24-week study assessed the efficacy and safety of the addition of sitagliptin in 353 patients treated

FIGURE 8.1 — Sitagliptin Added to Ongoing Metformin Therapy Enhanced Glycemic Control and β-Cell Function in Patients With Type 2 Diabetes

A. Mean (SE) A1C Over Time[a]

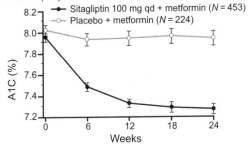

B. Mean (SE) Plasma Glucose Concentration (mg/dL) at Baseline and Week 24 Following 3-Point MTT[b,c]

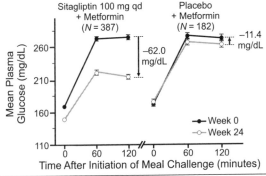

[a] LS mean difference between groups [95% CI] in A1C = –0.65% [–0.77, –0.53]; $P < 0.001$.

[b] Patients ingested a standardized meal consisting of two nutrition bars and one nutrition drink (–680 kcal; carbohydrates, 111g; fat, 14 g; protein, 26 g.

[c] LS mean difference between groups in change from baseline at week 24 in 2-hour postmeal glucose [95% CI] = –50.6 mg/dL [–60.5, –40.8]; $P < 0.001$.

Charbonnel B, et al. *Diabetes Care*. 2006;29:2638-2643.

with pioglitazone monotherapy. Patients were randomized (1:1) to receive placebo or sitagliptin 100 qd in addition to ongoing pioglitazone (**Figure 8.2**). After 24 weeks, sitagliptin/pioglitazone treatment resulted in significant placebo-subtracted reductions in A1C (−0.70%) (**Figure 8.2-A**) and FPG (−17.7 mg/dL). The effects on glycemic control were maintained over the 24-week treatment period. The percentage of patients achieving target A1C

FIGURE 8.2 — Efficacy and Safety of Sitagliptin Added to Ongoing Pioglitazone Therapy in Patients With Type 2 Diabetes

A. Mean (SE) A1C Over Time[a]

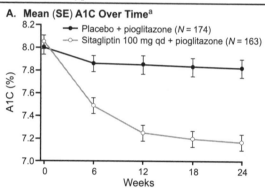

B. Proportion of Patients Achieving A1C Levels of <7.0% and <6.5% by Treatment Group[b]

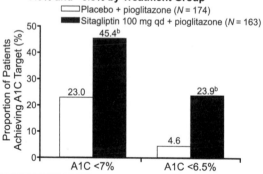

[a] LS mean difference between groups [95% CI] = −0.70% [−0.85, −0.59]; $P < 0.001$.

[b] $P < 0.001$ for sitagliptin 100 mg qd + pioglitazone vs placebo + pioglitazone.

Rosenstock J, et al. *Clin Ther*. 2006;28:1556-1568.

<7% was 45% and 23% in the sitagliptin/pioglitazone and placebo/pioglitazone groups, respectively (**Figure 8.2-B**). There was no between-group difference in mean body weight change. The overall incidence of AEs and hypoglycemia was similar in the two groups, although the incidence of abdominal pain was slightly higher in patients who received sitagliptin.

A 52-week, noninferiority trial compared the efficacy and tolerability of sitagliptin and glipizide in patients who had inadequate glycemic control with MET monotherapy. A total of 1172 patients were randomized to sitagliptin 100 mg qd or glipizide up to 20 mg daily (maximum titrated dose). There were significant similar mean reductions in A1C (0.67%) vs baseline in each treatment group in these patients with mildly elevated baseline A1C levels (mean 7.5%), and similar proportions of patients achieved A1C goal (<7%) in each group (63% with sitagliptin vs 59% with glipizide). At 52 weeks, the prespecified bounds for noninferiority of sitagliptin vs glipizide were achieved. Patients in the sitagliptin group experienced significant weight loss (mean, -1.5 kg) from baseline at 52 weeks, while those in the glipizide group experienced significant weight gain (mean, +1.1 kg). The between-group difference was statistically significant ($P<0.001$). Additionally, there was a significantly higher rate of hypoglycemia in glipizide-treated patients than in sitagliptin-treated patients (patients experiencing at least one hypoglycemic episode regardless of severity: 32.0% vs 4.9%, respectively).

The efficacy and tolerability of adding sitagliptin 100 mg once daily to ongoing treatment with glimepiride alone or glimepiride in combination with MET was assessed in a 24-week, randomized, placebo-controlled trial in 441 patients. Of these patients, 212 (48%) were on glimepiride ($\geq$4 mg/day) monotherapy and 229 (52%) were on glimepiride ($\geq$4 mg/day) plus MET ($\geq$1500 mg/day) combination therapy. After 24 weeks, sitagliptin significantly reduced A1C by 0.74% relative to placebo. In the subset of patients on glimepiride plus MET, sitagliptin reduced A1C by 0.89% relative to placebo, compared with a reduction of 0.57% in the subset of patients on glimepiride alone. The addition of sitagliptin reduced FPG by 20.1 mg/dL and increased homeostasis model assessment-β, a marker of β-cell function, by 12% compared with placebo. The addition of sitagliptin was generally well tolerated, with a modest increase in the incidence of hypoglycemia (12% vs 2% with placebo) and body weight (+0.8 kg vs −0.4 kg with placebo), consistent with glimepiride therapy and the observed degree of glycemic improvement.

A 24-week, randomized, double-blind, placebo-controlled study assessed the efficacy and safety of adding sitagliptin 100 mg in 641 patients who were inadequately controlled on stable doses of insulin (long-acting, intermediate-acting, or premixed) with or without concomitant MET. The addition of sitagliptin significantly reduced A1C by 0.6% compared with placebo (0.0%). A greater proportion of patients achieved an A1C level <7% with sitagliptin compared with placebo (13% vs 5%, respectively). The incidence of adverse experiences was higher with sitagliptin (52%) compared with placebo (43%), due mainly to the increased incidence of hypoglycemia (sitagliptin 16% vs placebo 8%). However, the number of hypoglycemic events meeting the protocol-specified criteria for severity was low with sitagliptin ($n=2$) and placebo ($n=1$).

A 54-week study in 1091 patients observed significant and comparable reductions from baseline in A1C levels with initial treatment with monotherapy with sitagliptin 100 mg (−0.8%), MET 1000 mg (−1.0%), MET 2000 mg (−1.3%) or the combination of sitagliptin 100 mg plus and MET 1000 mg (−1.4%) or sitagliptin 100 mg plus MET 2000 mg (−1.8%). Glycemic response was generally durable over time across treatments. Mean body weight decreased from baseline in the combination and MET monotherapy groups and was unchanged in the sitagliptin monotherapy group. The incidence of hypoglycemia was low (1% to 3%) across treatment groups. The incidence of GI adverse experiences with the combination of sitagliptin and MET was similar to that observed with MET alone.

Use in Patients With Renal Disease

Since sitagliptin is primarily renally excreted and its $AUC0-\infty$ is increased approximately 2- to 4-fold compared with healthy subjects in patients with moderate to severe renal insufficiency and ESRD, respectively, a randomized, placebo-controlled study assessed the safety of sitagliptin in type 2 diabetes patients with a CrCl <50 mL/minute. After diet/exercise and an antihyperglycemic drug washout period (except in patients on prior insulin therapy who remained on insulin), 91 patients (A1C 6.2% to 10.3%, mean 7.7%) were randomized (2:1) to sitagliptin or placebo for 12 weeks. Patients with moderate renal insufficiency (CrCl 30 to <50 mL/min) who were randomized to sitagliptin were treated with 50 mg qd and those with severe renal insufficiency (CrCl <30 mL/min) or ESRD received 25 mg qd in order to achieve drug exposure similar to that observed with 100 mg qd in patients with normal to mildly impaired renal function. At baseline, 10% were on insulin therapy and 43% had CrCl <30 mL/minute. The overall incidence of AEs was similar in the two groups. The incidences of drug-related AEs, serious AEs, and discontinuations due to AEs was modestly, but not meaningfully, higher in sitagliptin-treated patients. Furthermore, there were no differences in the percentage of patients who experienced hypoglycemia or GI AEs between groups. Body weight was unchanged in sitagliptin-treated patients. Although this was a safety study, after 12 weeks, mean A1C and FPG decreased by 0.59% and 25.5 mg/dL, respectively, in the sitagliptin groups (doses pooled) and by 0.18% and 3.0 mg/dL in the placebo group.

Adverse Events With Sitagliptin

Adverse reactions reported in ≥5% of patients treated with sitagliptin and more commonly than in patients treated with placebo are:

- Upper respiratory tract infection
- Nasopharyngitis
- Headache.

Hypoglycemia was also reported more commonly in patients treated with the combination of sitagliptin and an SFU, with or without MET, vs placebo. Sitagliptin is contraindicated in patient with a history of a serious hypersensitivity reaction to sitagliptin, including anaphylaxis and angioedema. There have been postmarketing reports of acute pancreatitis, including fatal and nonfatal hemorrhagic or necrotizing pancreatitis, in patients taking sitagliptin. If pancreatitis is suspected, sitagliptin should be discontinued promptly. It is unknown whether patients with a history of pancreatitis are at increased risk for the development of pancreatitis while using sitagliptin.

Prescribing Sitagliptin

In patients with type 2 diabetes, the recommended dose of sitagliptin is 100 mg qd as monotherapy or combination therapy. Sitagliptin can be taken with or without food. Sitagliptin should not be used in patients with type 1 diabetes or for the treatment DKA since it would not be effective in these settings. Dosage adjustment is recommended in patients with moderate (CrCl $\geq$30 to <50 mL/min) or severe (CrCl <30 mL/min) renal insufficiency and in patients with ESRD requiring hemodialysis or peritoneal dialysis. Since dosage adjustment based on renal function is needed, assessment of renal function is recommended prior to initiation of sitagliptin and periodically thereafter. Mean (SE) increases in serum creatinine were observed in patients treated with sitagliptin (0.12 mg/dL [0.04]) and in patients treated with placebo (0.07 mg/dL [0.07]). The clinical significance of this added increase in serum creatinine relative to placebo is not known.

■ Sitagliptin Fixed-Dose Combinations With Metformin (Janumet and Janumet XR)

Sitagliptin is also available in a fixed-dose, single-tablet formulation containing sitagliptin and MET (Janumet). Another fixed-dose, single-tablet formulation containing sitagliptin and MET is also available as an extended-release formulation (Janumet XR).

These combination formulations are indicated as an adjunct to diet and exercise to improve glycemic control in adult patients with type 2 diabetes mellitus who are not adequately controlled on MET or sitagliptin alone or in patients already being treated with the combination of sitagliptin and MET. Although neither of these fixed-dose, single-tablet combination of sitagliptin and MET have been studied specifically in patients with an inadequate response to insulin, the combination of sitagliptin with/without MET administered separately was shown to be effective in patients with an inadequate response to insulin.

Prescribing Janumet

The dosage of Janumet should be individualized on the basis of the patient's current regimen, effectiveness, and tolerability and should not exceed the maximum recommended daily dose of 100 mg sitagliptin and 2000 mg MET (**Table 8**.1).

Janumet should generally be given twice daily with meals, with gradual dose escalation, to reduce the GI side effects due to MET.

The starting dose of Janumet should be based on the patient's current regimen and should be given twice daily with meals. The following doses are available:

- 50 mg sitagliptin/500 mg MET
- 50 mg sitagliptin/1000 mg MET.

Prescribing Janumet XR

The dosage of Janumet XR should be individualized on the basis of the patient's current regimen, effectiveness, and tolerability and should not exceed the maximum recommended daily dose of 100 mg sitagliptin and 2000 mg MET XR.

Janumet XR should be administered once daily with food preferably in the evening, with gradual dose escalation, to reduce the GI side effects due to MET.

The starting dose of Janumet XR should be based on the patient's current regimen and should be given twice daily with meals. The following dosages are available:

- 50 mg sitagliptin/500 mg MET XR
- 50 mg sitagliptin/1000 mg MET XR
- 100 mg sitagliptin/1000 mg/1000 mg MET XR.

■ Saxagliptin (Onglyza)

Saxagliptin is approved for monotherapy and combination therapy as an adjunct to diet and exercise to improve glycemic control in adults with type 2 diabetes mellitus.

Saxagliptin is 10 times more potent than sitagliptin. The M2 metabolite is 2-fold less potent than saxagliptin. In healthy volunteers, mean C_{max} was 24 ng/mL for saxagliptin and 47 ng/mL for the M2 metabolite. Mean T_{max} was 2 hours for saxagliptin and 4 hours for M2. After an oral glucose load or a meal, there were 2- to 3-fold increases in circulating levels of active GLP-1 and

GIP, decreased glucagon concentrations, and increased glucose-dependent insulin secretion from pancreatic β cells. The increase in insulin and decrease in glucagon were associated with lower fasting glucose concentrations and reduced glucose excursions following an oral glucose load or a meal.

Monotherapy Trials

A 24-week, trial randomized 401 treatment-naïve patients to once-daily treatment with saxagliptin 2.5 mg, 5.0 mg, 10 mg, or placebo (main treatment cohort [MTC]). A separate open-label cohort (OLC) with 66 patients with baseline A1C >10% to <12% received saxagliptin 10 mg for 24 weeks. In the MTC, all three doses of saxagliptin demonstrated statistically significant decreases in mean A1C changes (all $P<0.0001$ vs placebo). Mean changes from baseline in FPG with saxagliptin also were significantly greater than with placebo. Mean changes from baseline in PPG at the 120-minutes time point were significantly lower with all three doses of saxagliptin compared with placebo. A greater proportion of saxagliptin-treated patients achieved A1C <7% at week 24 (35% [P=NS], 38% [P=0.0443], 41% [P=0.0133]) for saxagliptin 2.5, 5, and 10 mg, respectively, than placebo (24%). As in the MTC, clinically meaningful reductions in A1C, FPG, and PPG were observed in the OLC. Consistent with the higher baseline A1C (10.7%) in these patients, the mean decrease in A1C of 1.9% was greater than those observed in the MTC, as were changes in FPG (−33 mg/dL) and PPG at 120 min (−66 mg/dL). By week 24, an A1C <7% was achieved in 14% of patients.

Combination Trials

The efficacy of saxagliptin at doses of 2.5 mg or 5 mg once daily in combination with MET, an SFU (glyburide), or a TZD (pioglitazone or rosiglitazone) was studied in four large, 24-week, randomized, double-blind, placebo-controlled trials.

Saxagliptin With Metformin as Initial Therapy

The efficacy of initial combination therapy with saxagliptin plus MET vs saxagliptin or MET monotherapy was evaluated in 1306 treatment-naïve patients with type 2 diabetes and inadequate glycemic control. Patients were initially randomized to receive saxagliptin 5 mg plus MET 500 mg, saxagliptin 10 mg plus MET 500 mg, saxagliptin 10 mg plus placebo, or MET 500 mg plus placebo. From weeks 1 through 5, MET was uptitrated in 500-mg/day increments to 2000 mg/day maximum in the saxagliptin 5 mg plus MET, saxagliptin 10 mg plus MET, and MET plus placebo treatment groups.

At 24 weeks, saxagliptin 5 mg plus MET and saxagliptin 10 mg plus MET demonstrated statistically significantly greater decreases vs saxagliptin 10 mg and MET monotherapies in A1C and FPG (**Figure 8.3**). The proportion of patients achieving an A1C <7% was 60.3% and 59.7%, respectively, for saxagliptin 5 mg plus MET and saxagliptin 10 mg plus MET compared with 32.2% with saxagliptin monotherapy and 41.1% with MET monotherapy (all $P<0.0001$ vs both monotherapies).

Saxagliptin Added to Metformin

Saxagliptin 2.5, 5.0, or 10 mg once daily as add-on therapy was evaluated in 743 patients with type 2 diabetes with inadequate glycemic control with MET alone (1500-2500 mg/day). By week 24, all three doses of saxagliptin added to stable MET doses demonstrated statistically significant mean decreases from baseline vs placebo in A1C, FPG, and PPG (**Table 8.2**). More than twice as many patients achieved A1C <7.0% with 2.5, 5, and 10 mg saxagliptin compared with placebo. As in other clinical trials, β-cell function and postprandial C-peptide, insulin, and glucagon AUCs improved in all saxagliptin treatment groups. Reductions in body weight with saxagliptin were similar to that with placebo.

Saxagliptin Added to Glyburide

The addition of saxagliptin 2.5 mg or 5 mg once daily to a stable dose of glyburide (7.5 mg once daily) compared with uptitrated glyburide in 768 patients who had inadequate glycemic control on suboptimal dose of an SFU alone for ≥2 months (defined as less than the maximum approved dose for each SFU). During a single-blind, 4-week dietary and exercise run-in period, previous SFU therapy was discontinued and replaced with glyburide 7.5 mg once daily. Following the run-in

FIGURE 8.3 — Change in Glycemic Parameters After 24 Weeks With Saxagliptin Added to Metformin vs Saxagliptin or Metformin Monotherapy as Initial Therapy in Treatment-Naïve Patients

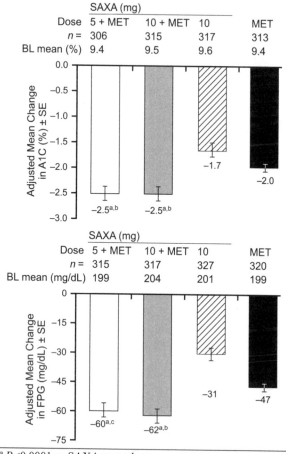

Jadzinsky M, et al. *Diabetes Obes Metab.* 2009;11:611-622.

TABLE 8.2 — Change From Baseline in Glycemic Parameters After 24 Weeks of Treatment With Saxagliptin as Add-On Therapy With Metformin

| Efficacy End Point | SAXA (mg) + MET | | | PBO + MET |
	2.5 (n=192)	5.0 (n=191)	10.0 (n=181)	(n=179)
A1C (%):				
Change from baseline	−0.59	−0.69	−0.58	+0.13
Difference from PBO	−0.73[a]	−0.83[a]	−0.72[a]	—
FPG (mg/dL):				
Change from baseline	−14.3	−22.0	−20.5	+1.2
Difference from PBO	−15.6[a]	−23.3[a]	−21.7[a]	—
A1C <7%:				
n (%)	69 (37.1)[a]	81 (43.5)[a]	80 (44.4)[a]	29 (16.6)
PPG at 120 min (mg/dL):				
Change from baseline	−61.5	−58.2	−49.8	−18.0
Difference from PBO	−43.5[a]	−40.3[a]	−31.8[a]	—

[a] $P \leq 0.0001$ vs PBO + MET.

Defronzo RA, et al. *Diabetes Care.* 2009;32(9):1649-1655.

8

95

period, patients were randomized to receive 2.5 mg or 5 mg of saxagliptin added to 7.5 mg glyburide or to placebo plus a 10-mg total daily dose of glyburide. Patients who received placebo were eligible for blinded glyburide uptitration to a total daily dose of 15 mg. At week 24, 92% of glyburide-only patients had been uptitrated to a total glyburide dose of 15 mg/day. Both doses of saxagliptin in combination with glyburide were associated with significant decreases from baseline in A1C, FPG, and 2-hour PPG. More than twice as many patients in both saxagliptin plus glyburide groups achieved A1C <7%. Mean body weight increased in all treatment groups and were significantly greater in each saxagliptin treatment group vs uptitrated glyburide (+0.7 kg [$P=0.0381$] and +0.8 kg [$P=0.0120$] for saxagliptin 2.5 and 5 mg, respectively, vs +0.3 kg for uptitrated glyburide].

Saxagliptin Added to Thiazolidinedione

A total of 565 patients with inadequate glycemic control despite at least 12 weeks of treatment with TZD monotherapy (pioglitazone 30 or 45 mg or rosiglitazone 4 or 8 mg) were treated with saxagliptin (2.5 or 5 mg once daily) or placebo, all in addition to a stable dose of TZD. The primary outcome measure was change in A1C from baseline to week 24. Secondary outcomes included change from baseline in FPG and proportion of patients achieving A1C <7. At week 24, there were significant reductions from baseline in A1C and FPG in both saxagliptin groups compared with placebo (**Figure 8.4**). A significantly greater proportion of patients in the saxagliptin 2.5 mg and 5 mg groups achieved an A1C <7% (42.2% and 41.8% respectively; both $P<0.05$ vs 25.6% with placebo). In addition, there were statistically significant reductions from baseline in PPG-AUC in both saxagliptin groups compared with the placebo group (both $P<0.0001$). A small increase from baseline in body weight occurred in all treatment groups (1.3, 1.4, and 0.9 kg for saxagliptin 2.5 and 5 mg, and placebo, respectively).

Long-Term Use

The long-term efficacy of saxagliptin added to MET was demonstrated by the preliminary results of an exten-

FIGURE 8.4 — Change in Glycemic Parameters After 24 Weeks With Saxagliptin Added to Thiazolidinedione

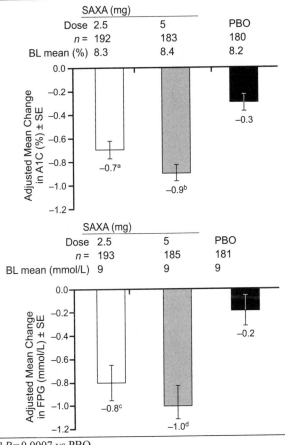

[a] $P = 0.0007$ vs PBO.
[b] $P < 0.0001$ vs PBO.
[c] $P = 0.0053$ vs PBO.
[d] $P < 0.0005$ vs PBO.

Modified from Hollander P, et al. *J Clin Endocrinol Metab.* 2009;94: 4810-4819.

sion of the 24-week study discussed above. After 102 weeks, the placebo-subtracted changes from baseline in A1C levels in patients who received saxagliptin 2.5 or 5 mg once-daily add-on therapy vs MET alone were 0.62% and 0.72%, respectively. During this period, 58% and 52% of patients treated with 2.5 or 5 mg of saxagliptin in combination with MET compared with 72% of those treated with MET monotherapy discontinued treatment or received rescue therapy for insufficient glycemic control.

Adverse Events With Saxagliptin

Saxagliptin as monotherapy or in combination with other OADs was generally well tolerated, with most adverse reactions being of mild or moderate intensity. In the above clinical trials, the incidence of treatment-emergent AEs were generally similar to that in patients who received other OADs or placebo. The most common AEs reported in $\geq 5\%$ of patients treated with saxagliptin and more commonly than in patients treated with placebo were:

- Upper respiratory tract infection
- Urinary tract infection
- Nasopharyngitis
- Headache.

The incidence of hypoglycemic events in patients treated with saxagliptin was generally similar to that in patients receiving placebo or other OADs. In patients treated with saxagliptin 2.5 or 5 mg as monotherapy, the incidence of hypoglycemic events was 4% and 6%, respectively (vs 4% of placebo recipients). When used as add-on therapy, the incidence was 9% and 8% with saxagliptin 2.5 or 5 mg, respectively (vs 7% of patients who received MET, glyburide, or a TZD).

Prescribing Saxagliptin

In patients with type 2 diabetes, the recommended dose of saxagliptin is 2.5 mg or 5 mg once daily taken regardless of meals. Saxagliptin should not be used in patients with type 1 diabetes or for the treatment DKA since it would not be effective in these settings. Saxagliptin has not been studied in combination with insulin.

No dosage adjustment for saxagliptin is recommended for patients with mild renal impairment (CrCl >50 mL/min). However, the recommended dose of saxagliptin is 2.5 mg qd for patients with moderate or severe renal impairment (CrCl ≤50 mL/min) or with ESRD requiring hemodialysis. Saxagliptin should be administered following hemodialysis. Because the dose of saxagliptin should be limited to 2.5 mg based upon renal function, assessment of renal function is recommended prior to initiation of saxagliptin and periodically thereafter. When coadministered with strong cytochrome P450 3A4/5 (CYP3A4/5) inhibitors (eg, ketoconazole, atazanavir, clarithromycin, indinavir, itraconazole, nefazodone, nelfinavir, ritonavir, saquinavir, and telithromycin), the recommended dose of saxagliptin is 2.5 mg qd.

■ Saxagliptin Fixed-Dose Combination With Metformin XR (Kombiglyze XR)

Saxagliptin is also available in a fixed-dose, single-tablet formulation containing saxagliptin and MET XR (Kombiglyze XR).

This combination formulation is indicated as an adjunct to diet and exercise to improve glycemic control in adults with type 2 diabetes mellitus when treatment with both saxagliptin and MET is appropriate. This fixed-dose, single-tablet combination of saxagliptin and MET XR has not been studied specifically in patients with an inadequate response to insulin. However, the combination of alogliptin with/without MET administered separately was shown to be effective in patients with an inadequate response to insulin.

Prescribing Kombiglyze XR

The dosage of Kombiglyze XR should be individualized on the basis of the patient's current regimen, effectiveness, and tolerability. It should generally be administered once daily with the evening meal, with gradual dose titration to reduce the GI side effects associated with MET. The following dosage forms are available:

- 5 mg saxagliptin and 500 mg MET XR
- 5 mg saxagliptin and 1000 mg MET XR
- 2.5 mg saxagliptin and 1000 mg MET XR.

The recommended starting dose of Kombiglyze XR in patients who need 5 mg of saxagliptin and who are not currently treated with MET is 5 mg saxagliptin/500 mg MET XR once daily with gradual dose escalation to reduce the GI side effects due to MET. The maximum daily recommended dose is 5 mg saxagliptin and 2000 mg MET XR.

■ Linagliptin (Tradjenta)

Linagliptin is indicated as an adjunct to diet and exercise to improve glycemic control in adults with type 2 diabetes mellitus. Linagliptin can be used as monotherapy or as add-on or combination therapy with other commonly prescribed OADs (eg, MET, SFU, or pioglitazone). Linagliptin is the first DPP-4 inhibitor approved at one dosage strength; no dose adjustment is recommended for patients with type 2 diabetes who have kidney or liver impairment.

Studies have shown that the pharmacokinetic parameters of linagliptin are similar in healthy subjects and in patients with type 2 diabetes. The absolute bioavailability of linagliptin is approximately 30%. Administration with a high-fat meal has a small, but not clinically relevant, effect on C_{max} and AUC; therefore, linagliptin may be administered with or without food. After once-daily dosing, a steady-state plasma concentration of linagliptin 5 mg is reached by the third dose. Unlike other DPP-4 inhibitors so far characterized, linagliptin is excreted unchanged mainly via feces (~80%) rather than by the renal route (~5%). Studies in healthy subjects and patients with type 2 diabetes with normal or various degrees of renal or hepatic function indicate that no dosage adjustment is necessary in patients with renal or hepatic impairment.

Monotherapy Trials

The efficacy and safety of linagliptin monotherapy were evaluated in two double-blind, placebo-controlled studies, one of 18-weeks duration and another of 24-weeks duration that enrolled 730 patients with type 2 diabetes with inadequate glycemic control (A1C, 7% to 10%). Before randomization in both studies, patients previously treated with OADs underwent a washout period of 6 weeks, which included a placebo run-in period during the last 2 weeks. Patients previously untreated with OADs underwent a 2-week placebo run-in period. In the 18-week study, treatment with linagliptin 5 mg once daily provided statistically significant improvements from baseline in A1C and FPG compared with placebo. By 18 weeks, 28% of linagliptin-treated patients achieved an A1C <7% compared with 15% of patients in the placebo-group.

In the 24-week study, 336 patients received lina-gliptin 5 mg once daily and 167 patients received placebo. Overall, the adjusted mean difference in the change in A1C comparing linagliptin with placebo was −0.69% ($P<0.0001$). Changes in adjusted mean A1C increased over time (−0.46% at 6 weeks to −0.69% at 24 weeks, all $P<0.0001$) (**Figure 8.5**). Reductions from baseline were smaller in patients previously treated with OADs than the difference between linagliptin and placebo in OAD-naïve patients. Patients treated with linagliptin were more likely to achieve a reduction in A1C of ≥0.5% at 24 weeks than those in the placebo arm (47.1% and 19.0%, respectively; $P<0.0001$). Fasting plasma glucose improved by −1.3 mmol/L ($P<0.0001$) with linagliptin vs placebo, and linagliptin produced an adjusted mean reduction from baseline after 24 weeks in 2-hour postprandial glucose of −3.2 mmol/L ($P<0.0001$). Linagliptin monotherapy was well tolerated and exhibited a safety profile comparable with that of placebo, with a very low incidence of hypo-glycemia (8.6% with linagliptin vs 22.8% with placebo in the 24-week study). There were no clinically significant changes in body weight between treatment groups.

Combination or Add-On Treatment

Linagliptin has been studied as combination or add-on treatment with MET, an SFU, or pioglitazone in randomized, parallel group, placebo-controlled studies of 18-weeks or 24-weeks duration. In these studies, patients were randomized after appropriate washout and placebo run-in periods.

Linagliptin Added to Metformin

Linagliptin as an add-on to MET was evaluated in 701 patients previously treated with MET alone or MET

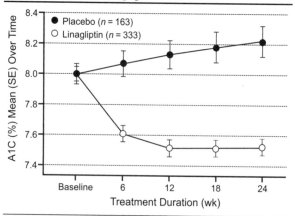

Differences in change from baseline in A1C between placebo and linagliptin are significant at each time point after baseline (*P*<0.0001).

Modified from Del Prato S, et al. *Diab Obes Metab*. 2011;13:258-267.

and other OADs. Eligible patients were randomized in a 3:1 ratio to treatment with either placebo or linagliptin 5 mg once daily. All patients continued to take their usual dosage of MET throughout the trial. After 24 weeks of treatment, linagliptin reduced the mean A1C level by 0.49%, whereas in the placebo group, A1C increased by 0.15%; a treatment difference of −0.64% (*P*<0.0001). The significant difference between treatments in mean A1C change increased over time from 6 weeks (−0.43%) to 18 weeks (−0.65%), then remained stable until the end of the 24 weeks (−0.64%) (**Figure 8.6**). The placebo-corrected reduction in A1C from baseline at 24 weeks was greater in patients who had previously been treated with an OAD in addition to MET compared with those who had not previously received an OAD in addition to MET (−0.79 vs −0.60%, respectively; but not significant). Linagliptin treatment also resulted in significant reductions vs placebo in FPG (−0.59 vs 0.58 mmol/L) and 2-hour PPG (−2.7 vs 1.0 mmol/L; all *P*<0.0001). Overall, linagliptin was well tolerated. AEs occurred at a similar

FIGURE 8.6 — Mean A1C (%) Over Time During Treatment With Linagliptin or Placebo Added to Metformin

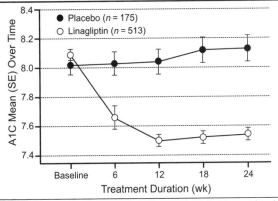

Differences in change from baseline in A1C between placebo and linagliptin are significant at each time point after baseline ($P<0.0001$).

Modified from Taskinen M, et al. *Diabet Obes Metab.* 2011;13:65-74.

rate in both groups. Hypoglycemia was rare, occurring in three patients (0.6%) treated with linagliptin and five patients (2.8%) in the placebo group. Body weight did not change significantly from baseline in either group.

Linagliptin Added to a Sulfonylurea

An 18-week, placebo-controlled study in a total of 245 patients with type 2 diabetes evaluated the efficacy of linagliptin added to an SFU. Patients on SFU mono-therapy ($n=142$) were randomized after completing a 2-week, single-blind, placebo run-in period. Patients on an SFU plus one additional OAD ($n=103$) were randomized after a washout period of 4 weeks and a 2-week single-blind placebo run-in period. Patients were randomized to the addition of linagliptin 5 mg or to placebo, each administered once daily. After 18 weeks, linagliptin in combination with an SFU provided statisti-cally significant improvement in A1C compared with placebo. Although FPG decreased by 8.2 mg/dL while it increased by 8.1 mg/dL, the difference compared with placebo was not significant. There was no significant difference between linagliptin and placebo in body weight.

Linagliptin Added to Metformin and a Sulfonylurea

The efficacy of linagliptin 5 mg added to a combination of MET and an SFU was assessed in 1058 patients with type 2 diabetes in a 24-week placebo-controlled study. The most common SFUs used by patients in the study were glimepiride (31%), glibenclamide (26%), and gliclazide (26%, not available in the United States). Patients previously treated with an SFU and MET with inadequate glycemic control were randomized to receive linagliptin 5 mg or placebo, each administered once daily. In combination with an SFU and MET, linagliptin provided statistically significant improvements in A1C and FPG compared with placebo (**Table 8.3**). Change from baseline in body weight did not differ significantly between the groups.

Linagliptin Added to Pioglitazone as Initial Therapy

Linagliptin plus pioglitazone as initial combination treatment was evaluated in a 24-week, placebo-controlled study in drug-naïve or previously treated patients with type 2 diabetes. After appropriate washout and placebo run-in periods, patients were randomized to receive pioglitazone 30 mg plus placebo or linagliptin 5 mg plus pioglitazone 30 mg, both once daily. After 24 weeks of treatment, the adjusted mean change in A1C from baseline for linagliptin plus pioglitazone was –1.1 compared with –0.6 for placebo plus pioglitazone. The difference in the adjusted mean A1C between the linagliptin and placebo groups was –0.5 ($P<0.0001$). Patients taking linagliptin plus pioglitazone compared with those receiving placebo plus pioglitazone were more likely to achieve an A1C of <7.0% (42.9% vs 30.5%, respectively; $P=0.0051$) and reduction in A1C of $\geq$0.5% (75.0% vs 50.8%, respectively; $P<0.0001$). Reductions in FPG were significantly greater for linagliptin plus pioglitazone than with placebo plus pioglitazone. Overall, the proportion of patients that experienced at least one AE was similar in both groups (52.5% and 53.1% in the linagliptin plus pioglitazone and placebo plus pioglitazone, respectively). Most AEs were of mild or moderate intensity. Weight

TABLE 8.3 — Glycemic Parameters in a 24-Week Placebo-Controlled Study of Linagliptin Added to Metformin and a Sulfonylurea

	Linagliptin + MET + SFU	PBO + MET + SFU
A1C (%)		
Patients (*N*)	778	262
Baseline (mean)	8.2	8.1
Change from baseline (adjusted mean)	-0.7	-0.1
Difference from PBO + pioglitazone (adjusted mean) (95% CI)	-0.6 (-0.7, -0.5)	—
Patients achieving A1C <7% (%)	31.2	9.2
FPG (mg/dL)		
Patients (*N*)	739	248
Baseline (mean)	159.2	162.6
Change from baseline (adjusted mean)	-4.6	+8.1
Difference from PBO (adjusted mean) (95% CI)	-12.7 (-18.1, -7.3)	—

Tradjenta [package insert]. Ridgefield, CT: Boehringer Ingelheim Pharmaceuticals, Inc; 2012.

8

increase, the most frequently reported drug-related AE, occurred in 2.3% and 0.8% of the linagliptin plus pioglitazone and placebo plus pioglitazone arms, respectively. Hypoglycemic events (mostly mild) occurred in 1.2% of the linagliptin plus pioglitazone group and in none of the patients receiving placebo plus pioglitazone.

Long-Term Treatment

The efficacy of linagliptin is being evaluated in a 104-week, double-blind, glimepiride-controlled, noninferiority trial in patients with type 2 diabetes with insufficient glycemic control despite MET therapy. Patients being treated with MET only entered a run-in period of 2-weeks duration, whereas patients pretreated with MET and one additional OAD entered a run-in treatment period of 6-weeks duration with MET monotherapy (dose of ≥1500 mg/day) and washout of the other agent. After an additional 2-week placebo run-in period, patients were randomized 1:1 to the addition of linagliptin 5 mg once daily or glimepiride. Glimepiride was given as an initial dose of 1 mg/day, then electively titrated over the next 12 weeks to a maximum dose of 4 mg/day as needed to optimize glycemic control. Thereafter, the glimepiride dose was to be kept constant, except for down-titration to prevent hypoglycemia. After 52 weeks, linagliptin and glimepiride both had reductions from baseline in A1C (–0.4% for linagliptin, –0.6% for glimepiride) from a baseline mean of 7.7%. Patients treated with linagliptin exhibited a significant mean decrease from baseline body weight compared with a significant weight gain in patients administered glimepiride (–1.1 kg vs +1.4 kg, $P<0.0001$).

Adverse Events With Linagliptin

In placebo-controlled clinical trials, nasopharyngitis was the most common adverse reaction, occurring in ≥5% of patients (5.8% vs 5.5% with linagliptin and placebo, respectively). Adverse reactions reported in ≥2% of patients treated with linagliptin in combination with pioglitazone, SFU, or MET and at least 2-fold more commonly than in patients in the placebo groups were nasopharyngitis (4.3% vs 1.2% when combined with an SFU), hyperlipidemia (2.7% vs 0.8% when combined with pioglitazone), cough (2.4% vs 1.1% when combined with MET), hypertriglyceridemia (2.4% vs 0.0% when combined with an SFU), and weight gain (2.3% vs 0.8% in combination with pioglitazone).

Prescribing Linagliptin

The recommended dose of linagliptin, as monotherapy or combination or add-on therapy, is 5 mg once daily. Linagliptin can be taken with or without food. When linagliptin is used in combination with an insulin secretagogue (eg, SFU), a lower dose of the insulin secretagogue may be required to reduce the risk of hypoglycemia. No dose adjustment is recommended for patients who have impaired renal or liver function.

■ Linagliptin Fixed-Dose Combination With Metformin (Jentadueto)

Linagliptin is also available in a fixed-dose, single-tablet formulation containing saxagliptin and MET (Jentadueto).

This combination formulation is indicated as an adjunct to diet and exercise to improve glycemic control in adults with type 2 diabetes mellitus when treatment with both linagliptin and MET is appropriate. This fixed-dose, single-tablet combination of linagliptin and MET has not been studied specifically in patients with an inadequate response to insulin with MET. However, the addition of linagliptin in patients with inadequate glycemic control despite insulin with/without MET and with/with pioglitazone was shown in a 24-week clinical trial. As a result, Jentadueto was recently approved in Europe as add-on treatment in patients receiving insulin.

Prescribing Jentadueto

The starting dosage of Jentadueto should be individualized on the basis of the patient's current regimen. Jentadueto should be given twice daily with meals, with gradual dose escalation to reduce the GI side effects due to MET. The maximum recommended dose is 2.5 mg linagliptin/1000 mg MET bid. The following dosage forms are available:

- 2.5 mg linagliptin/500 mg MET hydrochloride
- 2.5 mg linagliptin/850 mg MET hydrochloride
- 2.5 mg linagliptin/1000 mg MET hydrochloride.

■ Alogliptin (Nesina)

Alogliptin, the fourth selective DPP-4 inhibitor, was recently approved by the FDA as an adjunct to diet and exercise to improve glycemic control in adults with type 2 diabetes.

The pharmacokinetic parameters of alogliptin are similar in healthy subjects and in patients with type 2 diabetes. The absolute bioavailability of alogliptin is approximately 100%. Administration of alogliptin with a high-fat meal results in no significant change in total and peak exposure to alogliptin. Therefore, linagliptin may be administered with or without food. After administration of single oral doses up to 800 mg in healthy subjects, the peak plasma alogliptin concentration (median T_{max}) occurred 1 to 2 hours after dosing. At the maximum recommended clinical dose of 25 mg, alogliptin is eliminated with a mean terminal half-life of approximately 21 hours. Alogliptin does not undergo extensive metabolism and 60% to 71% of the dose is excreted as unchanged drug in the urine. Studies in healthy subjects and patients with type 2 diabetes with normal or various degrees of renal function indicate that dosage adjustment is necessary in patients with moderate or severe renal impairment. In patients with moderate renal impairment (CrCl ≥30 to <60 mL/min) an approximate 2-fold increase in plasma AUC of alogliptin was observed, and in those with severe renal impairment (CrCl ≥15 to <30 mL/min) and end-stage renal disease (CrCl <15 mL/min or requiring dialysis), an approximate 3- and 4-fold increase in plasma AUC of alogliptin were observed, respectively.

Efficacy

The glycemic efficacy of alogliptin was assessed in nine randomized, double-blind, placebo- or active-controlled studies as monotherapy and in combination with MET, an SFU, a TZD (either alone or in combination with MET or an SFU), and insulin (either alone or in combination with MET) in a total of 8673 patients with type 2 diabetes. Three trials were performed in patients with inadequate glycemic control with diet and exercise, while the patients in six trials had failed treatment with one or more antihyperglycemic agents. Overall, treatment with alogliptin resulted clinically meaningful and statistically significant improvements in A1C and FPG compared with placebo. The reductions in A1C and fasting plasma glucose appeared to be related to the degree of A1C elevation at baseline.

Patients with Inadequate Glycemic Control on Diet and Exercise

Three 26-week placebo- or active-controlled studies in a total of 1768 patients assessed the glycemic efficacy of alogliptin as monotherapy or in combination with MET or pioglitazone. All three studies had a 4-week, single-blind, placebo run-in period followed by a 26-week randomized treatment period. The mean changes from baseline in A1C, FPG, and proportion of patient achieving A1C ≤7% are summarized in **Table 8.4**.

Alogliptin Monotherapy

In one study, monotherapy with alogliptin 25 mg qd resulted in statistically significant placebo-subtracted reductions in A1C. A greater proportion of patients in the alogliptin group achieved the ≤7.0% A1C target. In addition, reductions in FPG were significantly greater with alogliptin compared with placebo (−16 mg/dL and +11, respectively; difference −28 mg/dL; $P < 0.01$). Improvements in A1C were not affected by gender, age, or baseline BMI. The mean change in body weight with alogliptin was similar to placebo.

Alogliptin Add-On to Metformin

In the second 26-week trial, patients were randomized to one of seven treatment groups: placebo; alogliptin 12.5 mg bid, MET 500 mg or 1000 mg bid, alogliptin 12.5 mg bid in combination with MET 500 mg bid or MET 1000 mg bid. Both combination regimens resulted in statistically significant improvements in A1C compared with their respective individual alogliptin and MET component regimens. Significantly greater proportions of patients in both combination regimens achieved the ≤7.0% A1C target compared with the alogliptin or MET monotherapy groups. Compared with alogliptin monotherapy, the combinations of alogliptin 12.5 mg bid with either MET 500 or 1000 mg bid resulted in significantly greater comparator-subtracted reductions

TABLE 8.4 — Summary of Changes From Baseline in A1C in 26-Week Phase 3 Studies With Alogliptin Monotherapy or Combination Therapy in Treatment-Naive Patients With Inadequate Glycemic Control With Diet and Exercise

Treatment	n	Mean Baseline A1C	Change From Baseline	Mean Difference	Patients Achieving A1C ≤7.0% (%)
Alogliptin Monotherapy					
Placebo	63	8.0	0	—	23
Alogliptin 25 mg	128	7.9	-0.6	-0.6[a]	44[a]
Alogliptin or MET Monotherapy or in Combination					
Placebo	102	8.5	0.1	—	4
Alogliptin 12.5 mg	104	8.4	-0.6	—	20
MET 500 mg	103	8.5	-0.9	—	27
MET 1000 mg	108	8.4	-1.1	—	34
Alogliptin 12.5 mg + MET 500 mg	102	8.5	-1.2	0.7[b] 0.6[c]	47[d]
Alogliptin 12.5 mg + MET 1000 mg	111	8.4	-1.6	1.0[b] 0.4[c]	59[d]

Alogliptin or Pioglitazone Monotherapy vs Combination

Alogliptin 25 mg	160	8.8	-1.0	—	24
Pioglitazone 30 mg	153	8.8	-1.2	—	34
Alogliptin 25 mg + Pioglitazone 30 mg	158	8.8	-1.7	-0.8[e] -0.6[f]	63[g]

[a] $P<0.01$ vs placebo.
[b] $P<0.05$ vs alogliptin alone.
[c] $P<0.05$ vs MET alone.
[d] $P<0.05$ vs alogliptin or MET alone.
[e] $P<0.01$ vs alogliptin 25 mg.
[f] $P<0.01$ vs pioglitazone 30 mg.
[g] $P<0.01$ vs alogliptin or pioglitazone alone.

Data from Bosi E, et al. *Diab Obes Metab.* 2011;13(12):1088-1096; DeFronzo RA, et al. *J Clin Endocrinol Metab.* 2012;97:1615-1622; Nauck MA, et al. *Int J Clin Pract.* 2009;63(1):46-55; Pratley RE, et al. *Curr Med Res Opin.* 2009;25(10):2361-2371; Pratley RE, et al. *Diab Obes Metab.* 2009;11:167-176; Rosenstock J, et al. *Diab Obes Metab.* 2009;11:1145-1152.

8

in FPG (–22 mg/dL and –36 mg/dL, $P<0.05$ for both). Similarly, compared with either MET monotherapy regimen, both combinations of alogliptin and MET produced significantly greater net decreases in FPG (–20 mg/dL with alogliptin bid + MET 500 bid and –14 mg/dL with alogliptin bid + MET 1000 bid; $P<0.05$ for both). In a subgroup of 193 patients who underwent a standard meal challenge, there were significantly greater reductions in 2-hour PPG levels compared with alogliptin alone (–25 mg/dL and –43 mg/dL with 12,5 mg alogliptin with MET 500 mg or 1000 mg bid, respectively, compared with alogliptin 12.5 mg bid) or MET alone (–19 mg/dL and –32 mg/dL with 12.5 mg alogliptin with MET 500 mg or 1000 mg bid, respectively, compared with MET 500 mg or 1000 mg bid).

Alogliptin With or Without Pioglitazone

In the third 26-week, active-controlled study, patients with a mean baseline A1C of 8.8% were treated with alogliptin 25 mg qd alone, pioglitazone 30 mg qd alone, or alogliptin 25 mg qd in combination with pioglitazone 30 mg qd. Coadministration of alogliptin 25 mg with pioglitazone 30 mg resulted in statistically significant ($P<0.01$) improvements from baseline both in A1C and FPG compared with either of the components alone. Almost twice the number of patients treated with the combination regimen achieved the ≤7% A1C target goal compared with alogliptin or pioglitazone monotherapy (63% vs 24% and 34%, respectively).

Patients With Inadequate Glycemic Control on One or More Agents

The efficacy of alogliptin in combination with MET, an SFU, a TZD (either alone or in combination with MET or an SFU), and insulin (either alone or in combination with MET) was assessed in six double-blind, placebo- and/or active-controlled studies. All patients entered a 4-week, single-blind, placebo run-in period prior to randomization. The mean changes from baseline in A1C are summarized in **Table 8.5**.

Alogliptin Added to MET

Two 26-week studies were performed in patients inadequately controlled on MET at a dose of at least 1500 mg per day or at the maximum tolerated dose. Patients were maintained on a stable dose of MET (median dose = 1700 mg) during the treatment period.

In the first placebo-controlled trial, the addition of alogliptin 25 mg qd to MET resulted in statistically significant improvements from baseline in A1C (placebo-subtracted change –0.5). The placebo-subtracted decrease in FPG with alogliptin also was statistically significant (17 mg/dL; $P<0.001$). Significantly more patients who received the combination of alogliptin and MET achieved the ≤7% target goal compared with those who received MET and placebo (44% vs 18%; $P<0.001$).

Alogliptin With/Without Pioglitazone Added to MET

In the second 26-week double-blind, placebo- and active-controlled study, patients already on MET were treated with either placebo; alogliptin 25 mg alone; 15 mg, 30 mg, or 45 mg of pioglitazone alone; or 12.5 mg or 25 mg of alogliptin in combination with 15 mg, 30 mg, or 45 mg of pioglitazone. Patients were maintained on a stable dose of MET. All three combination regimens of alogliptin and pioglitazone provided statistically significant improvements in A1C and the proportions of patients achieving the ≤7% target goal compared with placebo, to alogliptin alone, or to pioglitazone alone when added to background MET. In addition, all three combinations produced significant reductions in FPG (–38 mg/dL, –42 mg/dL, and –53 mg/dL with alogliptin 25 mg combined with pioglitazone 15 mg, 30 mg, or 45 mg, respectively (all $P<0.01$ compared with placebo and the corresponding dosages of alogliptin or pioglitazone).

Alogliptin or Pioglitazone and MET

In a 52-week, active-comparator study, patients inadequately controlled on a current regimen of pioglitazone 30 mg and MET (at least 1500 mg/day at the maximum tolerated dose) were randomized to receive the addition of alogliptin 25 mg, pioglitazone 15 mg, 30, or 45 mg, or combinations of alogliptin 25 mg with

TABLE 8.5 — Summary of Changes From Baseline in A1C in Phase 3 Studies With Alogliptin Alone or in Combination in Patients With Inadequate Glycemic Control With One or More Antihyperglycemic Agents

Treatment	n	Mean Baseline A1C	Change From Baseline	Mean Difference	Patients Achieving A1C ≤7.0% (%)
Alogliptin Add-On to MET					
Placebo/MET	103	8.0	-0.1	—	18
Alogliptin 25 mg/MET	203	7.9	-0.6	-0.5[a]	44[a]
Alogliptin Add-On to Pioglitazone + MET					
Pioglitazone 45 mg + MET	394	8.1	0.3	—	21
Alogliptin 25 mg + pioglitazone 30 mg + MET	397	8.2	0.7	0.4[b]	33[c]
Alogliptin and/or Pioglitazone Add-On to MET					
Placebo	121	8.5	-0.1	—	6
Alogliptin 25 mg + MET	123	8.6	-0.9	—	27
Pioglitazone 15 mg + MET	127	8.5	-0.8	—	26
Pioglitazone 30 mg + MET	123	8.5	-0.9	—	30
Pioglitazone 45 mg + MET	126	8.5	-1.0	—	36
Alogliptin 25 mg + pioglitazone 15 mg + MET	127	8.5	-1.3	-0.5[d]	55[d]
Alogliptin 25 mg + pioglitazone 30 mg + MET	124	8.5	-1.4	-0.5[d]	53[d]
Alogliptin 25 mg + pioglitazone 45 mg + MET	126	8.6	-1.6	-0.6[d]	60[d]

114

Treatment					
Alogliptin Add-On to Pioglitazone + MET ± SFU					
Placebo + pioglitazone ± MET ± SFU	95	8.0	-0.2	—	34
Alogliptin 25 mg + pioglitazone ± MET ± SFU	195	8.0	-0.8	-0.6[e]	49[e]
Alogliptin Add-On to Glyburide					
Placebo + glyburide	97	8.2	0	—	18
Alogliptin 25 mg qd + glyburide	197	8.1	-0.5	-0.5[f]	35[f]
Alogliptin Add-On to Insulin ± MET					
Placebo + insulin	126	9.3	-0.1	—	1
Alogliptin 25 mg + insulin	126	9.3	-0.7	-0.6[g]	8

[a] $P<0.001$ vs placebo.
[b] Noninferior and statistically superior to MET + pioglitazone at the 0.025 one-sided significance level.
[c] $P<0.001$ vs pioglitazone + MET.
[d] $P<0.01$ vs corresponding doses of alogliptin or pioglitazone.
[e] $P<0.01$ vs placebo + pioglitazone.
[f] $P<0.01$ vs placebo + glyburide.
[g] $P<0.05$ vs insulin ± MET.

Data from Bosi E, et al. *Diab Obes Metab.* 2011;13(12):1088-1096; DeFronzo RA, et al. *J Clin Endocrinol Metab.* 2012;97:1615-1622; Nauck MA, et al. *Int J Clin Pract.* 2009;63(1):46-55;Pratley RE, et al. *Curr Med Res Opin.* 2009;25(10):2361-2371; Pratley RE, et al. *Diab Obes Metab.* 2009;11:167-176; Rosenstock J, et al. *Diab Obes Metab.* 2009;11:1145-1152.

8

either pioglitazone or MET. Patients were maintained on a stable dose of MET (median dose = 1700 mg). When added to pioglitazone and MET, alogliptin 25 mg resulted in a statistically superior decrease in A1C (–0.4) and FPG (–15 mg/dL and –4 mg/dL; alogliptin add-on compared with pioglitazone/MET combination) at week 52.

Alogliptin Add-On to Pioglitazone and MET With/Without an SFU

In a 26-week, placebo-controlled study, patients inadequately controlled with a TZD alone or in combination with MET or an SFU (10 mg) were treated with alogliptin 25 mg qd or placebo. Patients were maintained on a stable dose of pioglitazone (median dose = 30 mg) during the treatment period; those who were also previously treated with MET (median dose = 2000 mg) or an SFU (median dose = 10 mg) prior to randomization were maintained on the combination therapy during the treatment period. The addition of alogliptin 25 mg qd to pioglitazone therapy resulted in statistically significant improvements from baseline in A1C and FPG compared with the addition of placebo to pioglitazone. A significantly greater proportion of patients achieved the ≤7% target goal.

Alogliptin Add-On to Glyburide

The efficacy of alogliptin as an add-on to an SFU was evaluated in a 26-week, placebo-controlled study in which patients inadequately controlled on an SFU were treated with alogliptin 25 mg qd or placebo as added to an SFU. Patients were maintained on a stable dose of glyburide (median dose = 10 mg) during the treatment period. The addition of alogliptin 25 mg to glyburide therapy resulted in statistically significant improvements from baseline in A1C (–0.5) and FPG (–11 mg/dL) compared with placebo.

Add-On to Insulin With/Without MET

Alogliptin as add-on in patients inadequately controlled on insulin alone (42%) or in combination with MET (58%) (mean baseline A1C = 9.3%) were treated with alogliptin 25 mg qd or placebo. Patients were maintained on their insulin regimen (median dose = 55 IU) upon randomization and those previously treated with insulin in combination with MET (median dose = 1700 mg) prior to randomization continued on the combination regimen. Patients entered the trial on short-, intermediate-, or long-acting (basal) insulin or premixed insulin. Alogliptin 25 mg qd added on to insulin therapy resulted in statistically significant placebo-subtracted improvement from baseline in A1C (–0.6) and FPG (–18 mg/dL). Clinically meaningful reductions in A1C were observed with alogliptin compared with placebo regardless of whether subjects were receiving concomitant MET and insulin (–0.2% placebo vs –0.8% alogliptin therapy or insulin alone (–0.1% placebo vs –0.7% alogliptin). Improvements in A1C were not affected by baseline insulin dose.

Adverse Events

Alogliptin as monotherapy or in combination with other OADs was generally well tolerated, with most adverse reactions being of mild or moderate intensity. In a pooled analysis of 14 controlled clinical trials, the overall incidence of AEs was 66% in patients treated with alogliptin 25 mg compared with 62% with placebo and 70% with an active comparator. The incidence of discontinuations due to AEs was 4.7% with alogliptin 25 mg compared with 4.5% with placebo or 6.2% with an active comparator. Adverse reactions reported in ≥4% of patients treated with alogliptin and more frequently than in patients who received placebo were:

- Nasopharyngitis
- Headache
- Upper respiratory tract infection.

The incidence of hypoglycemic events in patients treated with alogliptin in placebo- and active-controlled trials was generally low and the events were not considered to be severe except for one event in the add-on to insulin trial. The rate of hyperglycemia was highest when alogliptin was added to insulin with/without MET (27% vs 24% with placebo) and lowest when alogliptin was added to MET (0% vs 3% with placebo, respectively). The rates of hyperglycemia with alogliptin were lower than those with glipizide alone (5.4% vs 26%, respectively) and when alogliptin or glipizide was added to MET (1.4% vs 23.8%, respectively).

Prescribing Alogliptin

The recommended dose of alogliptin is 25 mg once daily in patients with normal renal function or mild renal impairment.

The dose should be adjusted in patients with moderate or severe renal impairment or ESRD:

- In moderate renal impairment (CrCl $\geq$30 to <60 mL/min) the recommended dose is 12.5 mg once daily.
- In severe/renal impairment/ESRD (CrCl <30 mL/min) the recommended dose is 6.25 mg once daily.

Alogliptin is available in three dosage strength tablets: 6.25 mg, 12.5 mg, and 25 mg.

■ **Alogliptin Fixed-Dose Combination With Metformin (Kazano)**

Alogliptin is also available in a fixed-dose, single-tablet formulation containing alogliptin and MET (Kazano).

This combination formulation is indicated as an adjunct to diet and exercise to improve glycemic control in adults with type 2 diabetes mellitus. This fixed-dose, single-tablet combination of alogliptin and MET has not been studied specifically in patients with an inadequate response to insulin. However, the combination of alogliptin with/without MET administered separately was shown to be effective in patients with an inadequate response to insulin (**Table 8.5**).

Prescribing Kazano

The starting dose of Kazano should be individualized on the basis of the patient's current regimen. Kazano should be taken twice daily with food. The dosage may be adjusted based on effectiveness and tolerability, while not exceeding the maximum recommended daily dose of 25 mg alogliptin and 2000 mg MET.

Kazano is available as tablets containing:
- 12.5 mg alogliptin and 500 mg MET
- 12.5 mg alogliptin and 1000 mg MET.

■ **Alogliptin Fixed-Dose Combination With Pioglitazone (Oseni)**

Alogliptin is also available in a fixed-dose, single-tablet formulation containing alogliptin and pioglitazone. It is currently the only single-tablet combination formulation of a DPP-4 inhibitor and pioglitazone.

This combination formulation is indicated as an adjunct to diet and exercise to improve glycemic control in adults with type 2 diabetes mellitus. The combination of alogliptin and pioglitazone administered separately or as a fixed-dose, single-tablet formulation has not been studied in patients with an inadequate response to insulin.

Prescribing Oseni

The starting dose of Oseni should be individualized on the basis of the patient's current regimen and concurrent medical condition but not to exceed a daily dose of alogliptin 25 mg and pioglitazone 45 mg.

- In patients with NYHA Class I or II heart failure, the initial dose of pioglitazone should limited to 15 mg once daily. Oseni should not be used in patients with established NYHA Class III or IV heart failure.
- In patients with moderate renal impairment (CrCl ≥ 30 to <60 mL/min), the recommended dosages are 12.5 mg alogliptin/15 mg pioglitazone, 12.5 mg alogliptin/30 mg pioglitazone, and 2.5 mg alogliptin/45 mg pioglitazone. Oseni is not recommended for patients with severe renal impairment or ESRD requiring dialysis.
- The maximum recommended dose of pioglitazone is 15 mg once daily in patients taking strong CYP2C8 inhibitors (eg, gemfibrozil).

Oseni is available as tablets containing:
- 25 mg alogliptin and 15 mg pioglitazone
- 25 mg alogliptin and 30 mg pioglitazone
- 25 mg alogliptin and 45 mg pioglitazone
- 12.5 mg alogliptin and 15 mg pioglitazone
- 12.5 mg alogliptin and 30 mg pioglitazone
- 12.5 mg alogliptin and 45 mg pioglitazone.

8

■ **Summary**

The introduction of DPP-4 inhibitors represents a significant advance in the treatment of type 2 diabetes. Not only are they effective in improving overall glycemic control as indicated by the FBG and PPG values and A1C, but at the same time they are either weight neutral or lead to weight loss. These effects on weight are very important since weight gain associated with intensification of therapy in an effort to normalize or near normalize A1C is a significant challenge in clinical practice. The combination of DPP-4 inhibitors with MET appears to be not only effective in terms of metabolic outcomes but also safe in terms of a lower risk of hypoglycemia. It also appears that the weight gain seen with SFUs and TZDs is blunted when these agents are combined with this new class of antidiabetic agents.

SGLT2 Inhibitors

In healthy individuals, glucose is filtered at the glomerulus and virtually 100% is reabsorbed in the proximal tubule of the nephron. Two sodium glucose co-transporters (SGLTs), SGLT1 and SGLT2, play an important role in renal glucose reabsorption. SGLT2 is expressed primarily in the S1 segment of the proximal tubule of kidney and is responsible for the majority of glucose reabsorption (~90%) (**Figure 8.7**). SGLT1 is expressed in the S2/S3 segment of the proximal tubule and participates to a lesser extent in renal tubular glucose reabsorption (~10%). SGLT1 also plays an important role in intestinal glucose and galactose absorption. Inhibition of SGLT2 reduces renal reabsorption of filtered glucose and increases urinary glucose excretion. Preclinical studies have shown that SGLT2 inhibitors increase glucose excretion and normalize plasma glucose in diabetic models. In addition to lowering plasma glucose concentrations, the increased urinary glucose excretion with SGLT2 inhibition also results in an osmotic diuresis, with the diuretic effect likely contributing to a reduction in systolic blood pressure (SBP). Furthermore, a loss of calories from glucose loss may translate to some reduction in body weight. Given these effects, agents that

FIGURE 8.7 — SGLT2 Mediates Glucose Reabsorption in the Kidney

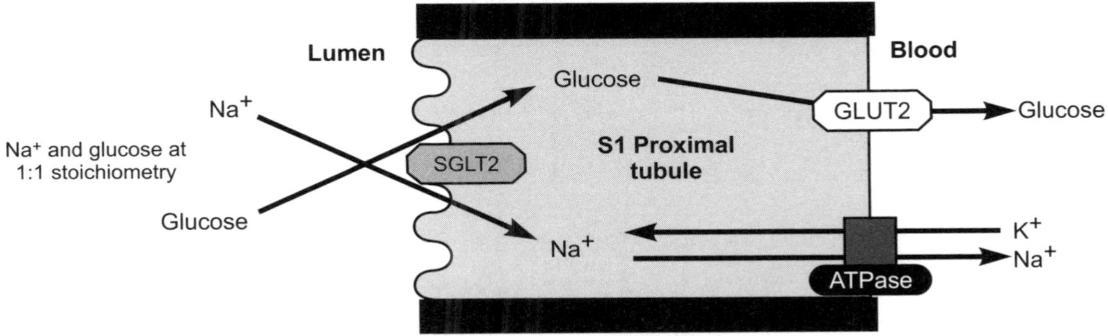

SGLT2 is a high-capacity and low-affinity glucose transporter expressed in the proximal renal tubules. Nearly all glucose filtered through the glomerulus is reabsorbed until SGLT2 reaches maximum reabsorptive capacity. Above the renal threshold for glucose (RTG), urinary excretion of glucose increases in proportion to the plasma glucose concentration.

Adapted from Robert Henry, MD, New Classes of Pharmacologic Agents for the Treatment of Hyperglycemia on the Horizon: Sodium Glucose Cotransporter (SGLT) - Type 2 Inhibitors; February, 2009.

inhibit SGLT2 represent a novel new class of antidiabetic agents.

Unlike most other approved non-insulin antidiabetic drugs currently indicated for the treatment of type 2 diabetes, the direct glucose-lowering effect of SGLT2 inhibitors does not depend on augmentation of endogenous insulin secretion or improvement of insulin sensitivity. It does, however, depend on the ability of the kidney to filter glucose, which in turn is correlated to both the prevailing plasma glucose level and the glomerular filtration rate. Therefore, the glucose-lowering effect of SGLT2 inhibition may be expected to wane with diminished renal function.

■ Canagliflozin (Invokana)

Canagliflozin is a SGLT2 inhibitor indicated as an adjunct to diet and exercise to improve glycemic control in adults with type 2 diabetes mellitus. It is not for treatment of type 1 diabetes mellitus or diabetic ketoacidosis.

In vitro, canagliflozin was shown to be 160-fold more selective for SGLT2 than for SGLT1. Following oral administration, C_{max} of canagliflozin is reached within 1 hour and the absolute oral bioavailability of canagliflozin is ~65%. Canagliflozin exhibits dose-proportional pharmacokinetics. Following once-daily administration of 100 mg and 300 mg doses, steady-state plasma concentrations of canagliflozin are attained in 4 to 5 days. Canagliflozin is extensively (99%) bound to plasma proteins (mainly albumin) and is metabolized to inactive glucuronide metabolites. In healthy adults, approximately 33% of an orally-administered dose is excreted in urine, most as metabolites, while 60% is excreted in feces. The elimination half-life canagliflozin is ~12 hours.

Efficacy

The efficacy and safety of canagliflozin were assessed in nine phase 3 randomized, double-blind, parallel-group, placebo- and/or active-controlled studies in which canagliflozin was used as monotherapy, and as add-on to MET, MET/pioglitazone, or MET/SFU. Three of these trials were performed in special populations: older adults, patients with moderate renal dysfunctions, and those with or at high risk of CV disease. **Table 8.6** provides an overview of the designs of these studies. Seven trials compared canagliflozin with placebo while two were noninferiority trials in which canagliflozin was compared with glimepiride or sitagliptin. Across these phase 3 trials, a total of 7803 patients with type 2 diabetes were randomized and received at least one dose of study drug. Of those who received study drug, 4994 received canagliflozin 100 mg ($n=2302$) or 300 mg ($n=2692$), 1583 received placebo, and 1226 were treated with an active comparator. The primary efficacy end point for these phase 3 studies was the percent change in A1C from baseline to the end of the study. Secondary end points included changes from baseline to the end of the study in FPG and 2-hour PPG, proportion of patients achieving an A1C target (eg, <7.0%) at the end of the study, and percent change from baseline to the end of the study in body weight, SBP, and fasting plasma lipids.

Glycemic Efficacy

As shown in **Table 8.7**, canagliflozin was effective in reducing A1C in a broad range of subjects, both as monotherapy and in dual or triple combinations. In each of the placebo-controlled studies/substudies, both dosages of canagliflozin were significantly superior to placebo in lowering A1C. Subgroup analysis of the monotherapy study by baseline A1C demonstrated substantially greater A1C lowering in patients with the highest baseline levels. In the substudy in patients with baseline A1C >10.0% to ≤12.0%, the mean changes in A1C from baseline to week 26 were –2.13% and –2.56% for the canagliflozin 100 mg and 300 mg groups, respectively. In the active-comparator trials, canagliflozin was shown to be noninferior to glimepiride and resulted in significant reduction in A1C compared with sitagliptin.

In the placebo-controlled studies, the proportion of patients reaching the A1C target of <7.0% was significantly greater in the canagliflozin groups compared with the placebo group and the difference relative to placebo was statistically significant for the canagliflozin 100 mg and 300 mg groups across studies (**Figure 8.8**). The treatment effect with canagliflozin was larger with the 300-mg dose than with the 100-mg dose. In the study in

8

TABLE 8.6 — Overview of Study Designs of Phase 3 Studies of Canagliflozin

Study Design	Treatment Period[a]	Treatment Arms (n)	Baseline A1C (%)
Canagliflozin Monotherapy			
Main Study	26 weeks (+ 26 weeks)	Placebo (192) Canagliflozin 100 mg (195) Canagliflozin 300 mg (197)	≥7 to ≤10
High A1C substudy	26 weeks	Canagliflozin 100 mg (47) Canagliflozin 300 mg (44)	>10 to ≤12
Canagliflozin Add-On to Other OAD Monotherapy			
Add-on to MET	26 weeks (+ 26 weeks)	Placebo (183) Canagliflozin 100 mg (368) Canagliflozin 300 mg (367) Sitagliptin 100 mg (366)	≥7 to ≤10.5
Add-on to MET[b]	52 Weeks (+ 52 Weeks)	Canagliflozin 100 mg (483) Canagliflozin 300 mg (485) Glimepiride (↑6/8 mg) (484)	≥7 to ≤9.5
Canagliflozin Add-On to Dual Combination OAD Therapy			
Add-on to MET/SFU	26 weeks (+ 26 weeks)	Placebo (156) Canagliflozin 100 mg (157) Canagliflozin 300 mg (156)	≥7 to ≤10.5

Add-on to MET/pioglitazone	26 weeks (+ 26 weeks)	Placebo (115) Canagliflozin 100 mg (113) Canagliflozin 300 mg (114)	≥7 to ≤10.5
Add-on to MET/SFU[b]	52 weeks (NA)	Canagliflozin 300 mg (377) Sitagliptin 100 mg (378)	≥7 to ≤10.5
Special Populations			
Older adults (≥55 to ≤80 years)	26 weeks (+ 78 weeks)	Placebo (237) Canagliflozin 100 mg (241) Canagliflozin 300 mg (236)	≥7 to ≤10
Moderate renal impairment (eGFR ≥30 to <50 mL/min)	26 weeks (+ 26 weeks) (NA)	Placebo (90) Canagliflozin 100 mg (90) Canagliflozin 300 mg (89)	≥7 to ≤10.5
High CV risk (interim safety)[c]	Event driven (ongoing)	Placebo (1441) Canagliflozin 100 mg (1445) Canagliflozin 300 mg (1441)	≥7 to ≤10.5
Insulin substudy[d]	18 weeks (NA)	Placebo (565) Canagliflozin 100 mg (566) Canagliflozin 300 mg (587)	≥7 to ≤10.5
SFU substudy[e]	18 weeks (NA)	Placebo (45) Canagliflozin 100 mg (42) Canagliflozin 300 mg (40)	≥7 to ≤10.5

Continued

8

125

TABLE 8.6 — *Continued*

[a] Duration to primary end point. *(Planned double-blind, placebo- or active-controlled extension period.)*

[b] Noninferiority trial; noninferiority margin of 0.3% used for comparisons of canagliflozin and comparator.

[c] Patients on currently available OADs with a history or high risk of CV disease.

[d] Patients on insulin ≥20 units/day as monotherapy in combination with other OAD(s).

[e] Patients on SFU monotherapy.

Data on file, Janssen Research and Development, LLC. Canagliflozin as an adjunctive treatment to diet and exercise alone or co-administered with other antihyperglycemic agents to improve glycemic control in adults with type 2 diabetes mellitus. JNJ-28431754 (Canagliflozin), NDA 204042. December 11, 2012: 1-184.

patients with GFR ≥30 to <50 mL/min, the decreases in A1C, although significant, were less compared with those observed in other studies.

Across the placebo-controlled studies, both dosages of canagliflozin produced significant reductions in FPG (**Figure 8.9**). The placebo-subtracted mean reductions ranged from −22.4 to −37.4 mg/dL with the 100-mg dose, and from −27.7 to −48.1 mg/dL with the 300-mg dose. Patients in the canagliflozin monotherapy and canagliflozin add-on to MET studies underwent a mixed meal tolerance test. The mean changes with canagliflozin in 2-hour PPG in the monotherapy trial (5.2, −42.9, and −58.6 mg/dL; placebo, 100 mg and 300 mg, respectively) and the add-on trial (−9.8, −47.9, and −57.1 mg/dL; placebo, 100 mg and 300 mg, respectively) were significantly greater with both dosages of canagliflozin compared with placebo.

Secondary End Points

Effect on Body Weight

Across the placebo-controlled phase 3 studies, the placebo-subtracted mean percent changes from baseline in body weight at time of primary efficacy assessment ranged from approximately −1.4% to −2.7% with the canagliflozin 100 mg group and from approximately −1.8% to −3.7% with the canagliflozin 300 mg group (**Figure 8.10**). The change in the high glycemic cohort of the monotherapy study was similar to that observed in the main study population. Body weight reduction with canagliflozin 300 mg was greater than with the 100 mg dosage. In the 52-week, add-on to MET study, weight loss was seen with both dosages of canagliflozin whereas body weight increased with glimepiride. In the 52-week add-on to MET/SFU, there was a loss of body weight with canagliflozin and a weight neutral effect with sitagliptin. In both of these studies, the reductions in body weight with canagliflozin were maintained over the 52-week treatment periods.

Effect on Blood Pressure

Both dosages of canagliflozin consistently lowered SBP across the placebo-controlled phase 3 studies

TABLE 8.7 — Summary of Changes From Baseline in A1C in Phase 3 Studies of Canagliflozin[a]

Study (Weeks)	Treatment	n	Baseline A1C Mean	Change From Baseline Mean±SE	CANA Minus Control	P Value
Canagliflozin Monotherapy						
Main Study (26)	Placebo	189	7.97	0.14±0.06		
	Canagliflozin 100 mg	191	8.06	-0.77±0.06	-0.91	<0.0001
	Canagliflozin 300 mg	193	8.01	-1.03±0.06	-1.16	<0.0001
High A1C substudy (26)	Canagliflozin 100 mg	46	10.59	-2.13	—	—
	Canagliflozin 300 mg	43	10.62	2.56	—	—
Canagliflozin Add-On to Other OAD Monotherapy						
Add-on to MET (26)	Placebo	181	7.96	-0.17±0.06		
	Canagliflozin 100 mg	365	7.94	-0.79±0.04	-0.62	<0.0001
	Canagliflozin 300 mg	360	7.95	-0.94±0.04	-0.77	<0.0001
Add-on to MET (52)[b]	Canagliflozin 100 mg	478	7.78	-0.82±0.04	-0.01	0.8074
	Canagliflozin 300 mg	474	7.79	-0.93±0.04	-0.12	0.0158
	Glimepiride	473	7.83	-0.82±0.04		

Canagliflozin Add-On to Dual Combination OAD Therapy					
Add-on to MET/SFU (26)	Placebo	150	8.12	-0.13±0.08		
	Canagliflozin 100 mg	155	8.13	-0.85±0.08	-0.71	<0.0001
	Canagliflozin 300 mg	152	8.13	-1.06±0.08	-0.92	<0.0001
Add-on to MET/pioglitazone (26)	Placebo	114	8.00	-0.26±0.07		
	Canagliflozin 100 mg	113	7.99	-0.89±0.07	-0.62	<0.0001
	Canagliflozin 300 mg	112	7.84	-1.03±0.07	-0.76	<0.0001
Add-on to MET/SFU (52)c	Canagliflozin 300 mg	365	8.13	-0.66±0.05	-0.37	<0.0001
	Sitagliptin 100 mg	374	8.12	-1.03 ± 0.05		
Special Populations						
Older adults (26)	Placebo	232	7.76	-0.03±0.06		
	Canagliflozin 100 mg	239	7.77	-0.06±0.06	-0.57	<0.0001
	Canagliflozin 300 mg	229	7.69	-0.73±0.06	-0.70	<0.0001
Moderate renal impairment (26)	Placebo	87	8.02	-0.03±0.09		
	Canagliflozin 100 mg	88	7.89	-0.32±0.09	-0.29	0.0131
	Canagliflozin 300 mg	89	7.97	-0.44±0.09	-0.42	0.0004
Insulin substudy (18)	Placebo	545	8.24	0.02±0.03		
	Canagliflozin 100 mg	551	8.34	-0.63±0.03	-0.65	<0.0001
	Canagliflozin 300 mg	572	8.27	-0.72±0.03	-0.74	<0.0001

Continued

TABLE 8.7 — *Continued*

Study (Weeks)	Treatment	n	Baseline A1C Mean	Change From Baseline Mean ± SE	CANA Minus Control	P Value
Special Populations *(continued)*						
SFU substudy (18)						
	Placebo	40	8.49	0.04 ± 0.15		
	Canagliflozin 100 mg	40	8.29	-0.70 ± 0.15	-0.74	<0.0005
	Canagliflozin 300 mg	39	8.28	-0.79 ± 0.15	-0.83	<0.0001

[a] Data from the modified intent-to-treat (mITT) LOCF population (all patients who received at least one dose of study drug) at completion of the protocol-specified duration.

[b] Canagliflozin noninferior to glimepiride.

[c] Canagliflozin noninferior to sitagliptin.

Data on file, Janssen Research and Development, LLC. Canagliflozin as an adjunctive treatment to diet and exercise alone or co-administered with other antihyperglycemic agents to improve glycemic control in adults with type 2 diabetes mellitus. JNJ-28431754 (Canagliflozin), NDA 204042. December 11, 2012: 1-184.

FIGURE 8.8 — Proportion of Patients With A1C <7.0% at Primary Assessment Time Point in Placebo-Controlled Phase 3 Studies

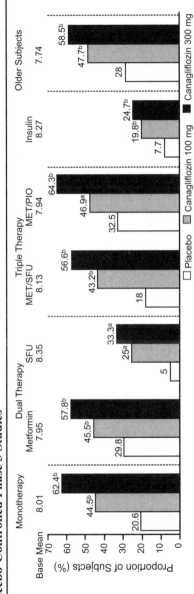

Data on file, Janssen Research and Development, LLC. Canagliflozin as an adjunctive treatment to diet and exercise alone or co-administered with other antihyperglycemic agents to improve glycemic control in adults with type 2 diabetes mellitus. JNJ-28431754 (Canagliflozin), NDA 204042. December 11, 2012: 1-184.

[a] P <0.05.
[b] P <0.001.

8

FIGURE 8.9 — Mean Changes From Baseline in Fasting Plasma Glucose From Baseline to Primary Assessment Time Point in Placebo-Controlled Phase 3 Studies

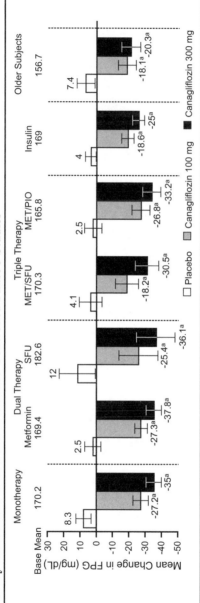

[a] $P<0.001$.

Data on file, Janssen Research and Development, LLC. Canagliflozin as an adjunctive treatment to diet and exercise alone or co-administered with other antihyperglycemic agents to improve glycemic control in adults with type 2 diabetes mellitus. JNJ-28431754 (Canagliflozin), NDA 204042. December 11, 2012: 1-184.

FIGURE 8.10 — Body Weight: Plasma Glucose LS Mean Changes From Baseline at Primary Assessment Time Point: Study-by-Study Comparison of Placebo-Controlled Phase 3 Studies

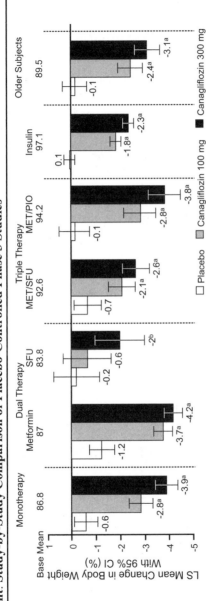

[a] Statistically significant ($P < 0.001$) [($P < 0.05$[b])] vs placebo.

Data on file, Janssen Research and Development, LLC. Canagliflozin as an adjunctive treatment to diet and exercise alone or co-administered with other antihyperglycemic agents to improve glycemic control in adults with type 2 diabetes mellitus. JNJ-28431754 (Canagliflozin), NDA 204042. December 11, 2012: 1-184.

(**Figure 8.11**). The placebo-subtracted mean changes from baseline in SBP at time of secondary efficacy assessment ranged from –2.2 to –5.7 mm Hg with canagliflozin 100 mg and from –1.6 to –7.9 mm Hg with canagliflozin 300 mg. Reductions were typically observed at the first measurement (week 6), and remained generally stable over the remainder of the treatment periods. In the study in patients with renal impairment, the mean change from baseline relative to placebo was –5.73 mm Hg with canagliflozin 100 mg and –6.12 mm Hg with canagliflozin 300 mg. In the active-comparator trials, canagliflozin was associated with larger mean decreases from baseline in SBP compared with glimepiride (between group differences relative to glimepiride of –3.48 and –4.76 mm Hg for the 100-mg and 300-mg doses, respectively) or compared with sitagliptin (between-group difference relative to sitagliptin of –5.91 mm Hg for the 300-mg dose).

Reductions in diastolic blood pressure (DBP) were also observed with both canagliflozin dosages in each of the phase 3 studies. The mean changes from baseline relative to placebo at the primary assessment time point across the studies ranged from –1.02 to –2.47 mm Hg with the 100-mg dosage and 0.53 to –3.22 mm Hg with the 300-mg dosage.

Safety

The incidences of AEs reported in the broad population of patients in the phase 3 clinical trials with canagliflozin are summarized in **Table 8.8**.

The incidence of patients who experienced any AE during the phase 3 trials was generally similar across treatment groups. The incidence of AEs considered related to study drug was higher in the canagliflozin 100 mg and 300 mg groups compared with the non-canagliflozin group. These differences largely reflected a higher incidence of AEs related to osmotic diuresis and a higher incidence of AEs related to female or male genital mycotic infections in the canagliflozin groups. The incidence of discontinuations due to AEs was higher in the canagliflozin groups relative to the non-canagliflozin group, with no notable difference in the incidence of serious AEs, serious AEs leading to discontinuation, or deaths. The incidence of subjects with serious AEs that

FIGURE 8.11 — Systolic Blood Pressure: Plasma Glucose LS Mean Changes From Baseline at Primary Assessment Time Point: Study-by-Study Comparison of Placebo-Controlled Phase 3 Studies

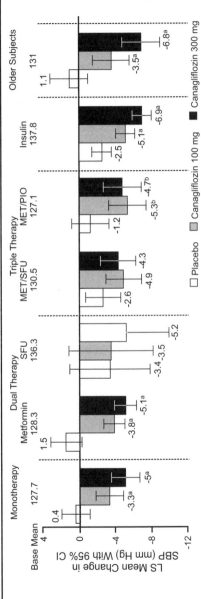

[a] Statistically significant ($P<0.001$) [($P<0.05^b$)] vs placebo.

Data on file, Janssen Research and Development, LLC. Canagliflozin as an adjunctive treatment to diet and exercise alone or co-administered with other antihyperglycemic agents to improve glycemic control in adults with type 2 diabetes mellitus. JNJ-28431754 (Canagliflozin), NDA 204042. December 11, 2012: 1-184.

8

TABLE 8.8 — Summary of Incidences of Adverse Events in Phase 3 Clinical Trials With Canagliflozin

Adverse Events	All Non-CANA (*n* = 3262) (%)	Canagliflozin		All (*n* = 6177) (%)
		100 mg (*n* = 3092) (%)	300 mg (*n* = 3085) (%)	
Any	75.8	76.6	77.0	76.8
Leading to discontinuation	5.0	5.6	7.3	6.4
Related to study drug[a]	21.8	29.4	33.6	31.5
Related to study drug[a] and leading to discontinuation	2.1	3.6	4.6	4.1
Serious	13.6	13.5	13.2	13.3
Serious, leading to discontinuation	2.2	2.0	1.7	1.9
Serious related to study drug[a]	0.8	1.1	1.1	1.1
Serious related to study drug[a] and leading to discontinuation	0.3	0.5	0.5	0.5
Deaths	1.1	0.8	0.8	0.8

[a] Possibly, probably, or very likely related to study drugs as determined by investigator.

Data on file, Janssen Research and Development, LLC. Canagliflozin as an adjunctive treatment to diet and exercise alone or co-administered with other antihyperglycemic agents to improve glycemic control in adults with type 2 diabetes mellitus. JNJ-28431754 (Canagliflozin), NDA 204042. December 11, 2012: 1-184.

were considered related to study drug was also low, with similar incidences in the combined canagliflozin and non-canagliflozin groups.

The incidence of specific AEs reported by ≥2% of patients in the four 26-week phase 3 placebo-controlled trials are shown in **Table 8.9**.

In pooled data from all phase 3 clinical trials, the incidence of hypoglycemia was low in both canagliflozin treatment arms and all non-canagliflozin treatments. However, in several trials, canagliflozin was administered as an add-on to other agents associated with hypoglycemia. A separate analysis was conducted based on patients in placebo-controlled trials that did not include such agents. In this pooled population, the incidence of hypoglycemic episodes was overall low, slightly higher in the canagliflozin 100-mg (3.8%) and 300-mg groups (4.3%) relative to the placebo group (2.2%). The event rates per subject-year exposure for the canagliflozin 100-mg and 300-mg groups were greater (0.22 and 0.18, respectively) relative to placebo group (0.10), and with no apparent dose-relationship. The incidence of severe hypoglycemia was low, with one subject in each canagliflozin group reported to have had a severe hypoglycemic episode.

In patients with moderate renal impairment, overall AE rates with canagliflozin 100 mg, canagliflozin 300 mg, or placebo were 77.8%, 74.2%, and 73.3%, respectively with serious AE rates of 11.1%, 11.2%, and 17.8%, respectively. Compared with placebo, canagliflozin 100 mg and 300 mg were associated with increases in serum creatinine (9% and 10% vs 4%) and BUN (9% and 6% vs 2%).

In the study in patients with moderate renal impairment (mean baseline eGFR 39.4 mL/min/1.73 m^2), the absolute decreases in eGFR were similar to those observed in the placebo-controlled studies. However, due to the lower baseline eGFR, there were larger decreases in percent mean change from baseline at week 26 (–8.3% and –8.9%, respectively, in the canagliflozin 100 mg and 300 mg groups, with a change from baseline in the placebo group of –3.8%).

In the 52-week trial in which canagliflozin 300 mg or sitagliptin 100 mg were added in patients receiving MET

TABLE 8.9 — Incidences of Specific Adverse Events Reported by ≥2% of Patients in Four 26-Week, Placebo-Controlled, Phase 3 Clinical Trials With Canagliflozin[a]

Adverse Events	Placebo (n = 646) (%)	Canagliflozin 100 mg (n = 833) (%)	Canagliflozin 100 mg (n = 834) (%)
Female genital mycotic infections[b]	3.2	10.4	11.4
Urinary tract infections[c]	4.0	5.9	4.3
Increased urination[d]	0.8	5.3	4.6
Male genital mycotic infections[e]	0.6	4.2	3.7
Vulvovaginal pruritus	0.0	1.6	3.0
Thirst[f]	0.2	2.8	2.3
Constipation	0.9	1.8	2.3
Nausea	1.5	2.2	2.3

[a] The four placebo-controlled trials included one monotherapy trial and three add-on combination trials with metformin, metformin and sulfonylurea, or metformin and pioglitazone.

[b] Includes: vulvovaginal candidiasis, vulvovaginal mycotic infection, vulvovaginitis, vaginal infection, vulvitis, and genital infection fungal.

c Includes: urinary tract infection, cystitis, kidney infection, and urosepsis.
d Includes: polyuria, pollakiuria, urine output increased, micturition urgency, and nocturia.
e Includes: balanitis or balanoposthitis, balanitis candida, and genital infection fungal.
f Includes: thirst, dry mouth, and polydipsia.

Invokana [package insert]. Titusville, NJ: Janssen Pharmaceuticals, Inc; 2013.

8

and SU, overall AE rates were similar with canagliflozin and sitagliptin (76.7% vs 77.5%) as were serious AEs (6.4% vs 5.6%). AEs consistent with superficial genital fungal infections were more frequent with canagliflozin than with sitagliptin (women, 15.3% vs 4.3%; men, 9.2% vs 0.5%) while incidences of urinary tract infections were similar. More patients had ≥1 hypoglycemic episode with canagliflozin (43.2%) than with sitagliptin (40.7%).

In the 52-week study in which canagliflozin or glimepiride were added to MET, overall AE rates were similar with canagliflozin 100 mg, canagliflozin 300 mg, and GLIM (64.2%, 68.5%, and 67.6%, respectively). Serious AE and AE-related discontinuation rates were low across groups. Treatment with canagliflozin 100 and 300 mg were associated with higher rates than glimepiride of AEs consistent with superficial genital fungal infections (women, 14.3% and 23.8% vs 3.7%; men, 6.7% and 8.3% vs 1.1%), urinary tract infections (6.4% for both vs 4.4%), and osmotic diuresis-related AEs (<3% per specific AE).

Because canagliflozin increases urinary glucose excretion, it acts as an osmotic diuretic with an increase in urine output. Therefore, in the placebo-controlled trials, the incidence of osmotic diuresis-related adverse events was higher in both canagliflozin treatment groups (6.8% and 7.1% with 100 mg and 300 mg, respectively) compared with placebo (1.9%). The incidence was not dose-dependent. The most frequently reported events were pollakiuria, thirst, and polyuria. None of the events were serious, and three canagliflozin-treated patients discontinued due to pollakiuria. In patients with moderate renal impairment, the incidence of osmotic diuresis-related adverse events was not higher than in the overall study population, However, the incidence of osmotic diuresis-related adverse events was slightly higher in the canagliflozin 100 mg treatment group (4.1%) compared with canagliflozin 300 mg (3.8%) or placebo (3.7%). None of the events were serious or led to discontinuation. Again, pollakiuria and thirst were the most commonly reported adverse events.

Prescribing Canagliflozin

Canagliflozin is supplied as 100-mg or 300-mg tablets. The recommended dosing and administration of canagliflozin is as follows:

- The recommended starting dose is 100 mg once daily, taken before the first meal of the day.
- Dose can be increased to 300 mg once daily in patients tolerating canagliflozin 100 mg once daily who have an eGFR of 60 mL/min/1.73 m^2 or greater and require additional glycemic control.
- Canagliflozin is limited to 100 mg once daily in patietns who have an eGFR of 45 to less than 60 mL/min/1.73 m^2
- Assess renal function before initiating canagliflozin. Do not initiate canagliflozin if eGFR is below 45 mL/min/1.73 m^2
- Discontinue canagliflozin if eGFR falls below 45 mL/min/1.73 m^2.

Thiazolidinediones

The TZDs work mainly to reduce insulin resistance in skeletal muscle, adipose tissue, and liver. At least some of their action involves stimulation of nuclear receptors called peroxisome proliferator-activated receptors (PPARs) that regulate gene transcription of a number of proteins involved in glucose and lipid metabolism. There are three types of PPAR receptors: PPARα, PPARβ/α, and PPARγ. The TZDs are synthetic activators of PPARγ; this activation is associated with a reduction in insulin resistance. The exact mechanism by which activation of PPARγ improves insulin action is unknown but involves modifications in the expression of specific gene products and activity of pivotal enzymes of insulin signaling. PPARγ is highly expressed in adipose tissue but is also found in other tissues including skeletal muscle, liver, pancreas, macrophages, monocytes, and other cells of the vasculature.

Since CV disease is the major cause of morbidity and mortality in type 2 diabetes, one intriguing observation was the ability of the TZDs to reduce CV risk factors, including markers of vascular inflammation (see *Effect on Cardiovascular Risk Factors* below). Although they have a positive effect on a broad range of CV risk factors, a correlation with a beneficial effect on CV events has not been consistently demonstrated (see *CVD and Mortality Risk* below). Currently, the two marketed TZDs are rosiglitazone and pioglitazone.

■ **Rosiglitazone (Avandia)**

Rosiglitazone (Avandia) is currently indicated for use as monotherapy and in combination with SFUs, MET, and insulin. Rosiglitazone is also available in fixed-dose single-tablet formulations with either MET (Avandamet) or a glimepiride (Avandaryl).

Although rosiglitazone and its combination formulations are still available in the United States, they currently are used rarely because of extensive restrictions, including a risk evaluation and mitigation strategy (REMS) program, safety concerns specified in the Black Box Warnings and Cautions, and the availability of an alternative drug in this class that does not have these restrictions on its use (see *CVD and Mortality Risk* below). The package insert should be consulted before prescribing. Dosage recommendations for Avandia, Avandamet, and Avandaryl are included in **Table 8.1**.

■ **Pioglitazone (Actos)**

Pioglitazone (Actos) is indicated for use as monotherapy or in combination with MET, SFUs, or insulin. Six registration studies (three monotherapy, three combination therapy) formed the basis of the FDA approval.

Monotherapy

The monotherapy studies included 865 patients with type 2 diabetes. In general, there was a −1.4% to −1.6% reduction in A1C observed with the highest dose of pioglitazone (45 mg/day) over a treatment period of 16 to 26 weeks. Greater reductions of A1C and FPG were observed in treatment-naïve patients with a short duration of diabetes. In another study, pioglitazone was compared head-to-head with MET in 206 drug-naïve type 2 diabetic patients (titrated to achieve FPG <126 mg/dL). Pioglitazone was equally as effective as MET in this double-blind 32-week trial (**Figure 8.12**).

FIGURE 8.12 — Head-to-Head, Double-Blind, 32-Week Trial Comparing Pioglitazone (30-45 mg/d) With Metformin (850-2550 mg/d) in 205 Drug-Naïve Type 2 Diabetic Patients (Titrated to Achieve FPG <126 mg/d)

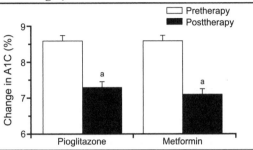

[a] $P<0.0001$ vs baseline.

Adapted from Pavo I, et al. *J Clin Endocrinol Metab*. 2003;88:1637-1645.

Combination Therapy

In the combination-therapy studies, pioglitazone or placebo was added to the regimen of patients in whom SFUs, MET, or insulin failed. In these studies, there was a significant 0.8% to 1.3% reduction in the A1C when pioglitazone 30 mg/day was used. **Figure 8.13** illustrates the lack of secondary failure with pioglitazone when used as monotherapy and combination therapy. When pioglitazone is added to MET, durable glycemic control is also seen. The combination of pioglitazone and MET is not only effective in reducing the A1C and preventing secondary failure over time, but also positively affects CV risk factors with minimal or no risk for hypoglycemia.

Pioglitazone Fixed-Dose Combinations (Actoplus Met, Actoplus Met XR, Duetact)

Pioglitazone is currently available in two different fixed-dose, single-tablet formulations containing pioglitazone and MET (Actoplus Met, Actoplus Met XR) or pioglitazone and glimepiride (Duetact).

Actoplus Met

This combination formulation is indicated to improve glycemic control in patients with type 2 diabetes who

FIGURE 8.13 — Durability (72 Weeks) of Glycemic Control With Pioglitazone in Five Double-Blind Trials[a]

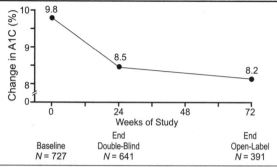

[a] Total trials, $N=727$; monotherapy, $N=56$; pioglitazone + sulfonylurea, $N=236$; pioglitazone + metformin, $N=154$; pioglitazone + insulin, $N=313$.

Rosenstock J, et al. *Int J Clin Pract.* 2002;56:251-257.

are already treated with a combination of pioglitazone and MET or whose diabetes is not adequately controlled with MET alone, and in those patients who have initially responded to pioglitazone alone and require additional glycemic control.

There have been no clinical efficacy studies conducted with Actoplus Met. However, the efficacy and safety of the separate components have been previously established and the coadministration of the separate components has been evaluated for efficacy and safety in two clinical studies that included patients receiving MET, either alone or in combination with another antihyperglycemic agent, who had inadequate glycemic control. As shown in **Table 8.10**, the combination of pioglitazone 30 mg and MET significantly reduced the mean A1C and mean FPG at week 16 compared with placebo and MET alone. In a 24-week study, both dosage regimens of pioglitazone produced significant reductions from baseline in A1C and FPG at week 24. The reduction in FPG with pioglitazone 45 mg was significantly greater than with pioglitazone 30 mg.

This combination formulation is indicated to improve glycemic control as an adjunct to diet and exercise in patients with type 2 diabetes who are already being treated with a combination of pioglitazone and an SFU or whose diabetes is not adequately controlled with an SFU alone and in those patients who have initially responded to pioglitazone alone and require additional glycemic control.

There have been no clinical efficacy studies conducted with Duetact. However, coadministration of pioglitazone and an SFU, including glimepiride, has been evaluated in two clinical studies in patients with type 2 diabetes receiving an SFU, either alone or in combination with another antihyperglycemic agent, who had inadequate glycemic control. In a 16-week study, the addition of pioglitazone 15 mg or 30 mg once daily to treatment with an SFU significantly reduced the mean A1C and the mean FPG compared with placebo and an SFU. In a 24-week study, both dosage regimens of pioglitazone plus an SFU significantly reduced mean A1C and FPG from baseline levels.

Effect on Lipid Levels

Pioglitazone used as monotherapy and in combination resulted in a significant mean percent decrease in triglycerides (up to 15%) and significant mean percent increases in HDL (up to 19%) with no change in the LDL and total cholesterol levels; however, many of the studies demonstrated a reduction in LDL as well. The difference in effects on the lipoprotein profile depends on the patient population studied and the effect of mechanisms of each drug on the PPAR system.

A randomized, 24-week, double-blind trial compared the differential effects of pioglitazone and rosiglitazone on serum lipoprotein particle concentrations in 735 diabetes patients with dyslipidemia. While both treatments increased LDL particle size, pioglitazone had a greater effect. Both treatments increased HDL cholesterol levels. However, pioglitazone increased both total HDL particle concentration and size but rosiglitazone decreased both.

TABLE 8.10 — Glycemic Control With Pioglitazone/Metformin Combination Therapy in Patients With Type 2 Diabetes Inadequately Controlled by Metformin Monotherapy

16-Week Study	PIO 30 mg + MET	MET + Placebo
FPG (mg/dL):	N=165	N=157
Baseline (mean)/change from baseline (mean)	254.4/−42.8[a,b]	259.9/−5.2
Difference in change between PIO/MET combination therapy vs MET + placebo	−37.7	—
Responder rate (patients achieving ≥30 mg/dL decrease from baseline) (%)	59.4	23.6
A1C (%):	N=161	N=153
Baseline (mean)/change from baseline (mean)	9.92/−0.64[a,b]	9.77/−0.19
Difference in change between PIO/MET combination therapy vs MET + placebo	−0.83	—
Responder rate (patients achieving an A1C ≤6.1% or a ≥0.6% decrease from baseline) (%)	54.0	21.6

24-Week Study	PIO 30 mg + MET	PIO 45 mg + MET
FPG (mg/dL):	N=399	N=399
Baseline (mean)/change from baseline (mean)	232.5/−32.8[a]	232.1/−50.7[a,c]
Responder rate (patients achieving ≥30 mg/dL decrease from baseline) (%)	52.3	63.7
A1C (%):	N=400	N=398
Baseline (mean)/change from baseline (mean)	9.88/−0.80[a]	9.81/−1.01[a]
Responder rate (patients achieving an A1C ≤6.1% or a ≥0.6% decrease from baseline) (%)	52.3	63.7

[a] $P \leq 0.05$ vs baseline.
[b] $P \leq 0.05$ vs MET + placebo.
[c] $P \leq 0.05$ vs 30 mg PIO + MET.

Adapted from Actoplus Met [package insert]. Deerfield, IL: Takeda Pharmaceuticals America, Inc; 2007.

Effect on Cardiovascular Risk Factors

Pioglitazone has also been shown to reduce traditional and nontraditional CV risk factors. Pioglitazone has also been shown to reduce PAI-1 levels and improve the procoagulant state. Consistent and sustained reductions in intimal medial thickness have been clearly demonstrated with pioglitazone.

Type 2 diabetes and coronary artery disease have both been identified as conditions associated with inflammation. In addition, pioglitazone, as well as rosiglitazone, has been shown to reduce CRP in patients with type 2 diabetes (**Figure 8.14**). Furthermore, A1C there were equivalent reductions in CRP value both in the patients who had a >1% decrease in the A1C value (responders) and those who did not have a large reduction in A1C value (nonresponders).

The PROactive Study

The Prospective Pioglitazone Clinical Trial In Macrovascular Events (PROactive) was designed to ascertain whether pioglitazone reduces macrovascular

FIGURE 8.14 — Pioglitazone Reduces C-Reactive Protein[a]

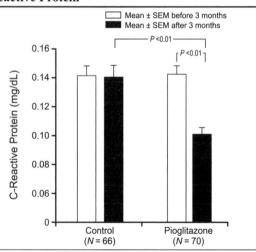

[a] Irrespective of antiglycemic effects.

Satoh N, et al. *Diabetes Care.* 2003;26:2493-2499.

morbidity and mortality in high-risk patients with type 2 diabetes. In this prospective, placebo-controlled trial, 5238 patients with type 2 diabetes who had evidence of macrovascular disease were randomized to receive pioglitazone ($N=2605$) titrated from 15 mg to 45 mg or placebo ($N=2633$). The primary end point was the composite of all-cause mortality, nonfatal MI (including silent MI), stroke, acute coronary syndrome, endovascular or surgical intervention in the coronary or leg arteries, and amputation above the ankle. The main secondary end point was the composite of all-cause mortality, nonfatal MI (excluding silent MI), and stroke. The average time of observation was 34.5 months.

Fewer patients in the pioglitazone group had at least one event more in the primary composite end point than did those in the placebo group (19.7% vs 21.7%, respectively; $P = 0.095$). In their discussion of the results, the investigators opined that the lack of a significant difference in the primary end point was likely related to the fact that when the protocol was designed, it was believed that the need for amputation or coronary or leg revascularization would respond to therapy in a similar way to stroke and MI. This hypothesis, however, did not prove correct in the case of cardiac and leg revascularization, perhaps because these end points are in part determined by the decision to intervene being based on local surgical or medical practice. Therefore, the study may have been underpowered to detect a significant difference in the primary composite end point.

Regarding the main secondary composite end point (the composite of all-cause mortality, nonfatal MI, and stroke), significantly fewer patients in the pioglitazone group (11.6%) than in the placebo group (13.3%) experienced at least one of these events (**Figure 8.15**).

Compared with patients in the placebo group, there was a rapid and sustained decrease in insulin doses in patients in the pioglitazone group who were receiving insulin at study entry (**Figure 8.16**). By study end, the mean insulin dose was significantly lower with pioglitazone (42 U/d) than with placebo (55 U/d); nevertheless, there was a greater decrease in A1C compared with placebo (−0.93% vs −0.45%). At final visit, insulin had

FIGURE 8.15 — Kaplan-Meier Curve of Time to Secondary End Point[a] in the PROactive Study

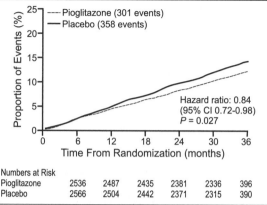

[a] All-cause mortality, nonfatal MI (including silent MI), stroke, acute coronary syndrome, endovascular or surgical intervention in the coronary or leg arteries, and amputation above the ankle.

Dormandy JA, et al. *Lancet.* 2005;366:1279-1289.

---

been discontinued in 9% of patients in the pioglitazone group vs 2% in the placebo group. Conversely, of the 3478 patients who were not receiving insulin at study entry, significantly fewer pioglitazone-treated patients than placebo-treated patients (11% vs 21%, respectively) began to use insulin permanently during the course of the study.

Overall safety and tolerability of pioglitazone were good and no changes in the safety profile of pioglitazone were observed, although edema and weight gain were more frequent compared with placebo. There were significantly more reports of heart failure in the pioglitazone group compared with the placebo group (417 vs 302, respectively); however, these reported events were not adjudicated and therefore possibly overreported. Despite the increase in reported heart failure among pioglitazone-treated patients, the number of deaths from heart failure was similar in both groups (25 and 22, respectively).

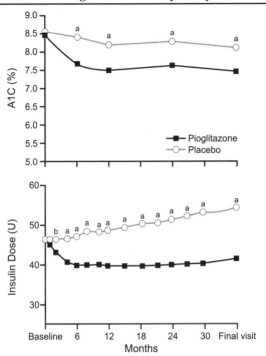

FIGURE 8.16 — Changes in A1C and Insulin Dose During the PROactive Study in Patients Receiving Insulin at Study Entry

[a] $P < 0.0001$ vs placebo.
[b] $P = 0.0371$ vs placebo.

Charbonnel B, et al. *J Clin Endocrinol Metab.* 2010;95:2163-2171.

Prescribing Pioglitazone

Dosing of pioglitazone should be titrated up to a maximum effective daily dose of 45 mg as monotherapy and in combination therapy. Pioglitazone is always administered once daily and can be taken without regard to the time of food ingestion. Onset of activity has been observed as early as 2 weeks, with maximum effects seen in 8 to 12 weeks. The FDA has eliminated the need for monitoring liver function every 2 months for the first year after initiating TZD therapy. The current recommendation for liver enzyme monitoring is prior to initiation of therapy and periodically thereafter.

Prescribing Actoplus Met

Actoplus Met is available in two tablet strengths: 15 mg pioglitazone/500 mg MET and 15 mg pioglitazone/850 mg MET.

In patients inadequately controlled on MET monotherapy, Actoplus Met may be initiated at either the 15 mg/500 mg or 15 mg/850 mg tablet strength qd or bid and gradually titrated after assessing adequacy of therapeutic response. In patients who initially responded to pioglitazone monotherapy but require additional glycemic control, Actoplus Met may be started at either the 15 mg/500 mg or 15 mg/850 mg tablet strength qd, and gradually titrated after assessing adequacy of therapeutic response.

Prescribing Duetact

Duetact is available in two tablet strengths: 30 mg pioglitazone/2 mg glimepiride or 30 mg pioglitazone/4 mg glimepiride.

In patients currently on glimepiride monotherapy, Duetact may be initiated at 30 mg/2 mg or 30 mg/4 mg tablet strengths qd, and adjusted after assessing therapeutic response. The usual starting dose of Duetact in patients currently on pioglitazone monotherapy is 30 mg/2 mg qd. When switching patients from combination therapy of pioglitazone plus glimepiride as separate tablets, Duetact may be initiated with 30 mg/2 mg or 30 mg/4 mg tablet strengths based on the dose of pioglitazone and glimepiride already being taken. Patients who are not controlled with pioglitazone 15 mg in combination with glimepiride should be carefully monitored when switched to Duetact. Since no exact dosage relationship exists between glimepiride and the other SFUs, the starting dose of Duetact should be limited to 30 mg/2 mg qd in patients currently receiving monotherapy with an SFU other than glimepiride.

■ Side Effects With TZDs

Liver Toxicity

After extensive use of rosiglitazone and pioglitazone in patients worldwide, liver toxicity does not appear to be an important clinical problem. Baseline LFTs should be done and if abnormal, an investigation should be initiated to determine the primary cause. Often steatohepatitis, or a fatty liver, may be the culprit.

Therapy with TZDs should not be initiated in patients with increased baseline liver enzyme levels (alanine aminotransferase [ALT] >2.5 times the upper limit of normal). In all patients, it is recommended that liver enzymes be monitored prior to initiation of TZD therapy and periodically thereafter. Patients with mildly elevated liver enzymes (ALT levels 1 to 2.5 times the upper limit of normal) at baseline or during therapy with TZDs should be evaluated to determine the cause of the liver enzyme elevation. Initiation or continuation of therapy with a TZD in patients with mild liver enzyme elevations should proceed with caution and include appropriate close clinical follow-up, including more frequent liver enzyme monitoring, to determine if the liver enzyme elevations resolve or worsen. If at any time ALT levels increase to >3 times the upper limit of normal in patients taking TZDs, liver enzyme levels should be rechecked as soon as possible. If ALT levels remain >3 times the upper limit of normal, TZD therapy should be discontinued.

CHF and Edema

The FDA has issued a boxed warning stating that, since TZDs can cause or exacerbate CHF, their use in patients with established NYHA Class III or IV heart failure is contraindicated. Furthermore, their use is not recommended in patients with symptomatic heart failure. Patients already receiving a TZD should be observed carefully for signs and symptoms of heart failure (including excessive, rapid weight gain, dyspnea, and/or edema). If these signs and symptoms develop, the heart failure should be managed according to current standards of care. Furthermore, discontinuation or dose reduction of the TZD must be considered.

In 2003, an ADA/American Heart Association (AHA) consensus conference was convened to discuss the issues of fluid retention and CHF as they relate to the use of TZDs. One of the most important statements from the conference was that the presence of edema does not always indicate the presence of CHF. When considering the use of TZDs in diabetic patients, it is always important to ascertain the potential presence of underlying cardiac disease by obtaining a good history of any past medical events (eg, MI) and use of medications associated with fluid retention (eg, vasodilators, nonsteroidal anti-inflammatory agents, or CCBs). Risk factors for heart failure in patients treated with TZDs are listed in **Table 8.11**.

TABLE 8.11 — Risk Factors for Heart Failure in Patients Treated With TZDs

- History of heart failure (either systolic or diastolic)
- History of prior myocardial infarction or symptomatic coronary artery disease
- Hypertension
- Left ventricular hypertrophy
- Significant aortic or mitral valve heart disease
- Advanced age (>70 years)
- Long-standing diabetes (>10 years)
- Preexisting edema or current treatment with loop diuretics
- Development of edema or weight gain on TZD therapy
- Insulin coadministration
- Chronic renal failure (creatinine >2.0 mg/dL)

Nesto RW, et al. *Circulation.* 2003;108:2941-2948.

A thorough physical examination is important to look for signs of CHF; documentation of the presence or absence of ankle edema is crucial for comparison after TZD therapy is initiated. Edema is not an absolute contraindication of TZDs and can be treated with a low-dose thiazide diuretic, especially if the blood pressure is not at goal levels.

The use of B-type natriuretic peptide (BNP), which is a marker of ventricular dysfunction, may prove to be valuable when initiating TZDs and in determining whether a patient is at risk for CHF and thus in need of long-term monitoring while taking a TZD.

TZDs have caused preload-induced cardiac hypertrophy in preclinical studies. However, in three FDA-required echocardiographic clinical studies in patients with type 2 no deleterious alterations in cardiac structure or function were observed. These studies were designed to detect a change in left ventricular mass $\geq 10\%$.

CVD and Mortality Risk

A meta-analysis of data from 42 trials that included nearly 28,000 patients indicated that the use of rosiglitazone produced a small but significant increased risk of MI and a small but not statistically significant increased risk of CV death. In November 2007, the FDA updated the Black Box warning in the label for rosiglitazone noting the increased risk of MI seen in that meta-analysis, while also stating that the research on the increased MI risk from rosiglitazone use is inconclusive. Subsequently, numerous other studies, meta-analyses, as well as retrospective "data-mining" studies, reported often-conflicting findings, which resulted in an ongoing controversy whether rosiglitazone is associated with an increased risk of CVD and mortality.

In contrast, the placebo-controlled, randomized, prospective PROactive trial (discussed above) reported a 10% trend in reduction in total CVD events with pioglitazone compared with placebo. The beneficial trends in events were not present until after 1 year of follow-up, pointing out one of the major limitations in some of the smaller trials with rosiglitazone. Additional data on the CV safety of pioglitazone comes from an independent analysis of the results from a total of 19 trials that enrolled 16,390 patients who were treated from 4 months to 3.5 years. The primary outcome, a composite of death, MI, or stroke, occurred in 375 of 8554 patients (4.4%) receiving pioglitazone and 450 of 7836 patients (5.7%) receiving control therapy (HR 0.82). Individual components of the primary end point were all reduced by a similar magnitude with pioglitazone treatment, with HRs ranging from 0.80 to 0.92. Serious heart failure was reported in 200 (2.3%) of the pioglitazone-treated patients and 139 (1.8%) of the control patients (HR 1.41).

On July 14, 2010, the FDA convened an advisory board that concluded that rosiglitazone may remain on the market with more supervision and stronger warnings. The FDA has concurred with the recommendations of the Advisory Board. The current FDA guidance on the prescription of Avandia, including the REMS program, can be found at the FDA website: http://www.fda.gov.

■ **Summary**

When used in the appropriate clinical situation, the TZD class of oral agents can have a significant impact on the metabolic management of type 2 diabetes. The novel mechanism of action of TZDs to improve insulin resistance has unique potential in new-onset type 2 diabetes. Many of the greatest benefits of these agents may occur in patients who are in the early stages of developing diabetes and premature CV disease. The expanded availability of fixed-dose, single-tablet formulations of combinations of a TZD and MET or an SFU (ie, glimepiride), provide more convenient administration and potential enhancement of therapy adherence.

Alpha-Glucosidase Inhibitors

Acarbose (Precose) and miglitol (Glyset) are alpha-glucosidase inhibitors that slow the breakdown of complex carbohydrates (disaccharides and polysaccharides) into monosaccharides or glucose. The enzymatic generation and subsequent absorption of glucose is delayed and the postprandial blood glucose values, which are characteristically high in patients with type 2 diabetes, are reduced with these agents. The PPG level is often overlooked but can significantly contribute to prolonged hyperglycemia. Acarbose and miglitol are excellent pharmacologic agents to "spread the calories," which is recommended by the ADA, and have been shown to smooth out daytime glycemia.

■ **Acarbose (Precose)**

Acarbose has been shown to reduce the mean PPG value by approximately 50 mg/dL and the fasting glucose by 10 to 20 mg/dL. Acarbose also lowers the postprandial integrated insulin levels, as less glucose is being presented to the pancreas at any one time. Acarbose does not stimulate insulin release and does not cause hypoglycemia when used alone. The average reduction in A1C is usually 0.5% to 1.0%. The reduction in glycemia is related to the carbohydrate content of the diet. Generally, the greater the complex carbohydrate content of the diet, the larger the reduction in postprandial hyperglycemia. In addition, a large-scale trial has demonstrated that when acarbose is given to patients with newly diagnosed diabetes (duration of up to 1 year) with poor metabolic control (baseline A1C >10%), a 3.0% to 4.6% reduction in A1C can be seen. Since acarbose primarily reduces the PPG and does not cause hypoglycemia, the drop in A1C is usually not as dramatic as one would see with the SFUs, which can cause hypoglycemia (the A1C is an average of the highs and lows of plasma glucose).

The combined use of acarbose with MET and/or insulin has been approved by the FDA. Acarbose has been used successfully with TZDs and repaglinide for the treatment of type 2 diabetes, although the latter two combinations are not yet approved by the FDA.

Side Effects of Acarbose

The main side effect of acarbose is flatulence. Soft stools or diarrhea and mild abdominal pain have also been reported. Many of the symptoms are dose-related and transient, occurring with the highest frequency during the first 8 weeks of therapy. The symptoms are probably caused by the osmotic effect of undigested carbohydrates in the distal bowel. The most important factor in avoiding side effects is to titrate acarbose slowly. Because acarbose is not absorbed systemically to any significant degree and does not cause hypoglycemia, it has been suggested that it may be safer than some of the other oral agents in patients with kidney disease, in the elderly, and in children with type 2 diabetes.

Prescribing Acarbose

The recommended maintenance dosage of acarbose is 50 mg to 100 mg orally 3 times a day with meals. The suggested starting dose of acarbose is 25 mg/day, which should be titrated up slowly to the maintenance dosage of 50 mg to 100 mg tid to avoid side effects (**Table 8.12**).

■ Miglitol (Glyset)

Miglitol is a similar compound to acarbose that also has AGI activity in the gut, thereby delaying or preventing the digestion and absorption of complex carbohydrates. In a similar fashion to acarbose, miglitol does not directly stimulate insulin secretion and does not cause hypoglycemia when used alone. The main clinical effect of miglitol is to lower the PPG value with additive

TABLE 8.12 — Acarbose/Miglitol Dosing Instructions for Patients

1. You have been given acarbose/miglitol because your blood sugar control needs to be improved. Acarbose/miglitol is a very safe medication that has been proven effective in improving overall blood glucose control in people with diabetes.
2. Acarbose/miglitol works by delaying the absorption of glucose in the gut or delaying the digestion of carbohydrates and subsequent absorption of glucose.
3. Acarbose/miglitol reduces the rise in blood sugar that typically occurs after eating. Marked elevation in blood sugar after eating is a common yet important problem that often is overlooked.
4. Acarbose/miglitol *may* cause flatulence (excess gas), mild stomach pain, and/or diarrhea. These side effects tend to occur at the beginning of therapy and can be lessened by starting with a low dose of acarbose/miglitol and increasing the dose very slowly.
5. Suggested dosing schedule:
   Step 1: Start with 25 mg[a] at breakfast only for 1 week
   Step 2: Take 25 mg with breakfast and dinner for 1 week
   Step 3: Take 25 mg with breakfast, lunch, and dinner for 1 week
   Step 4: Take 50 mg with breakfast and 25 mg with lunch and dinner for 1 week
   Step 5: Take 50 mg with breakfast and dinner, and 25 mg with lunch for 1 week
   Step 6: Take 50 mg with breakfast, lunch, and dinner[b]
6. Do not go to a higher step if you are having bothersome gas, stomach pain, or diarrhea. Stay at the current step or go to a lower step until your symptoms improve.
7. It is extremely important to take acarbose/miglitol with the beginning of your meal. Acarbose/miglitol will be less effective at lowering your blood sugar if you take it more than 15 minutes before you eat.

---

[a] Break the 50-mg pill in half or use a pill cutter.
[b] Do not increase your dose further until you talk with your caregiver.

---

effects of lowering postprandial insulin levels and a lesser reduction in the FPG values. The magnitude of reductions of the A1C values is on the same order of magnitude as seen with acarbose, although miglitol 50 mg tid has been shown to be equivalent to acarbose 100 mg tid in terms of efficacy. Miglitol can be safely added to all other oral agents on the market as well as combined with insulin.

Sides Effects of Miglitol

Flatulence is the main GI side effect experienced with miglitol therapy, although it may be better tolerated than other carbohydrate-absorption inhibitors.

Prescribing Miglitol

The recommended maintenance dosage of miglitol is 25 mg to 50 mg orally three times a day with meals. The suggested starting dose of miglitol is 25 mg/day, which should be titrated up slowly to the maintenance dosage of 25 mg to 50 mg tid to avoid side effects (**Table 8.12**).

Sulfonylureas

SFUs work primarily by chronically stimulating pancreatic insulin secretion, which in turn reduces hepatic glucose output and increases peripheral glucose disposal.

8

Four first-generation SFU compounds have been available in the United States for the treatment of type 2 diabetes for >20 years. They are:

- Acetohexamide
- Chlorpropamide
- Tolazamide
- Tolbutamide.

Two second-generation SFU compounds, glipizide and glyburide, were introduced in the United States in 1984 and another (glimepiride) more recently. Thus the second-generation compounds are:

- Glimepiride
- Glipizide
- Glyburide.

The efficacy of the first- and second-generation SFUs is similar, although second-generation agents are better formulated and have some advantages. Second-generation SFUs:

- Are more potent on a per-milligram basis
- Tend to produce fewer side effects
- Interact less frequently with other drugs.

Improved formulations of glipizide (Glucotrol XL) and glyburide (Glynase PresTab) are also available. In addition, the pharmacokinetics of some of these second-generation agents allow for more effective once-a-day dosing, which enhances compliance.

■ Side Effects of SFUs

Most of the side effects associated with SFU therapy are mild, infrequent, and occur less often with the second-generation agents; they include:

- Weight gain
- Hypoglycemia
- Mild GI upset
- Skin reactions:
    - Rashes
    - Purpura
    - Pruritus.

Hyponatremia, fluid retention, and an Antabuse-like reaction to alcohol have also been reported with the use of chlorpropamide. The major complication of SFU therapy is severe hypoglycemia, which has been more of a problem with chlorpropamide than with any other agent because of its long half-life and duration of action. Hypoglycemia is also more common in individuals who consume large amounts of alcohol and/or skip meals, and in the elderly. Other reactions are rare and include hematologic reactions (leukopenia, thrombocytopenia, and hemolytic anemia) and cholestasis (with and without jaundice).

■ Prescribing SFUs

In general, SFU therapy should be initiated at the lowest possible dose, especially in the elderly (**Table 8.1**). It is begun once daily, before breakfast, and increased progressively every 1 to 2 weeks until the desired therapeutic glycemic response is achieved or the maximum dose is reached. The dosing regimen is changed to twice daily when the daily dose approaches ≥50% of the maximum recommended dose. Dosing adjustments can also be made based on SMBG data. For example, if the patient's SMBG results show elevated FBG values, the evening dose should be titrated upward. If, on the other hand, the evening FBGs are elevated, the morning dose can be raised.

Clinicians should focus on achieving satisfactory glycemic control based on glucose and A1C levels and not concentrate solely on the patient's symptoms, which could lead to premature dosage discontinuation or dose reduction. In patients with glucose toxicity and markedly elevated glucose values (ie, >200-300 mg/dL), it may be necessary to use insulin temporarily to achieve glycemic control. Once glycemic control has been achieved for several days to weeks, the patient may be an appropriate candidate for oral-agent therapy alone. Patients who do not achieve appropriate glycemic control in response to one or more oral agents should be promptly switched to or have insulin therapy added to the existing oral regimen.

In general, SFUs should not be considered routinely as monotherapy for newly diagnosed obese patients with type 2 diabetes or in diabetic individuals in whom nonpharmacologic therapy has failed. Such patients usually have circulating hyperinsulinemia that can be further exacerbated if SFUs are used. SFUs also lead to weight gain and can cause hypoglycemia. There is also some evidence to suggest that the early use of SFUs may lead to premature β-cell exhaustion. In addition, concerns persist about the possible adverse effects of some SFUs on cardiac function.

■ Second-Generation SFUs

Glimepiride

Glimepiride (Amaryl) therapy has been shown to improve overall glucose control without producing clinically meaningful increases in fasting insulin and C-peptide levels. It is the only SFU with an FDA-approved indication for combination therapy with insulin. Studies have shown that glimepiride causes little or no weight gain or hypoglycemia.

The usual maintenance dosage is 1 mg to 4 mg once daily. The maximum recommended dosage is 8 mg once daily. After reaching a dose of 2 mg, further increases should be no more than 2 mg at 1- to 2-week intervals based on the patient's blood glucose response.

Glipizide

Glipizide (Glucotrol, Glucotrol XL) is a second-generation SFU that is metabolized by the liver mainly to inactive products, thereby reducing the risk of hypoglycemia. Glucotrol XL utilizes a controlled delivery system, and when compared with the immediate-release Glucotrol, the risk of hypoglycemia and the glucose and insulin responses to meals are similar although compliance is improved. Glipizide is particularly suited for the elderly or any patient with mild renal or liver dysfunction. Recommended dosing is normally 1 to 2 times daily for immediate-release glipizide. The long-acting extended-release formulation (Glucotrol XL) maintains therapeutic plasma levels effectively for 24 hours, and once-daily dosing is adequate in the majority of patients.

Glyburide

Glyburide (DiaBeta, Micronase, Glynase PresTab) is metabolized by the liver to mostly inert products that are excreted in the urine and bile. However, some of the by-products do have hypoglycemic activity and caution is advised, especially in patients with evidence of liver or kidney dysfunction. The duration of action is 16 to 24 hours, and recommended dosing is 1 to 2 times daily. A micronized particle formulation facilitates more rapid absorption (Glynase PresTab).

Glinides

■ Meglitinide

Repaglinide (Prandin)

Repaglinide (Prandin), a member of the meglitinide class of compounds, is chemically unrelated to the SFUs. It lowers blood glucose by blocking ATP-dependent potassium channels in pancreatic β-cells. This depolarizes the cell and results in the release of insulin in a glucose-dependent manner. Repaglinide monotherapy is indicated as an adjunct to diet and exercise in patients with type 2 diabetes mellitus whose hyperglycemia cannot be controlled satisfactorily by diet and exercise alone and also for combination therapy use (with MET or TZDs) in patients whose hyperglycemia cannot be controlled by monotherapy with MET, SFUs, repaglinide, or TZDs.

Repaglinide causes a rapid rise and fall of insulin secretion when ingested ≤30 minutes prior to a meal and mimics the normal postprandial insulin response that follows ingestion of food. Repaglinide is generally not recommended in combination with SFUs.

Repaglinide was studied in combination with MET in 83 patients with type 2 diabetes not satisfactorily controlled on exercise, diet, and MET alone. Repaglinide dosage was titrated for 4 to 8 weeks, followed by a 3-month maintenance period. Combination therapy with repaglinide and MET resulted in significantly greater improvement in glycemic control compared with repaglinide or MET monotherapy. The greater response in the combination group was achieved at a lower daily repaglinide dosage compared with repaglinide monotherapy. Monotherapy with repaglinide and nateglinide were compared in a 16-week clinical trial in 150 patients with type 2 diabetes. Doses of both agents were titrated up during the first 3 weeks to a maximum of 16 mg/day for repaglinide and 360 mg/day for nateglinide. At 16 weeks, patients on repaglinide achieved an average reduction in A1C of 1.67% while those on nateglinide achieved 1.08%; this difference was statistically significant. Furthermore, repaglinide and nateglinide in combination with MET were compared in a 16-week study in 192 patients with type 2 diabetes (**Figure 8.17**). All patients began MET therapy in the 4 weeks prior to the trial; 500 mg bid for 2 weeks followed by 1000 mg bid for 2 weeks. This was followed by a 2-week titration period and 14 weeks of maintenance therapy. Repaglinide in combination with MET exhibited a statistically significant (P <0.001) greater decrease in A1C (1.28%) than nateglinide with MET (0.67%).

Although not FDA approved, repaglinide works well with carbohydrate-absorption inhibitors, such as acarbose and miglitol, as well as with the TZDs. A potentially useful triple-combination oral antidiabetic regimen includes a TZD in the morning, repaglinide with each meal, and MET at bedtime. This triple combination addresses the three major physiologic abnormalities observed in the pathogenesis of hyperglycemia in type 2 diabetes (insulin resistance, impaired insulin secretion, and excessive hepatic glucose production).

FIGURE 8.17 — Reductions in A1C During 16 Weeks of Treatment With Repaglinide or Nateglinide Plus Metformin

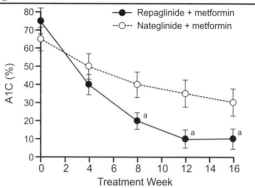

^a Fasting plasma glucose (FPG) values in the two treatment groups were significantly different ($P<0.05$).

Adapted from Raskin P, et al. *Diabetes Care*. 2003;26:2063-2068.

Prescribing Repaglinide

Repaglinide can be taken anytime between 30 minutes to immediately before a meal, but is usually taken 15 minutes prior to eating. The starting dose for patients who have not previously received an oral antidiabetic agent or those with an A1C <8% is 0.5 mg/meal. For patients who have previously used oral antidiabetic agents and have an A1C ≥8%, the starting dose is 1 mg/meal or 2 mg/meal. Repaglinide can be titrated up to 4 mg before each meal and a recommended maximum of 16 mg per day. Patients should be instructed that if they miss or add a meal they should omit or add the corresponding repaglinide dose. A maximum recommended daily dose is 16 mg.

Side Effects of Repaglinide

There is a small weight gain (3.3%) when a patient is treated with repaglinide as monotherapy and a low incidence of hypoglycemia. Since repaglinide is also cleared by the liver, it can be used in type 2 diabetic patients when renal impairment is present.

Repaglinide Fixed-Dose Combination

A fixed-dose, single-tablet formulation of repaglinide in combination with MET (PrandiMet) is available. PrandiMet is indicated as an adjunct to diet and exercise to improve glycemic control in adults with type 2 diabetes who are already treated with a meglitinide and MET or who have inadequate glycemic control on a meglitinide alone or MET alone. PrandiMet is available in tablets containing either 1-mg repaglinide/500-mg MET or 2-mg repaglinide/500-mg MET. The fixed-dose combination tablet of repaglinide and MET has been shown to be bioequivalent to concomitantly administered individual tablets of repaglinide and MET.

Treatment with PrandiMet should be individualized and initiated with 1-mg repaglinide twice daily unless the patient is already taking higher coadministered doses of repaglinide and MET. PrandiMet should be given in divided doses within 15 minutes prior to meals. The total daily dosage should not exceed 10-mg repaglinide/2500-mg MET or 4-mg repaglinide/1000-mg MET per meal.

■ D-Phenylalanine Derivative
Nateglinide

Nateglinide (Starlix), a member of the D-phenylalanine class of compounds, is structurally distinct from other available oral antidiabetic agents and, like repaglinide, exerts its glucose-lowering effect by rapid and transient effects on the ATP-sensitive potassium channels of pancreatic β-cells. Binding of nateglinide to SFU receptors leads to membrane depolarization and influx of calcium into the β-cell. The increased intracellular calcium stimulates insulin release from secretory granules. Nateglinide (Starlix) is approved for type 2 diabetes as initial monotherapy and in combination with MET. Nateglinide, when taken orally up to 30 minutes prior to meals, is rapidly and almost completely absorbed. It stimulates pancreatic insulin secretion within 20 minutes, reaching peak insulin levels within 1 hour, and returning to baseline levels within 4 hours of dosing. The extent of insulin secretion is glucose dependent so that more insulin is secreted when needed and its effects are rapidly reversed when glucose levels decrease. Thus insulin is secreted during the early phase after meals, reducing glucose spikes and minimizing prolonged insulin exposure and hypoglycemia.

Early insulin secretion released at the start of a meal suppresses hepatic glucose production and prevents exaggerated PPG levels. Early insulin secretion is impaired in patients with type 2 diabetes, leading to lack of suppression of hepatic glucose production and a rise in PPG levels. Nateglinide improves early insulin secretion through a fast-on, fast-off effect that mimics normal insulin secretion.

PPG or postmeal glucose excursions are a major component of A1C and are frequently increased yet untreated. When A1C is >7%, 90% of patients have a 2-hour plasma glucose >200 mg/dL. Elevated 2-hour PPG levels are also associated with an increased incidence of CV disease in diabetic individuals. Although there are as yet no outcome studies for targeted PPG levels, the general consensus is that 2-hour postmeal glucose should be <140 mg/dL to 160 mg/dL. These levels are now achievable with the new agents that target PPG control.

Studies have been conducted in both drug-naïve type 2 diabetic patients as well as those previously treated with other antidiabetic agents. In drug-naïve patients, 6 months' treatment with nateglinide 120 mg 3 times daily before meals achieved comparable reductions in A1C (1%) compared with placebo as 500 mg tid MET with meals (1.1%). In both drug-naïve and previously treated patients combined, A1C was reduced by nateglinide 0.8% and by MET 1.2% compared with placebo. When nateglinide and MET were combined for 6 months, the reduction in A1C (1.9%) compared with placebo was greater than either agent given alone. The preferential effect of nateglinide on PPG levels compared with that of MET was also evident in this study (**Figure 8.18**). Patients not achieving A1C target levels also benefit from addition of nateglinide. Nateglinide 120 mg 3 times daily before meals added to MET 1000 mg twice daily reduced A1C an additional 0.6% compared with addition of a placebo.

FIGURE 8.18 — Comparison of Nateglinide on PPG Levels Following Sustacal Challenge

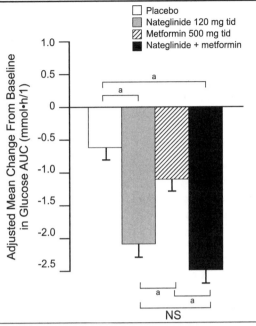

^a $P \leq 0.0001$.

Adapted from Horton ES, et al. *Diabetes Care*. 2000;23:1663.

Prescribing Nateglinide

Nateglinide is indicated as initial therapy, as an adjunct to diet and exercise, and in combination with MET. Patients in whom SFUs have failed do not achieve any additional benefit when nateglinide is switched or added. The recommended starting and maintenance dose of nateglinide, as monotherapy or in combination with MET, is 120 mg prior to each main meal. Unlike other antidiabetic agents, dose titration is usually not required. If a meal is skipped, nateglinide should not be given. If a patient is near the A1C goal, a 60-mg dose of nateglinide may be sufficient when initiated as monotherapy or in combination with MET. The dose also does not need to be adjusted in patients with mild to severe renal insufficiency or mild hepatic disease.

Side Effects of Nateglinide

AEs with nateglinide are similar to those with placebo. Small increases in mean uric acid levels (0.20-0.45 mg/dL) have been reported. During clinical trials, hypoglycemia was relatively uncommon (2.4% incidence vs placebo) and resulted in discontinuation of nateglinide in only 0.3% of patients. No severe hypoglycemia occurred requiring assistance of others. Minimal weight gain occurred with nateglinide, <1 kg from baseline values. Nateglinide is safe in elderly diabetic subjects and can be used in those with mild to severe renal insufficiency or mild hepatic insufficiency.

Bile Acid Sequestrant

■ **Colesevelam (Welchol)**

Colesevelam (Welchol), a specifically-engineered, non-absorbed polymer that binds bile acids in the intestine thereby impeding their resorption, is approved as an adjunct to diet and exercise to improve glycemic control adults with type 2 diabetes. It had been previously approved for treatment of primary hyperlipidemia as monotherapy or in combination with a hydroxymethyl-glutaryl-coenzyme A (HMG-A) reductase inhibitor ("statin") (also see *Chapter 14*).

Mechanism of Action

The mechanism(s) by which colesevelam and several of the older BASs improve glycemic control has not been elucidated, although several have been proposed. These include BAS-induced alterations in luminal bile acid composition, increases in incretins such as cholecystokinin, effects on hepatocyte nuclear factor 4 alpha 4, and "deactivation" of farsenoid X receptors by BAS, possibly resulting in an increase in pancreatic insulin secretion or an increase in pancreatic beta cell sensitivity to glucose.

Clinical Efficacy

The effect of colesevelam on glycemic control was first noted in a post hoc analysis of the results of safety data from a lipid-lowering trial in patients with dyslipidemia and type 2 diabetes during which colesevelam also reduced FPG levels by 12%. A subsequent small randomized, placebo-controlled pilot study in 65 patients with type 2 diabetes inadequately controlled (mean baseline A1C: 7.9% colesevelam, 8.1% placebo) on previous antidiabetic therapy demonstrated that colesevelam, added to stable oral antidiabetic drug (OAD) therapy, significantly reduced A1C by –0.5% compared with placebo, and by –1.0% in patients with a baseline A1C of ≥8.0%, as well as reducing FPG by 14 mg/dL. In addition, LDL-C was significantly reduced by –11.7% ($P = 0.007$) from baseline in the colesevelam group.

Subsequently, three larger phase 3 clinical trials were conducted in patients with type 2 diabetes who had not achieved A1C goals with insulin-containing therapy or OADs. One 16-week, double-blind, placebo-controlled trial evaluated the antihyperglycemic effects of colesevelam in 287 patients uncontrolled (A1C 7.5% to 9.5%, inclusive) on insulin alone or in combination with an OAD. Following a 2-week single-blind placebo run-in, subjects were randomized to either colesevelam 3.75 g/day or placebo (mean baseline A1C: 8.3% in both colesevelam and placebo groups). Daily mean insulin use was similar in both groups at baseline. Patients were maintained on existing oral agents and insulin doses were to remain within ±10% of the baseline dose. At week 16, the mean change from baseline in A1C was –0.41% for colesevelam and +0.09% for placebo (treatment effect –0.50%; $P < 0.0001$) (**Figure 8.19-A**). As expected, colesevelam-treated patients also experienced a reduction in mean LDL-C (12.8%, $P = 0.05$).

A second, 28-week, randomized, placebo-controlled study was conducted in 316 patients with inadequately controlled type 2 diabetes (mean baseline A1C: 8.2% and 8.1%, colesevelam and placebo groups, respectively) who were receiving a stable dose of MET or MET plus additional OADs for 3 months. After a 2-week, single-blind placebo run-in period, patients were randomized to 26 weeks' treatment with colesevelam 3.75 g/day or placebo added to their previous MET-based regimen. As shown in **Figure 8.19-B**, at week 26, colesevelam therapy resulted in significant mean placebo-corrected A1C reduction of –0.54% ($P < 0.001$), with a significant treatment difference as early as week 6 (–0.46%; $P < 0.001$). Mean LDL-C levels also decreased from baseline by 15.9% ($P = 0.01$).

FIGURE 8.19 — Mean Changes From Baseline in A1C With Colesevelam or Placebo in Patients With Type 2 Diabetes Inadequately Controlled With Insulin or Oral Antidiabetic Agents

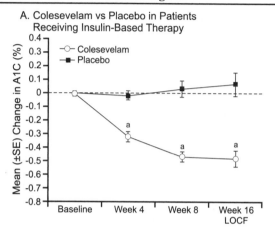

A. Colesevelam vs Placebo in Patients Receiving Insulin-Based Therapy

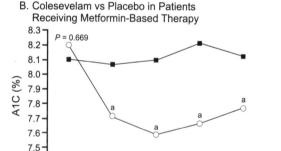

B. Colesevelam vs Placebo in Patients Receiving Metformin-Based Therapy

Continued

The third phase 3 trial also was a randomized, 28-week study conducted in 461 patients who were inadequately controlled (mean baseline A1C: 8.2% and 8.3%, colesevelam and placebo groups, respectively) while receiving a stable dose of an SFU alone or in combination with other OADs for 3 months. After the 2-week, placebo run-in period, patients were treated either with colesevelam (mean dose 3.75 g/day) or placebo added to their previous SFU-based regimen. After 26 weeks of treatment with colesevelam, there was a significant mean

FIGURE 8.19 — *Continued*

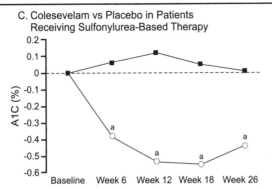

C. Colesevelam vs Placebo in Patients Receiving Sulfonylurea-Based Therapy

^a *P*<0.001.

Adapted from *(A)* Goldberg RB, et al. *Arch Intern Med*. 2008;168:1531-1540, *(B)* Bays HE, et al. *Arch Intern Med*. 1008;168:1975-1983, and *(C)* Fonseca VA, et al. *Diabetes Care*. 2008;31:1479-1484.

placebo-corrected A1C reduction of –0.54% (*P*<0.0001), and a significant treatment difference of –0.44% was seen as early as week 6 (*P*<0.001) (**Figure 8.19-C**). In addition, patients treated with colesevelam also had significantly greater reductions in FPG and fructosamine levels, and as expected, there were significant decreases in LDL-C (16.7%, *P* = 0.01) and apo B and increases in apo A-I and triglycerides.

Adverse Events

In double-blind, placebo-controlled trials in patients with type 2 diabetes, colesevelam was well-tolerated with no serious drug-related AEs. A total of 6.7% of colesevelam-treated patients and 3.2% of placebo-treated patients were discontinued from the diabetes trials due to AEs. This difference was due largely to GI adverse reactions, such as abdominal pain and constipation. The incidence of constipation was 8.7% with colesevelam and 2.0% with placebo. Dyspepsia was reported in 3.9% of colesevelam-treated patients compared with 1.4% of those who received placebo, while 3.0% of colesevelam-treated patients reported nausea and 1.4% of placebo patients reported nausea. Hypoglycemia occurred in 3% of patients receiving colesevelam and in 2.3% of those who received placebo. Although, like the older BASs, colesevelam may increase triglycerides, the increases were significant only in two of the phase 3 trials.

Prescribing Colesevelam

The recommended dose of colesevelam to improve glycemic control in patients with type 2 diabetes is 3750 mg/day administered as 6 tablets (625 mg) once daily or 3 tablets twice daily taken with a meal or liquid. A sugar-free, oral-suspension formulation is also available and may be more convenient to take (vs multiple tablets) for many patients. One packet containing 3750 mg of colesevelam mixed with water can be taken once daily. Colesevelam is contraindicated in patients with a history of bowel obstruction, serum triglyceride concentrations >500 mg/dL, and a history of hypertriglyceridemia-induced pancreatitis. Colesevelam should not be used for glycemic control in patients with type 1 diabetes as monotherapy or for treating diabetic ketoacidosis (DKA). It had not been extensively studied in combination with a DPP-4 inhibitor or in combination with a TZD.

Dopamine Receptor Agonist

■ Bromocriptine Mesylate (Cycloset)

The ergot derivative, bromocriptine mesylate (Cycloset) is approved by the FDA as an adjunct to diet and exercise to improve glycemic control in adults with type 2 diabetes mellitus.

Mechanism of Action

The mechanism by which bromocriptine mesylate improves glycemic control is not well understood. However, morning administration of bromocriptine mesylate has been shown to improve glycemic control in patients with type 2 diabetes without increasing plasma insulin concentrations. This may be related to the circadian peak in central dopaminergic tone in the brain areas that regulate peripheral fuel metabolism (including glucose, lipid metabolism, and protein metabolism) provided by morning administration of the quick-release bromocriptine formulation. This circadian peak in central dopaminergic tone that normally occurs at this time of day in healthy individuals has been linked to preservation and/or induction of normal insulin sensitivity and glucose metabolism in preclinical studies.

Clinical Efficacy

The approval of bromocriptine mesylate for the treatment of patients with type 2 diabetes was based on the results of four randomized, double-blind, placebo-controlled clinical trials that enrolled 3723 patients; a 24-week monotherapy trial, two 24-week trials in which bromocriptine mesylate was added to an SFU, and a 52-week safety trial in which patients also received various oral antidiabetic agents. In all four clinical trials, patients assigned to treatment with bromocriptine mesylate received an initial dose of 0.8 mg once daily, which was increased by 0.8 mg each week for 6 weeks (4.8 mg/day final dose) if no intolerance occurred or until the maximum tolerated dose ≥1.6 mg/day was reached. In these trials, treatment with bromocriptine mesylate resulted in clinically and statistically significant improvements in A1C.

In the monotherapy trial, the mean changes from baseline A1C were –0.1% and –0.3% in the bromocriptine mesylate and placebo groups, respectively. In one of the add-on to SFU trials, the mean changes in A1C were –0.4% and +0.3% with bromocriptine mesylate and placebo, respectively. In the second add-on to SFU trial, the changes in A1C were –0.1% and +0.4% in the bromocriptine mesylate and placebo groups, respectively. In these trials, treatment with bromocriptine mesylate also resulted in significant mean reductions in FPG compared with placebo. In these trials, there were small increases in body weight with both bromocriptine mesylate and placebo that were not significantly different (eg, +0.2 kg and 0.5 kg, respectively, in the monotherapy trial).

Adverse Events

In the pooled phase 3 clinical trials (bromocriptine mesylate $n = 2298$; placebo $n = 1266$), the most commonly reported AEs (nausea, fatigue, vomiting, headache, dizziness) lasted a median of 14 days and were more likely to occur during the initial titration. AEs leading to discontinuation of study drug occurred among 24% of the bromocriptine mesylate-treated patients and 15% of the placebo-treated patients. This between-group difference was driven mostly by GI AEs, particularly nausea. The incidence of hypoglycemia was slightly higher in bromocriptine mesylate-treated patients than in those who received placebo. In the monotherapy trial, hypoglycemia was reported in 2 (3.7%) and 1 (1.3% in the bromocriptine mesylate and placebo groups, respectively. In the two add-on to SFU trials, the incidence of hypoglycemia was 8.6% and 5.2% with bromocriptine mesylate and placebo, respectively. In the 52-week safety trial, the incidence of hypoglycemia was 6.9% and 5.3%, respectively. Bromocriptine mesylate can cause hypotension, including orthostatic hypotension and syncope, particularly when administered with antihypertensive medications.

The Cycloset Safety Trial studied the risk of adverse CV events with this drug. The 52-week study randomized 3095 patients with type 2 diabetes 2:1 to bromocriptine-QR or placebo in conjunction with the patient's usual diabetes therapy. The use of this quick-release formulation of bromocriptine was associated with a 42% relative risk reduction in the composite CVD end point of time to first event following randomization of MI, stroke, coronary revascularization, hospitalization for unstable angina, or hospitalization for CHF.

Prescribing Bromocriptine Mesylate

The administration of bromocriptine mesylate is time-sensitive. It should be taken once daily with food within 2 hours after waking in the morning. The initial dose is 1 tablet (0.8 mg) daily increased weekly by 1 tablet until maximal tolerated daily dose of 1.6 to 4.8 mg is achieved. Bromocriptine mesylate is contraindicated in patients with hypersensitivity to ergot-related drugs and in those with syncopal migraines. It should not be given to nursing women since it may inhibit lactation.

SUGGESTED READING

Action to Control Cardiovascular Risk in Diabetes Study Group; Gerstein HC, Miller ME, Byington RP, et al. Effects of intensive glucose lowering in type 2 diabetes. *N Engl J Med*. 2008;358:2545-2559.

American Diabetes Association. *Medical Management of Type 2 Diabetes*. 6th ed. Alexandria, VA: American Diabetes Association; 2008.

Aronoff S, Rosenblatt S, Braithwaite S, Egan JW, Mathisen AL, Schneider RL. Pioglitazone hydrochloride monotherapy improves glycemic control in the treatment of patients with type 2 diabetes: a 6-month randomized placebo-controlled dose-response study. The Pioglitazone 001 Study Group. *Diabetes Care*. 2000;23:1605-1611.

Aschner P, Katzeff HL, Guo H, et al; Sitagliptin Study 049 Group. Efficacy and safety of monotherapy of sitagliptin compared with metformin in patients with type 2 diabetes. *Diabetes Obes Metab*. 2010;12: 252-261.

Bays HE, Cohen DE. Rationale and design of a prospective clinical trial program to evaluate the glucose-lowering effects of colesevelam HCl in patients with type 2 diabetes mellitus. *Curr Med Res Opin*. 2007;23:1673-1684.

Bays HE, Goldberg RB. The 'forgotten' bile acid sequestrants: is now a good time to remember? *Am J Ther*. 2007;14;567-580.

Bays HE, Goldberg RB, Truitt K, Jones MR. Colesevelam hydrochloride therapy in patients with type 2 diabetes mellitus treated with metformin: glucose and lipid effects. *Arch Intern Med*. 2008;168:1975-1983.

Bosi E, Ellis GC, Wilson CA, Fleck PR. Alogliptin as a third oral antidiabetic drug in patients with type 2 diabetes and inadequate glycaemic control on metformin and pioglitazone: a 52-week, randomized, double-blind, active-controlled, parallel-group study. *Diabetes Obes Metab*. 2011;13(12):1088-1096.

Buse J, Hart K, Minasi L. The PROTECT Study: final results of a large multicenter postmarketing study in patients with type 2 diabetes. Precose Resolution of Optimal Titration to Enhance Current Therapies. *Clin Ther*. 1998;20:257-269.

Cefalu WT, Leiter LA, Niskanen L, et al. Efficacy and safety of canagliflozin, a sodium glucose co-transporter 2 inhibitor, compared with glimepiride in patients with type 2 diabetes on background metformin. *Diabetes*. 2012;61(suppl 1A):LB10. Abstract 38-LB.

Chacra AR, Tan GH, Apanovitch A, et al; CV181-040 Investigators. Saxagliptin added to a submaximal dose of sulphonylurea improves glycaemic control compared with uptitration of sulphonylurea in patients with type 2 diabetes: a randomised controlled trial. *Int J Clin Pract*. 2009;63:1395-1406.

8

Charbonnel B, DeFronzo R, Davidson J, et al; PROactive investigators. Pioglitazone use in combination with insulin in the prospective pioglitazone clinical trial in macrovascular events study (PROactive19). *J Clin Endocrinol Metab*. 2010;95(5):2163-2171.

Choi D, Kim SK, Choi SH, et al. Preventative effects of rosiglitazone on restenosis after coronary stent implantation in patients with type 2 diabetes. *Diabetes Care*. 2004;27:2654-2660.

Chou HS, Palmer JP, Jones AR, et al. Initial treatment with fixed-dose combination rosiglitazone/glimepiride in patients with previously untreated type 2 diabetes. *Diabetes Obes Metab*. 2008;10:626-637.

Dandona P, Aljada A. Endothelial dysfunction in patients with type 2 diabetes and the effects of thiazolidinedione antidiabetic agents. *J Diabetes Complications*. 2004;18:91-102.

Davidson J, Garber A, Mooradian A, Schneider S, Henry D. Metformin/glyburide tablets as first-line treatment in type 2 diabetes: distribution of A1C response. *Diabetes*. 2000;49(suppl 1):A356.

Deeg MA, Buse JB, Goldberg RD, et al. Pioglitazone and rosiglitazone have different effects on serum lipoprotein particle concentrations and sizes in patients with type 2 diabetes and dyslipidemia. *Diabetes Care*. 2007;30:2458-2464.

DeFronzo RA, Burant CF, Fleck P, Wilson C, Mekki Q, Pratley RE. Efficacy and tolerability of the DPP-4 inhibitor alogliptin combined with pioglitazone, in metformin-treated patients with type 2 diabetes. *J Clin Endocrinol Metab*. 2012;97(5):1615-1622.

DeFronzo RA, Goodman AM. Efficacy of metformin in patients with non-insulin-dependent diabetes mellitus. The Multicenter Metformin Study Group. *N Engl J Med*. 1995;333(9):541-549.

Defronzo RA, Hissa MN, Garber AJ, et al; for the Saxagliptin 014 Study Group. The efficacy and safety of saxagliptin when added to metformin therapy in patients with inadequately controlled type 2 diabetes on metformin alone. *Diabetes Care*. 2009;32:1649-1655.

Defronzo RA, Hissa MN, Garber AJ, et al. Once-daily saxagliptin added to metformin provides sustained glycemic control and is well-tolerated over 102 weeks in patients with T2D. Presented at: 69th Scientific Sessions of the American Diabetes Association; June 5-9, 2009; New Orleans, LA. Abstract 547-P.

Del Prato S, Barnett AH, Huisman H, Neubacher D, Woerle HJ, Dugi KA. Effect of linagliptin monotherapy on glycaemic control and markers of β-cell function in patients with inadequately controlled type 2 diabetes: a randomized controlled trial. *Diabetes Obes Metab*. 2011;13: 258-267.

Derosa G, Maffioli P, Salvadeo SA, et al. Effects of sitagliptin or metformin added to pioglitazone monotherapy in poorly controlled type 2 diabetes mellitus patients. *Metabolism*. 2010;59(6):887-895.

Devineni D, Morrow L, Hompesch M, et al. Canagliflozin improves glycaemic control over 28 days in subjects with type 2 diabetes not optimally controlled on insulin. *Diabetes Obes Metab.* 2012;14(6):539-545.

Dhillon A, Weber J. Saxagliptin. *Drugs.* 2009;69:2103-2114.

Dormandy JA, Charbonnel B, Eckland DA, et al; on behalf of the PROactive Investigators. Secondary prevention of macrovascular events in patients with type 2 diabetes in the PROactive Study (PROspective pioglitazone clinical trial In macrovascular Events): a randomized controlled trial. *Lancet.* 2005;366;1279-1289.

Duckworth W, Abraira C, Moritz T, et al; VADT Investigators. Glucose control and vascular complications in veterans with type 2 diabetes. *N Engl J Med.* 2009;360:129-139.

Einhorn D, Rendell M, Rosenzweig J, Egan JW, Mathisen AL, Schneider RL. Pioglitazone hydrochloride in combination with metformin in the treatment of type 2 diabetes mellitus: a randomized, placebo-controlled study. The Pioglitazone 027 Study Group. *Clin Ther.* 2000;22:1395-1409.

Fonseca V, Rosenstock J, Patwardhan R, Salzman A. Effect of metformin and rosiglitazone combination therapy in patients with type 2 diabetes mellitus: a randomized controlled trial. *JAMA.* 2000;283:1695-1702.

Fonseca VA, Rosenstock J, Wang AC, et al. Colesevelam HCL improves glycemic control and reduces LDL cholesterol in patients with inadequately controlled type 2 diabetes on sulfonylurea-based therapy. *Diabetes Care.* 2008;31:1479-1484.

Garber AJ, Donovan DS Jr, Dandona P, Bruce S, Park JS. Efficacy of glyburide/metformin tablets compared with initial monotherapy in type 2 diabetes. *J Clin Endocrinol Metab.* 2003;88:3598-3604.

Gaziano JM, Cincotta AH, O'Connor CM, et al. Randomized clinical trial of quick-release bromocriptine among patients with type 2 diabetes on overall safety and cardiovascular outcomes. *Diabetes Care.* 2010;33:1503-1508.

Goldberg RB, Fonseca VA, Truitt KE, Jones MR. Efficacy and safety of colesevelam in patients with type 2 diabetes and inadequate glycemic control receiving insulin-based therapy. *Arch Intern Med.* 2008; 168:1531-1540.

Gomis R, Espadero RM, Jones R, Woerle HJ, Dugi KA. Efficacy and safety of initial combination therapy with linagliptin and pioglitazone in patients with inadequately controlled type 2 diabetes: a randomized, double-blind, placebo controlled study. *Diabetes Obes Metab.* 2011;13(7):653-661.

Gross JL, Schernthaner G, Fu M, et al. Efficacy and safety of canagliflozin, a sodium glucose co-transporter 2 inhibitor, compared with sitagliptin in patients with type 2 diabetes on metformin plus sulfonylurea. *Diabetes.* 2012;61(suppl 1A):LB13. Abstract 50-LB.

8

Hoelscher D, Chu PL, Lyness W. Fixed-dose combination tablet of repaglinide and metformin is bioequivalent to concomitantly administered individual tablets of repaglinide and metformin: randomized, single-blind, three-period crossover study in healthy subjects. *Clin Drug Investig*. 2008;28:573-582.

Hollander P, Li J, Allen E, Chen R; CV181-013 Investigators. Saxagliptin added to a thiazolidinedione improves glycemic control in patients with type 2 diabetes and inadequate control on thiazolidinedione alone. *J Clin Endocrinol Metab*. 2009;94:4810-4819.

Home PD, Pocock SJ, Beck-Nielsen H, et al; RECORD Study Team. Rosiglitazone evaluated for cardiovascular outcomes in oral agent combination therapy for type 2 diabetes (RECORD): a multicentre, randomised, open-label trial. *Lancet*. 2009;373:2125-2135.

Horton ES, Clinkingbeard C, Gatlin M, Foley J, Mallows S, Shen S. Nateglinide alone and in combination with metformin improves glycemic control by reducing mealtime glucose levels in type 2 diabetes. *Diabetes Care*. 2000;23:1660-1665.

Inzucchi SE, Bergenstal RM, Buse JB, et al. Management of hyperglycemia in type 2 diabetes: a patient-centered approach. Position statement of the American Diabetes Association (ADA) and the European Association for the Study of Diabetes (EASD). *Diabetes Care*. 2012;35: 1364-1379.

Jadzinsky M, Pfützner A, Paz-Pacheco E, et al; CV181-039 Investigators. Saxagliptin given in combination with metformin as initial therapy improves glycaemic control in patients with type 2 diabetes compared with either monotherapy: a randomized controlled trial. *Diabetes Obesity Metab*. 2009;11:611-622.

Juurlink DN, Gomes T, Lipscombe LL, et al. Adverse cardiovascular events during treatment with pioglitazone and rosiglitazone: population based cohort study. *BMJ*. 2009;339:b2942.

Kahn SE, Haffner SM, Heise MA, et al; for the ADOPT Study Group. Glycemic durability of rosiglitazone, metformin, or glyburide monotherapy. *N Engl J Med*. 2006;355:2427-2443.

Kipnes MS, Krosnick A, Rendell MS, Egan JW, Mathisen AL, Schneider RL. Pioglitazone hydrochloride in combination with sulfonylurea therapy improves glycemic control in patients with type 2 diabetes mellitus: a randomized, placebo-controlled study. *Am J Med*. 2001;111:10-17.

Komajda M, McMurray JJ, Beck-Nielsen H, et al. Heart failure events with rosiglitazone in type 2 diabetes: data from the RECORD clinical trial. *Eur Heart J*. 2010;31(7):824-831.

Koshiyama H, Shimono D, Kuwamura N, Minamikawa J, Nakamura Y. Rapid communication: inhibitory effect of pioglitazone on carotid arterial wall thickness in type 2 diabetes. *J Clin Endocrinol Metab*. 2001;86:3452-3456.

Lincoff AM, Wolski K, Nicholls SJ, Nissen SE. Pioglitazone and risk of cardiovascular events in patients with type 2 diabetes mellitus: a meta-analysis of randomized trials. *JAMA*. 2007;298:1180-1188.

Mathisen A, Geerlof J, Houser V, the Pioglitazone 026 Study Group, Takeda America Research and Development Center, Inc. The effect of pioglitazone on glucose control and lipid profile in patients with type 2 diabetes. *Diabetes*. 1999;48(suppl 1):A102-A103.

Moses RG. Achieving glycosylated hemoglobin targets using the combination of repaglinide and metformin in type 2 diabetes: a reanalysis of earlier data in terms of current targets. *Clin Ther.* 2008;30:552-554.

Nathan DM, Buse JB, Davidson MB, et al. Management of hyperglycemia in type 2 diabetes: a consensus algorithm for the initiation and adjustment of therapy. A consensus statement from the American Diabetes Association and the European Association for the Study of Diabetes. *Diabetes Care*. 2006;29:1963-1972.

Nauck MA, Ellis GC, Fleck PR, Wilson CA, Mekki Q; Alogliptin Study 008 Group. Efficacy and safety of adding the dipeptidyl peptidase-4 inhibitor alogliptin to metformin therapy in patients with type 2 diabetes inadequately controlled with metformin monotherapy: a multicentre, randomised, double-blind, placebo-controlled study. *Int J Clin Pract*. 2009;63(1):46-55.

Nesto RW, Bell D, Bonow RO, et al. Thiazolidinedione use, fluid retention, and congestive heart failure. A consensus statement from the American Heart Association and American Diabetes Association. *Circulation*. 2003;108:2931-2948.

Nicolle LE, Capuano G, Ways K, Usiskin K. Effect of canagliflozin, a sodium glucose co-transporter 2 (SGLT2) inhibitor, on bacteriuria and urinary tract infection in subjects with type 2 diabetes enrolled in a 12-week, phase 2 study. *Curr Med Res Opin*. 2012;28(7):1167-1171.

Nissen SE, Wolski K. Effect of rosiglitazone on the risk of myocardial infarction and death from cardiovascular causes. *N Engl J Med*. 2007;356:2457-2471.

Pantalone KM, Kattan MW, Yu C, et al. The risk of developing coronary artery disease or congestive heart failure, and overall mortality, in type 2 diabetic patients receiving rosiglitazone, pioglitazone, metformin, or sulfonylureas: a retrospective analysis. *Acta Diabetol*. 2009;46:145-154.

Patel J, Anderson RJ, Rappaport EB. Rosiglitazone monotherapy improves glycemic control in patients with type 2 diabetes: a twelve-week, randomized, placebo-controlled study. *Diabetes Obes Metab*. 1999;1:165-172.

Pavo I, Jermendy G, Varkonyi TT, et al. Effect of pioglitazone compared with metformin on glycemic control and indicators of insulin sensitivity in recently diagnosed patients with type 2 diabetes. *J Clin Endocrinol Metab*. 2003;88:1637-1645.

Pratley RE, Kipnes MS, Fleck PR, Wilson C, Mekki Q; Alogliptin Study 007 Group. Efficacy and safety of the dipeptidyl peptidase-4 inhibitor alogliptin in patients with type 2 diabetes inadequately controlled by glyburide monotherapy. *Diabetes Obes Metab.* 2009;11(2):167-176.

Pratley RE, McCall T, Fleck PR, Wilson CA, Mekki Q. Alogliptin use in elderly people: a pooled analysis from phase 2 and 3 studies. *J Am Geriatr Soc.* 2009;57(11):2011-2019.

Pratley RE, Reusch JE, Fleck PR, Wilson CA, Mekki Q; Alogliptin Study 009 Group. Efficacy and safety of the dipeptidyl peptidase-4 inhibitor alogliptin added to pioglitazone in patients with type 2 diabetes: a randomized, double-blind, placebo-controlled study. *Curr Med Res Opin.* 2009;25(10):2361-2371.

Rosenstock J, Aggarwal N, Polidori D, et al; Canagliflozin DIA 2001 Study Group. Dose-ranging effects of canagliflozin, a sodium-glucose cotransporter 2 inhibitor, as add-on to metformin in subjects with type 2 diabetes. *Diabetes Care.* 2012;35(6):1232-1238.

Rosenstock J, Rendell MS, Gross JL, Fleck PR, Wilson CA, Mekki Q. Alogliptin added to insulin therapy in patients with type 2 diabetes reduces HbA(1C) without causing weight gain or increased hypoglycaemia. *Diabetes Obes Metab.* 2009;11(12):1145-1152.

Raskin P. Oral combination therapy: repaglinide plus metformin for treatment of type 2 diabetes. *Diabetes Obes Metab.* 2008;10:1167-1177.

Raskin P, Klaff L, McGill J, et al. Efficacy and safety of combination therapy: repaglinide plus metformin versus nateglinide plus metformin. *Diabetes Care.* 2003;26:2063-2068.

Rosenstock J, Hassman DR, Madder RD, et al. Repaglinide versus nateglinide monotherapy: a randomized, multicenter study. *Diabetes Care.* 2004;27:1265-1270.

Satoh N, Ogawa Y, Usui T, et al. Antiatherogenic effect of pioglitazone in type 2 diabetic patients irrespective of the responsiveness to its antidiabetic effect. *Diabetes Care.* 2003;26:2493-2499.

Scott LJ. Alogliptin: a review of its use in the management of type 2 diabetes mellitus. *Drugs.* 2010;70(15):2051-2072.

Smith SA, Porter LE, Biswas N, Freed MI. Rosiglitazone, but not glyburide, reduces circulating proinsulin and the proinsulin:insulin ratio in type 2 diabetes. *J Clin Endocrinol Metab.* 2004;89(12):6048-6053.

Staels B, Kuipers F. Bile acid sequestrants and the treatment of type 2 diabetes mellitus. *Drugs.* 2007;67:1383-1392.

Taskinen MR, Rosenstock J, Tamminen I, et al. Safety and efficacy of linagliptin as add-on therapy to metformin in patients with type 2 diabetes: a randomized, double-blind, placebo-controlled study. *Diabetes Obes Metab.* 2011;13:65-74.

Vilsbøll T, Rosenstock J, Yki-Järvinen H, et al. Efficacy and safety of sitagliptin when added to insulin therapy in patients with type 2 diabetes. *Diabetes Obes Metab*. 2010;12:167-177.

Wilcox R, Kupfer S, Erdmann E; Proactive Study investigators. Effects of pioglitazone on major adverse cardiovascular events in high-risk patient with type 2 diabetes: results from Prospective Pioglitazone Clinical Trial In Macrovascular Events (Proactive 10). *Am Heart J*. 2008;155:712-717.

Williams-Herman D, Johnson J, Teng R, et al. Efficacy and safety of initial combination therapy with sitagliptin and metformin in patients with type 2 diabetes: a 54-week study. *Curr Med Res Opin*. 2009;25:569-583.

Yale JF, Bakris G, Cariou B, et al. Efficacy and safety of canagliflozin in subjects with type 2 diabetes and chronic kidney disease. *Diabetes Obes Metab*. 2013;15(5):463-473.

Yang WS, Jeng CY, Wu TJ, et al. Synthetic peroxisome proliferator-activated receptor-gamma agonist, rosiglitazone, increases plasma levels of adiponectin in type 2 diabetic patients. *Diabetes Care*. 2002;25:376-380.

Zieve FJ, Kalin MF, Schwartz SL, Jones MR, Bailey WL. Results of the glucose-lowering effect of WelChol study (GLOWS): a randomized, double-blind, placebo-controlled pilot study evaluating the effect of colesevelam hydrochloride on glycemic control in subjects with type 2 diabetes. *Clin Ther*. 2007;29:74-83.

8

9

Insulin Therapy

Insulin therapy most commonly is reserved for patients in whom an adequate trial of diet, exercise, and oral antidiabetic agents has failed. However, institution of insulin therapy is commonly delayed inappropriately for months to years in such patients. Both physicians and patients are hesitant to start "the needle" because of fear, ignorance, and time constraints. There is no question that the benefits of improved glycemic control outweigh the initial hassles and risks of insulin therapy. We encourage early use of insulin soon after it is evident that oral antidiabetic agents are failing.

Many insulin regimens are recommended, although it is not clear from the literature which regimen is best. This chapter will focus on the different insulin regimens commonly used to normalize glucose levels and A1C in patients with type 2 diabetes mellitus.

Based on the natural history of type 2 diabetes, many patients will eventually require therapy with insulin. The period of time before insulin is required tends to be highly variable and is based on numerous factors. The most important explanation is the extent of β-cell exhaustion resulting in relative endogenous insulinopenia. This leads to progressive loss of compensatory hyperinsulinemia, which is required to achieve and maintain a sufficient degree of glycemic control, especially in patients taking oral hypoglycemic agents. In other cases, obesity, pregnancy, or any number of medications, as well as a variety of illnesses, may exacerbate the insulin-resistant state and convert a patient previously well controlled on an oral-agent regimen to one requiring insulin.

In addition to the natural history of type 2 diabetes, there is heterogeneity in its pathophysiology, which may influence when patients require insulin. Some patients diagnosed with type 2 diabetes may actually be closer to insulin-dependent or type 1 diabetes with severe insulinopenia. Many of these patients have been shown to have islet cell antibody (ICA) positivity or antibodies to glutamic acid decarboxylase (GAD), with a decreased

C-peptide response to glucagon stimulation and a propensity for primary oral medication failure. Latent autoimmune diabetes in adults, or LADA, is the term coined by the ADA to label this type of patient. There are also wide geographic and racial differences that may influence the need for insulin therapy. For example, Asian patients with type 2 diabetes tend to be thinner, to be diagnosed with diabetes at an earlier age, to experience failure of oral hypoglycemic agents much sooner, and to be more sensitive to insulin therapy than the classic centrally obese Caucasian patient.

Insulin therapy can improve or correct many of the metabolic abnormalities present in patients with type 2 diabetes mellitus. Exogenous insulin administration significantly reduces glucose levels by suppressing hepatic glucose production, increasing PPG utilization, and improving the abnormal lipoprotein levels commonly seen in patients with insulin resistance. Insulin therapy may also decrease or eliminate the effects of glucose toxicity by reducing hyperglycemia to improve insulin sensitivity and β-cell secretory function.

Selecting an Insulin Preparation

There are three types of insulin: animal, human, and insulin analogues. Although purified insulins from animal sources, (eg, beef and pork) were the original type, they are no longer manufactured in the United States. Currently, human insulin is the predominant form used. More recently, a number of insulin analogues have been developed. These include the fast-acting analogues, lispro (Humalog), aspart (Novolog), and glulisine (Apidra) (**Figure 9.1**), as well the long-acting analogues, insulin detemir (Levemir), and insulin glargine (Lantus). In addition, there are several premixed formulations containing a rapid-acting or short-acting insulin or analogue and a short- or intermediate-acting insulin (Humalog Mix 75/25, Humalog 50/50, Novolog Mix 70/30, Novolin 70/30) (see below for further discussion of these preparations). Therefore, the insulin preparations available to control blood glucose in patients with type 2 diabetes mellitus include:

- Fast-acting insulin analogues (lispro, aspart, glulisine)
- Short-acting preparations (regular insulin)
- Intermediate-acting insulins (NPH)
- Long-acting insulins (glargine and detemir)
- Premixed preparations (lispro + lispro protamine suspension, aspart + aspart protamine suspension).

The fast-acting insulin analogues are preferential to regular insulin due to their favorable clinical features. Administration is convenient as they can be given immediately prior to or with meals. Their faster onset of action limits postprandial hyperglycemic peaks by matching serum insulin availability to appearance of meal-derived glucose into the circulation. Their shorter duration of action also reduces development of late postprandial hypoglycemia. The analogues are used to control PPG and need to be given in concert with basal insulin replacement regimens.

Short/fast-acting insulins, as well as long-acting insulin preparations, are needed to mimic the pattern of insulin delivery that normally controls blood glucose in nondiabetic individuals. Basal insulin therapy with long-acting insulin is required to suppress hepatic glucose production overnight and between meals, while short/rapid insulin preparations are needed as bolus insulin to prevent hyperglycemia after meals.

Human insulin is particularly useful for patients with:

- Insulin allergy
- Severe insulin resistance caused by insulin antibodies
- Lipotrophy
- A requirement for intermittent insulin therapy (ie, during pregnancy and acute problems such as infection, MI, and emergency surgery).

Many of the complications of insulin therapy are now uncommon because of the advent of more purified human preparations and insulin analogues.

Selecting an appropriate insulin preparation also depends on the desired time course of action or pharmacokinetics. The values shown in **Table 9.1** are general

**FIGURE 9.1 — Fast-Acting Insulin Analogues:
Lispro (Humalog), Aspart (Novolog), and
Glulisine (Apidra)**

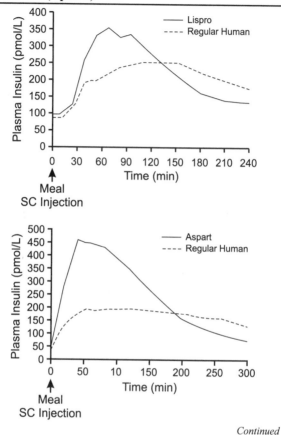

Continued

guidelines that can vary considerably among individuals,
especially those with type 2 diabetes. Other factors that
influence the action of insulin in an individual include:
- Dose
- Site and depth of injection
- Local tissue blood flow
- Skin temperature
- Exercise.

FIGURE 9.1 — *Continued*

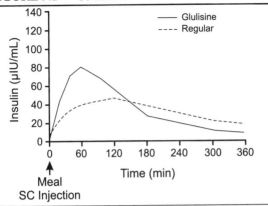

Heinemann L, et al. *Diabet Med*. 1996;13:625-629; Mudaliar SR, et al. *Diabetes Care*. 1999;22:1501-1506; Apidra [package insert]. Bridgewater, NJ: Aventis Pharmaceuticals, Inc; 2004.

The time courses of action of the various insulins are shown graphically in **Figure 9.2**. The recommended interval between an injection of regular or fast-acting insulin and mealtime is 30 to 45 and 5 minutes, respectively, when the preprandial blood glucose is adequate (<140 mg/dL). The patient should wait longer if the blood glucose is higher. Proper timing of the premeal injection can markedly improve the postprandial blood glucose level and possibly reduce the incidence of delayed hypoglycemia. Eating within a few minutes of the injection, or before the injection of regular insulin, markedly reduces the ability of the insulin to prevent a rapid rise in blood glucose and may increase the risk of delayed hypoglycemia. The fast-acting insulins have alleviated much of this problem because of their rapid onset and short duration of activity. Common insulin regimens used in adult diabetes are listed in **Table 9.2**.

Application of Intensive Insulin Therapy

The goals of therapy should be individually tailored. Candidates for intensive management should be:

TABLE 9.1 — Time Course of Action of Insulin Preparations[a]

Insulin Preparation	Onset of Action	Peak Action	Duration of Action
Mealtime Insulins			
Short-Acting			
Regular	30 minutes	2-3 hours	6-8 hours
Fast-Acting			
Aspart (Novolog)[b]	Minutes	1-3 hours	3-5 hours
Glulisine (Apidra)[b]			
Lispro (Humalog)[b]			
Basal Insulins			
Intermediate-Acting			
Isophane (NPH)	2-3 hours	6-8 hours	16-20 hours
Long-Acting			
Detemir (Levemir)[b]	0.8-2 hours	Relatively flat	Up to 24 hours
Glargine (Lantus)[b]	1-2 hours	Peakless	24 hours

Biphasic Insulin: Fixed Mixtures[c]

Humalog Mix 75/25, 50/50[b] (75% [50%] lispro suspension/25% [50%] lispro injection)	Minutes	2 peaks: ~1 hour and 6-8 hours	16-20 hours
Humulin 70/30, 50/50[b] (70% [50%] human insulin suspension/ 30% [50%] human insulin injection)	30 minutes	2 peaks: 2-3 h and 6-8 hours	16-20 hours
Novolog Mix 70/30[a] (70% aspart suspension/30% aspart injection)	10-29 minutes	2 peaks: 1 hour and 4 hours	Up to 24 hours
Novolin 70/30 (70% NPH suspension/30% regular insulin injection)	0.5 hour	2 peaks: 2 hours and 12 hours	Up to 24 hours
U-500	30-90 minutes[d]	3-4 hours[d]	6-8 hours[d]

9

FIGURE 9.2 — Peak Action of Insulin Compared With Peak Rise in Glucose After Eating

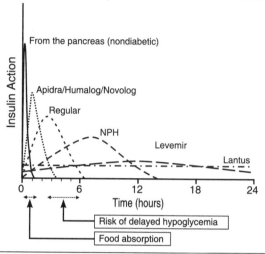

The time course of action (pharmacokinetics) for the fast-acting insulin analogues (Apidra, Humalog, Novolog) is not as fast as insulin from the pancreas of a nondiabetic individual, but it is much more physiologic than the older Regular insulin preparations. Also shown is the time course of action of the intermediate-acting insulin NPH and long-acting insulins Lantus and Levemir.

- Motivated
- Compliant
- Educable
- Without other medical conditions and physical limitations that preclude accurate and reliable self-monitoring of blood glucose (SMBG) and insulin administration.

In addition, caution is advised in patients who are elderly or who are unaware of the signs of hypoglycemia. Other limitations to achieving normoglycemia may include high titers of insulin antibodies, especially in those patients with a prior history of intermittent insulin use of animal origin. The site of insulin injection may also change the pharmacokinetics, and

TABLE 9.2 — Common Insulin Regimens Used in Adult Diabetes

Regimen	Administration	Comment
Single-injection insulin	NPH alone or with Apidra/Humalog/Novolog or regular insulin, or Humalog Mix/Novolog Mix/ Novolin at breakfast, supper, or bedtime, depending on HGM results	Glucose control usually inadequate with single-injection therapy
Insulin and oral agents	Detemir, glargine, or NPH at bedtime or premixed preparations (eg, Humalog 75/25; Novolog Mix 70/30) before supper added to oral antidiabetic agents	Total oral dose of the antidiabetic agents can be given before breakfast if predinner blood glucose values remain elevated
Multiple-injection insulin	Detemir, glargine, or NPH with regular insulin pre-breakfast and supper; regular insulin or Apidra/ Humalog/Novolog insulin before meals; and NPH at bedtime or late afternoon	Humalog 75/25 or Novolog Mix 70/30 prebreakfast and predinner are useful, especially in obese patients with high insulin requirements
Pump-therapy insulin	Apidra, Humalog, or Novolog insulin given as bolus and basal rates on a conventional insulin regimen	Effective strategy for patients with inflexible work hours and/or who are not doing well

9

absorption can be highly variable, especially if lipohypertrophy is present. The periumbilical area has been shown to be one of the more desirable areas in which to inject insulin because of the rapid and consistent absorption kinetics observed at this location.

Prior to initiating insulin therapy, the patient should be well educated in the:

- Technique of SMBG
- Proper techniques of mixing insulins and administration
- Self adjustment of insulin dose if appropriate
- Dietary and exercise strategies.

The patient and family members also need to be informed about hypoglycemia prevention, recognition, and treatment. Initial and ongoing education by a diabetes management team is crucial for long-term success and safety.

There is no one insulin that fits all patients with insulin-requiring type 2 diabetes. There is a natural progression of regimens that can be used as a general algorithm when considering insulin therapy. **Figure 9.3** demonstrates that when oral-agent therapy fails, an easy and often effective regimen can be combination therapy followed by a split-mixed regimen and then a basal bolus multiple-injection regimen.

Combination Therapy

Combination therapy usually refers to the use of oral antidiabetic agents (daytime) together with a single injection of intermediate-acting or long-acting insulin at bedtime. The rationale for using an evening-insulin strategy is based on the pathophysiology of fasting hyperglycemia in type 2 diabetes. The underlying tenet for combination therapy assumes that if evening insulin lowers the fasting glucose level to normal levels, the daytime oral agent will be more effective at controlling postprandial hyperglycemia and maintaining euglycemia throughout the day. Metabolic profiles in type 2 diabetes have clearly demonstrated that the FBG is a major determinant or predictor of glycemic control throughout the day. The FBG level is highly correlated with the degree

FIGURE 9.3 — General Algorithm When Considering Insulin Therapy

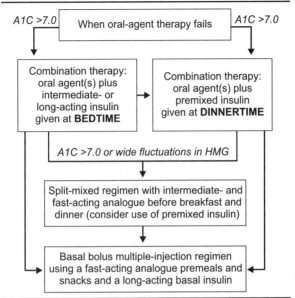

of hepatic glucose production during the early morning hours, which is suppressed by bedtime insulin. In addition, bedtime intermediate-acting insulin's peak action coincides with the onset of the dawn phenomenon (early morning resistance to insulin caused by diurnal variations in growth hormone and possibly norepinephrine levels), which usually occurs between 3 and 7 AM.

Patient selection is very important when considering combination therapy. The question of whether a patient is still responding in a satisfactory manner to oral antidiabetic agent(s), such as SFUs, is of primary importance. Patients also have a higher likelihood of success using daytime oral agents and bedtime insulin if they:

- Are obese
- Have had overt diabetes for <10 to 15 years
- Are diagnosed with type 2 diabetes after the age of 35
- Do not have FBG values consistently >250 to 300 mg/dL

- Have evidence of endogenous insulin secretory ability.

Although standard measurement conditions and levels for C-peptide have not been established for this clinical situation, a fasting (0.2 nmol/L or 0.6 ng/mL) or glucagon-stimulated (>0.40 nmol/L or 1.2 ng/mL) C-peptide value indicates some degree of endogenous insulin secretory ability. Patients with type 2 diabetes diagnosed under the age of 35 more often have atypical forms of diabetes. Subjects with diabetes longer than 10 to 15 years in duration tend to have a greater chance of β-cell exhaustion and thus be less responsive to the oral antidiabetic agents.

Thin patients are more likely to be hypoinsulinemic and often respond inadequately to oral SFUs, which leads to combination-therapy failure. In addition, when the fasting glucose level becomes markedly elevated, this is often associated with a concomitant decrease in endogenous insulin secretory ability, which renders oral agents less effective. The actual number of patients who might fit into this category and possibly respond to combination therapy is unknown but is estimated to be between 20% and 30% of all patients in whom maximum doses of oral-agent therapy fail.

There are also a number of practical reasons why combination therapy may be beneficial (**Table 9.2**):
- The patient does not need to learn how to mix different types of insulin
- Hospitalization is not required
- Patient compliance and acceptance are better with single rather than multiple injections of insulin
- The patient does not need to take injections during work or other activities
- It enables the patient to be initiated to insulin in a simple straightforward manner.

Combination therapy also requires a lower total dose of exogenous insulin than a full regimen of two or three injections per day. This usually contributes to less weight gain and peripheral hyperinsulinemia.

Calculation of the initial bedtime intermediate-acting insulin dose can be based on clinical judgment or on various formulas using FBG level or body weight. For example, one can divide the average FBG (mg/dL) by 18 or divide the body weight in kilograms by 10 to calculate the initial dose of NPH, Lente, or glargine to be started at bedtime. One can also safely start 5 to 10 units of intermediate-acting or long-acting insulin (NPH, Lente, or glargine) for thin patients and 10 to 15 units for obese patients at bedtime as an initial estimated dose. In either case, the dose is increased in 2- to 5-unit increments every 3 to 4 days until the morning FBG level is consistently in the range of 80 to 140 mg/dL (**Table 9.3**).

TABLE 9.3 — Guidelines for Dosing Insulin in Combination Therapy

1. To calculate insulin dose (NPH, detemir, or glargine): divide average fasting blood glucose (mg/dL) by 18 or divide body weight (kg) by 10 to calculate initial dose of NPH or long-acting insulin for bedtime (10:00 PM to midnight)
2. Initial bedtime dose for lean patients: 5-10 U intermediate-acting insulin
3. Initial bedtime dose for obese patients: 10-15 U intermediate-acting insulin
4. Increase dose of insulin in increments of 2-5 U every 3-4 days until the AM fasting blood glucose level is consistently 70-140 mg/dL (reliable patients can make their own adjustments using results from home glucose monitoring)
5. Patients continue taking the maximum dose of their oral agents; if daytime glucose levels become too low (<100 mg/dL), the dose of the oral agent must be decreased.
6. If the oral agent cannot maintain daytime euglycemia, other oral agents can be used or conventional insulin therapy started

The ideal time to give the evening injection of intermediate-acting or long-acting insulin is between 10 PM and midnight. Many reliable patients can make their own adjustments using SMBG. **Table 9.4** demonstrates a patient self-instruction sheet for bedtime insulin adjustments. Once the FBG levels are consistently in a desirable range, the prelunch, predinner, and bedtime blood glucose must be monitored to determine if the oral hypoglycemic agents are maintaining daytime euglycemia. If

TABLE 9.4 — Patient Self-Adjustment of Evening Insulin

1. Begin with a dose of _____ units of _____ insulin administered just before bedtime (NPH, Lente, glargine).
2. If the prebreakfast blood sugar is >140 mg/dL for 3 days in a row, then increase the evening _____ insulin dose by _____ units.
3. If the prebreakfast blood sugar is <80 mg/dL for 2 days in a row, then decrease the evening insulin by _____ units.
4. Remember not to increase the insulin dose more frequently than every 3 days.
5. If you have any questions, please call me at _____.
6. Provider's name:_____.

_____
Physician/Nurse Practitioner

glucose toxicity is present, the patient should wait for a few weeks of normal or near-normal prebreakfast blood glucose values before monitoring for daytime control.

Based on the results of SMBG, combination therapy can be altered to reduce hyperglycemia at identified times during the day. For example, a common situation seen with daytime SFUs and bedtime intermediate-acting or long-acting insulin is an improvement in the fasting, prelunch, and predinner blood glucose, although the postdinner blood glucose level remains excessively high (>200 mg/dL). In this clinical situation, an injection of premixed fast-acting analogue and intermediate-acting insulin (ie, Humalog Mix 75/25 or Novolog Mix 70/30) predinner instead of the bedtime dose of intermediate-acting insulin may be more efficacious (**Table 9.5**). This regimen will often improve the postdinner blood glucose values, because the premixed insulin contains rapidly acting regular insulin yet will still allow overnight glucose control secondary to the intermediate-acting component. With this regimen, however, one must be more cautious of early morning hypoglycemia because the intermediate insulin given before dinner will exert its peak effect earlier. The latter concern has not been a major clinical problem in patients with type 2 diabetes compared with those with type 1 diabetes.

TABLE 9.5 — Instructions for Adding Predinner Premixed Insulin to Daytime Oral Medication(s)[a]

- Start with a dose of **10** units of Humalog Mix 75/25 or Novolog Mix 70/30 just before dinner
- If the morning blood glucose level is >130 mg/dL for >3 consecutive days, increase the predinner Humalog Mix 75/25 or Novolog Mix 70/30 dose by **3** units
- If the morning blood glucose level is <80 mg/dL for 2 consecutive days, decrease predinner Humalog Mix 75/25 or Novolog Mix 70/30 dose by **3** units
- It is extremely important to not increase the dose of insulin more frequently than every 3 days

[a] Regimen must be tailored for the specific patient by the caregiver.

It is recommended that after addition of evening insulin, patients remain on their maximum dose of oral antidiabetic agent. If the daytime blood glucose levels start to become excessively low, the dose of oral medication must be adjusted downward, especially SFUs. This is not an uncommon scenario because glucose toxicity may be reduced as a result of improved glucose control, leading to enhanced sensitivity to both oral agents and insulin. If the prelunch and predinner blood glucose levels remain excessively high on combination therapy, the oral antidiabetic agent is likely not contributing significantly to glycemic control throughout the day. In this situation, use of other oral antidiabetic agents can be utilized or a more conventional regimen of two injections per day can be employed while discontinuing the oral antidiabetic agents.

In summary, combination therapy can be a simple and effective tool to normalize glycemia and A1C levels in selected patients with type 2 diabetes mellitus in whom oral antidiabetic agents fail. The most common clinical situation in which combination therapy can be successful is in the patient in whom oral antidiabetic therapy fails but with some evidence of responsiveness to the oral agents. Bedtime intermediate-acting or long-acting insulin is given and progressively increased so as to normalize the FBG level. When the FBG level is brought under control, the success of combination therapy is dependent upon the ability of the daytime oral antidiabetic agents to maintain euglycemia. If this cannot be achieved, other oral antidiabetic agents can be used or conventional insulin regimens employed.

■ Treat-to-Target Studies

The Treat-to-Target Study demonstrated the ease of administration and effectiveness of combination therapy with oral agents during the day and one injection of insulin glargine or NPH given at night in >400 patients (age ~55 years, ~BMI 32, duration of diabetes ~8 years). In 15 weeks of combination therapy, the average A1C for the two groups decreased from 8.6% to <7.0%, using an aggressive titration schedule for the bedtime insulin with a goal of an FBG <100 mg/dL (**Figure 9.4**). Both treatment arms were equally effective; however, the insulin glargine group experienced significantly less hypoglycemia during the night (**Figure 9.5**). In another study that used an aggressive treat-to-target titration protocol, insulin detemir and NPH were equally effective in controlling blood glucose levels when used twice daily as basal insulin, but detemir was associated with fewer hypoglycemic events, especially nocturnal hypoglycemia, in comparison with NPH, and 70% of patients achieved an A1C ≤7%.

FIGURE 9.4 — Mean A1C Level During Study (Both Treatment Groups)

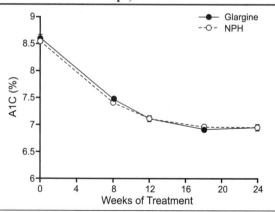

Riddle MC, et al. *Diabetes Care*. 2003;26:3080-3086.

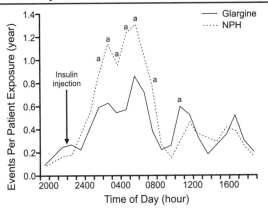

FIGURE 9.5 — Symptomatic Hypoglycemia by Time of Day

[a] $P<0.05$ (between treatment).

Riddle MC, et al. *Diabetes Care*. 2003;26:3080-3086.

Multiple-Injection Regimens   9

One of the more common insulin regimens utilized in type 2 diabetes mellitus is a split-mixed regimen consisting of a prebreakfast and predinner dose of an intermediate- and a fast-acting insulin. This split-mixed regimen of two injections per day is often inadequate for patients with type 1 diabetes mellitus and results in persistent early morning hypoglycemia and fasting hyperglycemia. Such problems do not appear to occur as frequently in type 2 diabetes. This is likely because of pathophysiologic differences between type 1 and type 2 diabetes, particularly in:

- Endogenous insulin secretory ability
- Insulin resistance
- Counterregulatory mechanisms.

There are a number of important aspects of intensive glucose control with insulin in obese patients with type 2 diabetes:

- First, the average daily dose of insulin needed to aggressively control such patients may approximate one unit per kilogram of body weight.

- Second, the total daily insulin requirement can successfully be split equally between the prebreakfast and predinner injections.
- Third, obese patients will require approximately 70% of their total insulin requirement as NPH with the remainder as a mealtime insulin, such as Humalog, Novolog, Apidra, or regular insulin.
- Fourth, the split-mixed regimen in obese patients with type 2 diabetes is usually devoid of the common problems seen with this regimen in type 1 diabetes, particularly early morning hypoglycemia and fasting (preprandial) hyperglycemia.
- Fifth, mild and severe hypoglycemic events are much less frequent in patients with type 2 diabetes mellitus compared with patients with type 1 diabetes undergoing intensive insulin therapy.
- Sixth, the use of fast-acting insulin analogues instead of the older regular insulins may be helpful in terms of reducing prolonged postprandial hyperglycemia, A1C, and the incidence of delayed hypoglycemia.
- Finally, weight gain with peripheral hyperinsulinemia frequently occurs in type 2 diabetes when glucose control is intensified with insulin therapy.

There are several acceptable methods to initiate insulin therapy in type 2 diabetes. A simple alternative method to initiating a split-mixed regimen in obese patients uses Novolog Mix 70/30 or Humalog Mix 75/25 with an initial total daily insulin dose (0.4 to 0.8 units/kg) equally split between the prebreakfast and predinner injections. Adjustments are made based on SMBG results, which may dictate the need to change the ratio of intermediate- to fast-acting insulin either upward or downward or transitioning to a multiple-daily-injection (MDI) regimen. For morbidly obese patients, the insulin requirements rise dramatically as ideal body weight increases above 150%. In contrast, caution should be used when starting thin patients with type 2 diabetes on insulin, especially premixed insulins with fixed doses of fast-acting insulin (initial total daily dose 0.2 to 0.5 units/kg). This group tends to be more sensitive to the glucose-lowering effects and thus more prone to severe hypoglycemia.

More intensive insulin regimens with MDIs will be needed for those patients who do not achieve glycemic goals with combination therapy and the split-mixed, two-injections-per-day regimen. The basal bolus insulin strategy, which can be utilized in patients with either type 1 or type 2 diabetes, incorporates the concept of providing continuous basal insulin secretion throughout the day and night, with brief increases in insulin levels at the time of meal ingestion via bolus doses. A strategy that provides for some flexibility is the mealtime administration of the rapid-acting insulin analogues administered immediately prior to meals, and as intermediate- and long-acting insulins (eg, NPH, glargine, detemir) as the basal insulin. NPH, which exhibits peak action 5 to 7 hours after administration, has also been utilized in combination with rapid-acting insulin analogues. It is commonly given twice daily, although the disadvantages of NPH used in this manner are similar to those previously associated with Ultralente. Because of its time to peak action, NPH should be given every 6 hours (4 times per day) to be effective as a basal insulin in many patients.

9

Improved mealtime glucose control with the rapid-acting analogues has exposed the gaps in basal insulin coverage provided by therapy with the traditional intermediate-acting and long-acting insulin preparations. A once-daily basal insulin analogue (eg, insulin glargine or detemir) with a relatively smooth pharmacokinetic profile would result in a more physiologic pattern of basal insulin replacement. Both insulin glargine and detemir in combination with rapid-acting insulin has demonstrated effective glycemic control and a lower incidence of nocturnal hypoglycemia than with other insulin preparations currently used for basal insulin supplementation.

In summary, there is not a perfect insulin regimen for all insulin-requiring patients with type 2 diabetes. There is a natural progression of insulin regimens as there is a natural history of type 2 diabetes. Combination therapy with a bedtime intermediate-acting or long-acting insulin is an easy first step when initiating insulin therapy. If glycemic goals are not met with the split-mixed regimen, considering premixed insulin can be an easy transition and can be especially effective in obese patients. A natural transition from the more simple regimens is the basal bolus MDI regimen, with a fast-acting analogue before meals and a long-acting basal insulin (eg, glargine) given once a day.

Insulin-Pump Therapy

Insulin-pump therapy has been traditionally used for people with type 1 diabetes. People with type 1 diabetes usually do not have insulin resistance, therefore, they require low basal rates and small insulin boluses. Because type 2 diabetics have the underlying defect of insulin resistance in addition to β-cell failure, they have increased insulin requirements. Insulin-pump therapy is extremely valuable in patients with insulin-requiring type 2 diabetes who have not achieved glycemic control with subcutaneous (SC) injections, who are experiencing wide fluctuations in blood glucose levels complicated by hypoglycemia, or who are seeking a more flexible lifestyle. All of the benefits of pump therapy that are enjoyed by patients with type 1 diabetes discussed previously also apply to people with type 2 diabetes. There are other potential advantages to pump therapy. A patient with type 2 diabetes should be treated with the minimal amount of insulin possible to improve glucose control because excess insulin administration could cause further weight gain. When the pump is used, the number of hypoglycemic events decreases. Therefore, there is less overeating to compensate for hypoglycemia and weight gain may be less of an issue.

Many older patients with the diagnosis of insulin-requiring type 2 diabetes have true late-onset type 1 diabetes. It has been documented in the literature that when large groups of patients with insulin-requiring type 2 diabetes mellitus were tested for anti-GAD antibodies, approximately 5% to 8% were positive. Such individuals are thinner at the time of diagnosis, generally do not respond well to oral agents, and require insulin, although they do not present with severe DKA. This condition is now formally called LADA. This is another group that could potentially benefit from insulin-pump therapy. In general, if a patient with insulin-requiring type 2 diabetes cannot achieve glycemic control with an intensive insulin-injection regimen, insulin-pump therapy should be considered.

Newer Insulins

■ Insulin Lispro

Lispro (Humalog) was the first fast-acting insulin analogue introduced in 1995. It is an effective agent for improving glycemic control while minimizing delayed hypoglycemia. The rapid onset of action appears to be mainly due to its faster absorption (peaking at approximately 30 to 60 minutes compared with 60 to 120 minutes for regular insulin) when injection is SC. Its unique absorption and action properties are the result of a reversal in the two adjacent amino acids: lysine at position 28 and proline at position 29 on the β-chain.

Some of the drawbacks of the older regular insulin preparations have been their slow onset of action as well as delayed clearance, resulting in inefficient control of postprandial excursions in blood glucose levels. With the faster rise and fall of the serum insulin level following a lispro injection, it is easier to coordinate the timing of insulin injections with the subsequent meal. Another advantage to this fast-acting insulin is that it does not have as prolonged an action as the currently available regular insulin, thereby reducing the incidence of delayed hypoglycemic reactions.

■ Insulin Aspart

Insulin aspart (Novolog) is another fast-acting insulin analogue developed by substituting proline with aspartate on the β-chain of the insulin molecule. The substitution of proline with aspartic acid in insulin aspart reduces its tendency to form hexamers like regular insulin. Insulin aspart has more rapid absorption and faster onset of action, within 10 to 20 minutes, than regular insulin, although both are absorbed to a similar extent. Insulin aspart peaks between 1 and 3 hours and has a duration of action of 3 to 5 hours. Because of its rapid onset and short duration, insulin aspart should be used in regimens along with intermediate- or long-acting insulin or with external pumps for subcutaneous insulin infusion. It may also be administered intravenously if under close medical supervision to monitor blood glucose and potassium levels. Differences in pharmacodynamics between insulin aspart and regular human insulin are not associated with differences in overall glycemic control. Insulin aspart has been studied in the pediatric population and been found to be comparable with regular insulin. It is also available in a premixed 70/30 mix disposable pen *(see below)*.

■ Insulin Glulisine

Insulin glulisine (Apidra) is also a fast-acting insulin analogue that was developed by replacing the asparagine in position B3 by lysine, and lysine at position B29 by glutamic acid. Final stages of clinical trials have been completed and it has been approved for therapeutic use in insulin-requiring diabetics.

■ Premixed Formulations

Insulin lispro and insulin aspart are also available in single premixed suspensions: Humalog Mix 75/25 (75% insulin lispro protamine suspension and 25% insulin lispro injection), Humalog mix 50/50 (50% insulin lispro protamine suspension and 50% insulin lispro injection), and NovoLog Mix 70/30 (70% insulin aspart protamine suspension and 30% insulin aspart injection). Because of the rapid onset of action of these new mixtures, they can be given anytime within 15 minutes before a meal and also can be effective if taken 15 minutes after a meal. These new mixtures are available in easy-to-use disposable insulin pens, each holding 300 units insulin. Another premixed formulation, Novolin 70/30, contains 70% NPH insulin Isophane suspension and 30% regular insulin.

The benefits of using the premixed formulations containing the fast-acting insulin analogues include:
- Reduction of postprandial hyperglycemia with the use of lispro/aspart
- No need to wait 30 to 45 minutes between an injection and mealtime
- Improved dosing accuracy in a pen compared with a syringe
- Lowered incidence of delayed hypoglycemia with the shorter-acting lispro or aspart in the mixture.

Several studies have compared regimens of twice-daily (prebreakfast and presupper) premixed dual peak formulations containing a fast-acting insulin analogue with once-daily basal insulin glargine. In one study in insulin-naïve patients with type 2 diabetes who were not adequately controlled with MET monotherapy, twice-daily Novolog Mix 70/30 plus MET achieved A1C targets in significantly more patients than once-daily insulin glargine plus MET. The incidence of minor hypoglycemia and weight gain were slightly higher with Novolog Mix 70/30. Another study in diabetic patients starting insulin therapy compared twice-daily Humalog Mix 75/25 plus MET and once-daily insulin glargine plus MET. Again, more patients on Humalog 75/25 achieved an A1C <7% than those on glargine. The overall rate of hypoglycemia in the Humalog Mix 75/25 group also increased slightly with the exception of nocturnal hypoglycemia. A third study in patients with type 2 diabetes inadequately controlled with intermediate insulin or insulin plus oral agent combination therapy found that patients in the Humalog Mix 75/25 plus MET group improved A1C levels, lower PPG levels, and experienced fewer episodes of nocturnal hypoglycemia vs once-daily insulin glargine with MET.

The disadvantage of premixed insulin is that the ratio of fast-acting to intermediate-acting insulin is fixed. The intermediate-acting dose must be given at dinnertime rather than at bedtime and there is no coverage at lunch. In addition, a patient cannot use carbohydrate counting or a correction factor to adjust the dose.

Patients with type 2 diabetes new to insulin might be considered good candidates for these new mixtures. In addition, patients already on the older 70/30, NPH insulin alone, or oral agents but who remain out of control or who have delayed hypoglycemia may benefit from these mixtures.

■ Insulin Detemir

Insulin detemir (Levemir) is the latest basal insulin to be approved for once- or twice-daily treatment of adult and pediatric patients with type 1 diabetes and adult patients with type 2 diabetes who require basal (long-acting) insulin. Produced by recombinant DNA technology, it differs from human insulin in that one amino acid (threonine) has been omitted on one chain and a fatty acid has been attached to the other chain. Its slow absorption and long duration of action are mediated by its strong self-association and extensive binding with albumin (approximately 98% bound) respectively. Compared with NPH insulin, detemir has slower, more prolonged absorption. Insulin detemir has a dose-dependent onset of action ranging from 0.8 hours at the highest dose to 2 hours at the lowest dose. Its time action profile is relatively flat with a duration of action that ranges from 5.7 hours at the lowest dose to 23.2 hours at the highest dose and a C_{max} between 6 and 8 hours. Insulin detemir (100 units per mL [U-100]) is currently available in a 10-mL vial and a 3-mL prefilled disposable insulin pen that can deliver 1 to 60 units of insulin in 1-unit increments.

The prolonged duration of action of insulin detemir (~6 to 23 hours, depending on dose) is mediated by slow absorption from the injection site and slow distribution to target tissues due to strong self-association and albumin binding. Clinical trials in which insulin detemir was compared with NPH insulin using a basal-bolus regimen in patients with type 1 diabetes and patients with type 2 diabetes who were insulin-naïve or receiving oral antihyperglycemic agents showed effects on A1C and blood glucose levels comparable to those with NPH insulin with somewhat less variation in blood glucose levels and somewhat less weight gain.

■ Insulin Glargine

Insulin glargine (Lantus) is the first peakless long-acting basal insulin analogue. Produced by recombinant DNA technology, it differs from human insulin through a change in one amino acid on the insulin α chain and two amino acids on the β chain. It exists in an acidic form and cannot be mixed in the same syringe with other insulins. After SC injection, insulin glargine forms microcrystalline precipitates that gradually release insulin. Glargine has its onset of action at 4 to 6 hours and a duration of action of >24 hours without a peak. The rate of absorption does not differ for different injection sites and the pharmacokinetics within subjects is fairly consistent.

Initial studies in patients with both type 1 and type 2 diabetes mellitus have shown that the drug is effective when either regular insulin or insulin lispro is used as adjunctive mealtime insulin. Glargine has also been studied as an additive agent in patients with type 2 diabetes who are taking oral agents. The Treat-to-Target Study is comparing the effects of NPH or glargine at bedtime in patients failing oral agents discussed above. Following are several clinical suggestions for glargine use.

Switching a Patient From the Traditional Split-Mixed Regimen to Detemir or Glargine

The recommended changeover suggests that the total NPH or Lente dose be reduced by 20% to determine the nighttime dose of detemir or glargine. It is important, however, to remember that a fast-acting insulin should be used before each meal, including lunch, with this new regimen. The total amount of insulin on the new long-acting/fast-acting insulin regimen should approximate the total split-mixed regimen dose. An example would be a 29-year-old white male who is taking 15 units of NPH and 5 to 10 units of Humalog, Novolog, or Apidra before breakfast and 10 units of NPH and 5 to 10 units of Humalog, Novolog, or Apidra before dinner. We recommend starting with an initial detemir or glargine dose of approximately 20 units at bedtime but also add in a prelunch injection of Humalog, Novolog, or Apidra of 5 to 10 units. Further adjustments should be based on the results of premeal and postmeal SMBG.

Switching a Patient From a Regimen of Ultralente Twice a Day Plus Fast-Acting Insulin (Multiple Daily Injections) to Detemir or Glargine

In this scenario, the conversion is slightly easier. Take the total Ultralente dose and subtract 0% to 5% to get the initial detemir or glargine dose. If the A1C value is fairly good on the Ultralente regimen, subtract 5%, and if the degree of control is not adequate, use the total Ultralente dose to calculate the detemir or glargine dose. The premeal doses of Humalog, Novolog, or Apidra that are being used would be the same.

When Converting a Patient From an Insulin Pump to a Detemir or Glargine Regimen or Vice Versa

Patients with type 2 diabetes are candidates for converting from an insulin pump or vice versa. To do so, we would take the amount of insulin used for the basal rate of the pump and use that for the initial detemir or glargine dose and vice versa when initiating pump therapy from a long-acting/fast-acting insulin regimen. In our experience, we have achieved fairly good success with using similar total doses without any reductions. Obviously, the premeal dose of Humalog, Novolog, or Apidra does not change when converting to this regimen. On the first night of the detemir or glargine injection when initiating pump therapy, we ask the patient to take the dose of long-acting insulin earlier in the evening, ie, 5 PM or 6 PM, and continue the basal rate of the pump until bedtime in order to avoid hyperglycemia the next morning.

Other Issues Regarding the Use of Glargine

It was originally recommended that glargine be taken at bedtime, although it is now approved to be taken at any time that is convenient for the patient. A patient who goes from an insulin pump to a glargine regimen may forget to take the injection of glargine at night during the first few weeks after initiating therapy, leading to morning hyperglycemia. Methods to avoid forgetting should be implemented, such as leaving a note or some type of reminder near the bedside clock or nightstand.

Glargine can cause burning when injected, although we have not found this to be a problem. Occasionally, a patient may state that he or she feels that glargine has a peak and is causing hypoglycemia to develop approximately 12 hours after injecting. If this is true, the time of injection can be changed, and the home glucose monitoring data should be reviewed after several days. A very small percentage of individuals will benefit from splitting the glargine dose.

Splitting the dose of Lantus is rarely needed and should be based on home or continuous glucose monitoring results and not on an arbitrary dosage amount.

Complications of Insulin Therapy

Weight gain and hypoglycemia are the most frequently reported complications of insulin therapy. Both can be minimized with appropriate preventive measures and dosage adjustments. It is important to emphasize that the benefits of improved glycemic control far outweigh any adverse effects of weight gain in a patient with poorly controlled diabetes.

■ Weight Gain

Hyperinsulinemia caused by large amounts of exogenous insulin can lead to marked increases in weight, which is a real concern in type 2 diabetes. Obesity itself is an insulin-resistant state that contributes to a cycle of worsening insulin resistance, increasing insulin requirements, and further weight gain. Some patients, particularly the obese, may require large doses of insulin to normalize glycemia in order to overcome the insulin resistance that is typical of type 2 diabetes. The additional exogenous insulin can result in hyperinsulinemia and an average increase in body weight of 3% to 9%. Excessive weight gain can be minimized by using the lowest possible dose of insulin to achieve target glycemic goals and encouraging the patient to decrease caloric intake and increase exercise. Insulin detemir has consistently demonstrated less weight gain compared with NPH insulin in clinical trials in patients with both type 1 and type 2 diabetes. Studies of patients with type 2 diabetes have reported less weight gain with insulin detemir (up to 2.6 lb) than with NPH insulin (up to 6.2 lb).

■ Hypoglycemia

The incidence of hypoglycemic reaction increases with insulin therapy, particularly intensive regimens, and the thin and the elderly are most affected by such episodes. Obese patients with type 2 diabetes tend to have much less hypoglycemia than those with type 1 diabetes. Severe hypoglycemia is rare in obese patients with type 2 diabetes and is usually related to causal factors such as:

- Overinsulinization
- Underfeeding
- Unplanned strenuous physical activity
- Excessive alcohol
- Incorrect dose of insulin or oral agents taken by patient.

Frequent SMBG by the patient with adjustment in the dose or type of insulin can significantly reduce the likelihood of hypoglycemia.

Edelman SV, Henry RR. Insulin therapy for normalizing the glycosylated hemoglobin in type II diabetes: applications, benefits and risks. *Diabetes Review*. 1994;3:308-334.

Haak T, Tiengo A, Draeger E, et al. Lower within-subject variablity of fasting blood glucose and reduced weight gain with insulin detemir compared to NPH insulin in patients with type 2 diabetes. *Diabetes Obes Metab*. 2005;7:56-64.

Hermansen K, Davies M, Derezinski T, Martinez Ravn G, Clauson P, Home P. A 26-week, randomized, parallel, treat-to-target trial comparing insulin detemir with NPH insulin as add-on therapy to oral glucose-lowering drugs in insulin-naive people with type 2 diabetes [published correction appears in *Diabetes Care*. 2007;30(4):1035]. *Diabetes Care*. 2006;29:1269-1274.

Home P, Kurtzhals P. Insulin detemir: from concept to clinical experience. *Expert Opin Pharmacother*. 2006;7:325-343.

Kolendorf K, Ross GP, Pavlic-Renar I, et al. Insulin detemir lowers the risk of hypoglycaemia and provides more consistent plasma glucose levels compared with NPH insulin in type 1 diabetes. *Diabet Med*. 2006;23:729-735.

Malone JK, Kerr LF, Campaigne BN, Sachson RA, Holcombe JH. Combined therapy with insulin lispro Mix 75/25 plus metformin or insulin glargine plus metformin: a 16-week, randomized, open-label, crossover study in patients with type 2 diabetes beginning insulin therapy. *Clin Ther*. 2004;26:2034-2044.

Malone JK, Bai S, Campaigne BN, Reviriego J, Augendre-Ferrante B. Twice-daily pre-mixed insulin rather than basal insulin therapy alone results in better overall glycaemic control in patients with type 2 diabetes. *Diabet Med*. 2005;22:374-381.

Mudaliar S, Edelman SV. Insulin therapy in type 2 diabetes. *Endocrinol Metab Clin North Am*. 2001;30:935-982.

Owens DR, Coates PA, Luzio SD, Tinbergen JP, Kurzhals R. Pharmacokinetics of 125I-labeled insulin glargine (HOE 901) in healthy men: comparison with NPH insulin and the influence of different subcutaneous injection sites. *Diabetes Care*. 2000;23:813-819.

Raskin P, Klaff L, McGill J, et al. Efficacy and safety of combination therapy: repaglinide plus metformin versus nateglinide plus metformin. *Diabetes Care*. 2003;26:2063-2068.

Raskin P, Allen E, Hollander P, et al. Initiating insulin therapy type 2 diabetes: a comparison of biphasic and basal insulin analogs. *Diabetes Care*. 2005;28:260-265.

Rave K, Heise T, Heinemann L, et al. Inhaled Technosphere insulin in comparison to subcutaneous regular human insulin: time action profile and variability in subjects with type 2 diabetes. *J Diabet Sci Technol.* 2008;2:205-212.

Richardson PC, Boss AH. Technosphere insulin technology. *Diabet Technol Therapeut.* 2007;9:S65-S72.

Riddle MC, Rosenstock J, Gerich J; Insulin Glargine 4002 Study Investigators. The Treat-to-Target Trial. Randomized addition of glargine or human NPH insulin to oral therapy of type 2 diabetic patients. *Diabetes Care.* 2003;26:3080-3086.

Rosenstock J, Hassman DR, Madder RD, et al. Repaglinide versus nateglinide monotherapy: a randomized, multicenter study. *Diabetes Care.* 2004;27:1265-1270.

9

10 Glucoregulatory Hormones

The quest for more physiologic approaches to augment insulin treatment prompted investigation of glucoregulatory hormones. These include the gut-derived hormones, such as the potent incretins glucagon-like polypeptide-1 (GLP-1) and gastric inhibitory peptide (GIP), and the β-cell hormone amylin,

Incretins

A potential role for intestinal peptides in the treatment of type 2 diabetes was based on the observation that insulin responses to an oral glucose load exceeded those after IV glucose administration measured at the same blood glucose concentration. This so-called incretin effect is attributed to the insulinotropic action of gut hormones, particularly:

- Glucose-dependent insulinotropic polypeptide (GIP)
- Glucagonlike peptide 1 (GLP-1).

Since the glucose-lowering effects of GIP have been shown to be impaired in patients with type 2 diabetes, interest has focused on developing antidiabetic therapies based upon the actions of GLP-1 and GIP, the response to which remains intact.

GLP-1 is produced by the tissue-specific cleavage of proglucagon into several smaller peptides in the L-cells of the intestinal mucosa and GIP is synthesized by K cells found in the intestinal mucosa (**Figure 10.1**). The insulinotropic functions of GLP-1 are mediated through interaction with GLP-1 receptors expressed on pancreatic β cells. The release of GLP-1 in response to a meal is rapid (within 10 minutes) and highly correlated with the release of insulin and amylin. In healthy subjects, postprandial levels of GLP-1 rise, whereas patients with diabetes or IGT exhibit reduced levels of meal-stimulated circulating GLP-1.

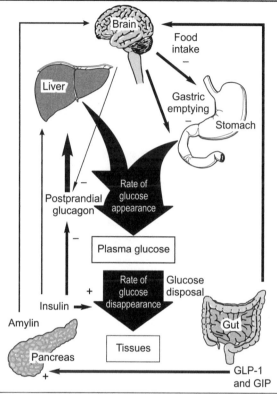

The multihormonal control of glucose homeostasis is regulated by a complex interplay of several gut and islet hormones, including insulin, amylin, glucagon, and incretins.

Exogenous GLP-1 has the potential to normalize fasting and PPG levels in patients with type 2 diabetes. One study in patients with type 2 diabetes demonstrated that intravenously administered GLP-1 significantly reduced FBG and, in a glucose-dependent manner, both enhanced insulin secretion and suppressed glucagon secretion (**Figure 10.2**). Another study found that subcutaneously (SC) administered GLP-1 normalized PPG, enhanced glucose-mediated insulin secretion, and delayed gastric emptying. Importantly, the insulinotropic

FIGURE 10.2 — Plasma Glucose, Insulin, and Glucagon Responses to the IV Administration of GLP-1 or Placebo in Patients With Type 2 Diabetes

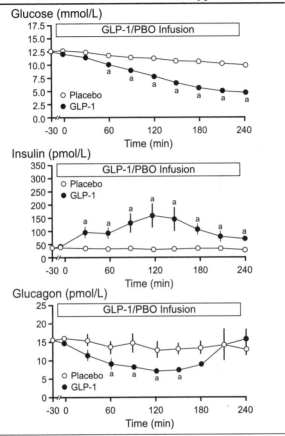

Data are mean ± SE.

[a] $P<0.05$.

Nauck MA, et al. *Diabetologia*. 1993;36:741-744.

and glucagonostatic actions of GLP-1 are strictly glucose dependent. Therefore, GLP-1 should not induce hypoglycemia when administered alone or with other antidiabetic agents that do not cause hypoglycemia, such as MET, TZDs, and AGIs.

Significant acute reductions in appetite and food intake after IV administration of GLP-1 both in healthy individuals and in patients with type 2 diabetes have been demonstrated. The weight effects of GLP-1 therapy are potentially significant for the treatment of type 2 diabetes, in which excessive caloric intake and weight management are important issues that are difficult to control.

In addition to these well-characterized metabolic activities, a number of novel biologic functions of GLP-1 have been shown to occur in animals and include:

- Regulation of β-cell genes involved in glucose sensing and insulin biosynthesis and secretion
- Expansion of β-cell mass through the proliferation and neogenesis of pancreatic cells
- Potentiation of glucose uptake in peripheral tissues.

Whether these effects occur in humans treated with GLP-1 agonists or analogues remains to be determined, although studies that looked at surrogate markers of β-cell health are promising.

The collective glucoregulatory actions of GLP-1 make this peptide a potential powerful agent for the treatment of diabetes. Despite these features, the therapeutic potential of GLP-1 has been limited by its rapid and extensive degradation. In humans, the half-life of GLP-1 is <2 minutes due to rapid degradation as a result of N-terminal cleavage by the ubiquitous enzyme, DPP-4. Elimination is principally via the kidneys.

GLP-1 Analogues

One approach to utilizing the therapeutic potential of GLP-1 has been the development of incretin mimetics. This has resulted in the production of GLP-1 analogues and GLP-1–like compounds that exhibit increased resistance to DPP-4 degradation. Several GLP-1 analogs and a GLP-receptor agonist that exhibit increased resistance to DPP-4 degradation, as well as DPP-4 inhibitors, have been developed. The GLP-1 receptor agonist exenatide (synthetic exendin-4) was the first agent of the incretin mimetic class to be approved by the FDA. More recently, the GLP-1 analog liraglutide also has been approved.

■ Exenatide (Byetta)

Exendin-4 is a naturally occurring incretin mimetic that was originally isolated from the salivary secretions of the lizard *Heloderma suspectum* (Gila monster). Exendin-4 and mammalian GLP-1 have an approximately 50% amino acid sequence identity. However, exendin-4 and GLP-1 are transcribed from distinct genes and, therefore, the exendin-4 gene is not the Gila monster homologue of the mammalian proglucagon gene from which GLP-1 is expressed. In mammals, exendin-4 exhibits antidiabetic activities similar to those of native GLP-1 but is resistant to degradation by DPP-4, and this contributes to its longer half-life compared with GLP-1.

Exenatide is indicated as monotherapy or adjunctive therapy to improve glycemic control in patients with type 2 diabetes mellitus who are taking MET, an SFU, a TZD, a combination of MET and an SFU, or a combination of MET and a TZD, but who have not achieved adequate glycemic control.

Phase 3 Clinical Trials

Three 30-week, double-blind, placebo-controlled trials were conducted to evaluate the safety and efficacy of exenatide in patients with type 2 diabetes unable to achieve adequate glycemic control with MET alone, an SFU alone, or MET in combination with an SFU. A total of 1446 patients were randomized in these three trials. The mean A1C values at baseline for the trials ranged from 8.2% to 8.7%. After a 4-week placebo lead-in period, patients were randomly assigned to receive exenatide 5 mcg bid, exenatide 10 mcg bid, or placebo before the morning and evening meals, in addition to their current oral antidiabetic agent. All patients randomized to exenatide began a treatment initiation period with 5 mcg bid for 4 weeks. After 4 weeks, those patients either continued to receive exenatide 5 mcg bid or had their dose increased to 10 mcg bid. Patients assigned to placebo received placebo bid throughout the study. The primary end point in each study was mean change from baseline A1C at 30 weeks. The results of the 30-week pivotal trials are summarized in **Table 10.1**.

The average reduction in A1C across the three phase 3 pivotal trials in patients completing the 30-week

TABLE 10.1 — Results of 30-Week Pivotal Phase 3 Trials of Exenatide

In Combination With:	Placebo			Exenatide 5 mcg bid			Exenatide 10 mcg bid		
	MET	SFU	MET + SFU	MET	SFU	MET + SFU	MET	SFU	MET + SFU
ITT population (N)	113	123	247	110	125	245	113	129	241
Mean baseline A1C (%)	8.2	8.7	8.5	8.3	8.5	8.5	8.2	8.6	8.5
Change at week 30 (%)	+0.1	+0.1	+0.2	−0.4[a]	−0.5[a]	−1.6	−0.8[b]	−0.9[†]	−1.6
Proportion achieving A1C ≤7% (%)	13.0	8.8	9.2	31.6[a]	32.6[a]	27.4[b]	46.4[a]	41.3[b]	33.5[b]
Mean baseline body weight (kg)	99.9	99.1	99.1	100.0	94.9	96.9	100.9	95.2	98.4
Change at week 30 (kg)	−0.3	−0.6	−0.9	−1.6	−0.9	−1.6[a]	−2.8[b]	−1.6[a]	−1.6[a]

[a] $P \leq 0.05$ vs placebo.
[b] $P \leq 0.0001$ vs placebo.

studies on the highest dose of exenatide (10 mg twice daily) approached 1%. Additionally, approximately 40% of these patients achieved A1C measurements ≤7%. On average, subjects in the phase 3 trials on the highest dose of exenatide also showed statistically significant reductions in body weight of approximately 2 kg. Exenatide was generally well tolerated and the most common adverse event reported was mild-to-moderate nausea, which occurred most frequently early in the study. Patients taking exenatide in combination with an SFU had an increased risk of hypoglycemia. When exenatide was used in combination with MET, no increase in hypoglycemia was seen over that of placebo in combination with MET. In general, hypoglycemia rates were consistent with exenatide's glucose-dependent action, with no difference between the placebo and drug arms. In all three pivotal trials, observed antibody formation to exenatide was consistent with data reported to date. These data do not suggest an influence of antibody formation on exenatide's glucose-lowering effect.

A randomized, placebo-controlled, double-blind trial was performed in 233 subjects with elevated A1C (in spite of therapy) with a TZD alone (20%) or with a TZD and MET (80%). Patients were randomized to receive SC injections of placebo or exenatide 5 mcg for 4 weeks then 10 mcg bid for 16 weeks in addition to their previous regimen (**Figure 10.3**). Exenatide therapy decreased A1C by −0.8 from a baseline of 7.9% (**Figure 10.3-A**). With exenatide, 62% of subjects achieved A1C ≤7% vs 16% with placebo (**Figure 10.3-B**). Fasting serum glucose with exenatide was −1.5 mmol/L (-27 mg/dL) lower than with placebo). Exenatide also significantly reduced body weight from baseline compared with placebo (−1.5 kg vs −0.2 kg respectively) (**Figure 10.3-C**). Nausea was the most frequent adverse event (40% vs 15%, exenatide vs placebo). There was no significant difference in the incidence of hypoglycemia between the two treatments.

Comparative and Long-Term Open-Label Trials

Exenatide vs Insulin Glargine

A 26-week, randomized, active-controlled noninferiority study was performed to determine if exenatide

FIGURE 10.3 — Adjunctive Treatment With Exenatide or Placebo in Patients With Type 2 Diabetes Not Adequately Controlled With a Thiazolidinedione Alone or in Combination With Metformin

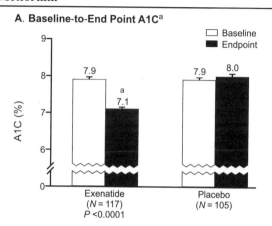

A. Baseline-to-End Point A1C[a]

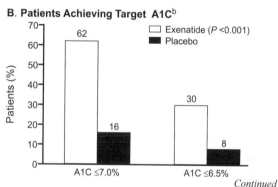

B. Patients Achieving Target A1C[b]

Continued

could be used safely and effectively as an alternative to basal insulin glargine in 551 patients being treated with MET and an SFU. Patients were randomized to receive exenatide (5 mcg bid for the first 4 weeks, then 10 mcg bid for the remainder of the study) or insulin glargine qd (one daily dose titrated to maintain FBG levels of 5.6 mmol/L [<100 mg/dL]). At end point, similar A1C reductions were achieved with exenatide and glargine (−1.1% and −1.1%, respectively) consistent

FIGURE 10.3 — *Continued*

C. Time Course of Change in Body Weight[a,c]

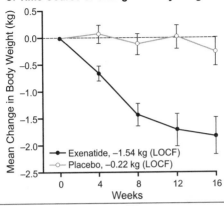

[a] ITT patient sample; mean + SE.

[b] Per-protocol patient sample: randomized patients who had no protocol violations and either completed the protocol or received at least 16 weeks of treatment. Baseline A1C >7% or 6.5%.

[c] Baseline body weight (mean ± SD): exenatide, 97.5 ± 18.9 kg; placebo, 96.9 ± 19.0 kg.

Zinman B, et al. *Ann Intern Med.* 2007;146:477-485.

with the noninferiority study design (**Figure 10.4-A**). As measured by 7-point glucose monitoring, exenatide reduced postprandial excursions following breakfast and dinner, whereas the predominant effect of glargine was a reduction of fasting glucose. Mean weight changes from baseline were –2.5 kg (5.5 lb) with exenatide and +1.8 kg (3.9 lb) with glargine (**Figure 10.4-B**). GI symptoms were more common in the exenatide group than in the insulin glargine group, including nausea (57.1% vs 8.6%), vomiting (17.4% vs 3.7%), and diarrhea (8.5% vs 3.0%). Nausea (57%), generally mild to moderate with a decreasing incidence during the study, was the most common adverse event with exenatide and resulted in a 6% discontinuation rate. The rates of symptomatic hypoglycemia were similar with the two treatments except that nocturnal hypoglycemia was significantly less common with exenatide (0.9 vs 2.4 mean events/patient/year).

FIGURE 10.4 — Exenatide/Insulin Glargine Comparator Trial

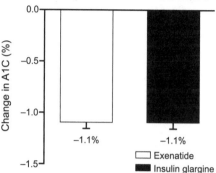

A. Achieved Equivalent Reductions in A1C

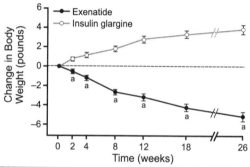

B. Exenatide Resulted in Progressive Weight Reductions

Intent-to-treat population; mean ± SE shown.

[a] $P<0.0001$, exenatide vs insulin glargine at same time point.

Heine RJ, et al. *Ann Intern Med.* 2005;143:559-569.

The ability of exenatide to improve glycemic control with minimal weight gain in overweight patients with type 2 diabetes compared with insulin glargine was assessed in the Helping Evaluate Exenatide in Overweight Patients With Diabetes Compared With Long-Acting Insulin (HEELA) study. Patients (mean BMI 34.1 kg/m²) inadequately controlled on two or three OADs and with elevated CV risk factors were randomized to open-label add-on treatment with exenatide 5-10 mcg bid ($n = 118$) or insulin glargine qd titrated to fasting plasma glucose ≤ 5.6 mmol/L ($n = 117$). The primary outcome was a composite of A1C $\leq 7.4\%$ and weight gain ≤ 1 kg. After 26 weeks, a significantly greater proportion of patients in the exenatide group achieved the composite end point compared with those in the insulin glargine group (53.4% vs 19.8%, respectively). Although there was no significant difference in the reductions in A1C with exenatide and insulin glargine (-1.25% and -1.26%, respectively), whereas mean body weight decreased in the exenatide group but increased in the insulin glargine group (-2.71 vs $+2.98$ kg, respectively). There were more treatment-related adverse events with exenatide but a lower incidence of nocturnal hypoglycemia, with no differences in overall or severe hypoglycemia.

A 1-year, randomized, open-label study in 69 MET-treated patients with type 2 diabetes found that exenatide significantly improved β-cell function (as assessed by arginine-stimulated hyperglycemic clamp) during 1 year of treatment compared with titrated insulin glargine. After cessation of both exenatide and insulin glargine therapy, the β-cell function, A1C, and body weight returned to pretreatment values, suggesting that ongoing treatment is necessary to maintain the beneficial effects of either therapy.

82-Week Studies

Several published analyses reported the effects of exenatide on A1C and weight over 82 weeks in patients with type 2 diabetes who had participated in prior 30-week phase 3 clinical trials and a subsequent 52-week open-label extension. One post hoc analysis examined changes in A1C and weight in 393 patients. During the open-label extensions, all patients received exenatide 5 mcg bid for 4 weeks followed by exenatide 10 mcg bid. All patients continued their MET, SFU, or MET plus SFU. In patients who were treated with exenatide 10 mcg bid for a total of 82 weeks, the reduction from baseline of A1C was -1.1% and the progressive reduction in weight was -4.5 kg or 9.9 lb (**Figure 10.5**). At week 82, patients who received placebo during the first 30 weeks prior to subsequent exenatide 10 mcg bid had reductions in A1C

FIGURE 10.5 — Open-Label Extension[a]: Sustained A1C Reductions and Progressive Body Weight Reductions With Exenatide Therapy Over 82 Weeks

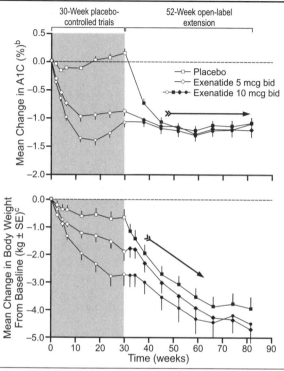

Mean (SE); $N=393$; completer population; 82-week data.

[a] All subjects received exenatide 10 mcg bid.

[b] Baseline A1C 8.3% in all three groups.

[c] Weight change was a secondary end point. Baseline weight: placebo, 98 kg; 5 mcg, 98 kg; 10 mcg, 100 kg.

Data on file: Amylin Pharmaceuticals, Inc.

of −1.2% as well as reductions in weight of −3.3 kg from their 30-week baseline.

Another analysis examined pooled data from a larger cohort of 314 overweight patients (weight 99 ± 21 kg, BMI 34 ± 6 kg/m^2) with type 2 diabetes who received exenatide in addition to an SFU and/or MET in a 30-week placebo-controlled trial and subsequently in an additional 52-week open-label uncontrolled extension study. Patients continued their SFU and/or MET regimens throughout. In these 314 patients who completed 82 weeks of exenatide treatment, reduction in A1C from baseline to week 30 (−0.9%) was sustained to week 82 (−1.1%), with 48% of patients achieving A1C ≤7% at week 82. At week 30, exenatide reduced body weight from baseline (−2.1 kg), with progressive reduction at week 82 (−4.4 kg) (**Figure 10.6**). In addition, patients who completed 82 weeks of exenatide showed statistically significant improvement in some CV risk factors.

Dosage and Administration

Exenatide therapy should be initiated at 5 mcg administered twice daily at any time within the 60-minute period before the morning and evening meals (or before the two main meals of the day, approximately 6 hours or more apart) (**Table 10.2**). Exenatide should not be administered after a meal. Based on clinical response, the dose of exenatide can be increased to 10 mcg twice daily after 1 month of therapy. Each dose should be administered as an SC injection in the thigh, abdomen, or upper arm. Exenatide is not recommended in patients with ESRD or severe renal impairment (CrCl <30 mL/min).

■ Exenatide Extended-Release Formulation

An extended-release formulation of exenatide (Bydureon) was recently approved by the FDA as an adjunct to diet and exercise to improve glycemic control in adults with type 2 diabetes in multiple clinical settings. Whereas the regular exenatide formulation is administered twice daily, this extended-release formulation is administered every 7 days.

Extended-release exenatide has been studied as monotherapy and in combination with MET, an SFU, a TZD, a combination of MET and an SFU, or a combination of MET and a TZD. The concurrent use of extended-release exenatide with insulin has not been studied and cannot be recommended.

The efficacy and safety of extended-release exenatide 2 mg once every 7 days and regular exenatide 10 mcg twice daily were compared in a 24-week, randomized, open-label trial in 252 patients with type 2 diabetes and

FIGURE 10.6 — Changes in Body Weight Over 82 Weeks of Treatment With Exenatide and Metformin, a Sulfonylurea, or Both in Patients Who Previously Participated in 30-Week Phase 3 Trials

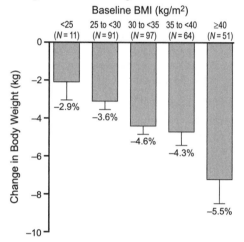

Weight Reductions by Baseline BMI

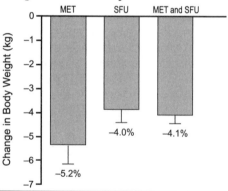

Weight Reductions by Concomitant Medication

Blonde L, et al. *Diabetes Obes Metab.* 2006:8:436-447.

TABLE 10.2 — Dosing With GLP-1 Agonists

Generic Name	Trade Name	Recommended Starting Dose	Recommended Daily Maximum Dose	Dose Frequency
GLP-1 Analogue				
Exenatide	Byetta	5 mcg	10 mcg	bid 60 min prior to a meal; doses ≥6 hours apart
Liraglutide	Victoza	0.6 mg	1.8 mg	qd at any time of day regardless of meals

Modified from: *Physicians' Desk Reference 2011.* 65th ed. Montvale, NJ: PDR Network, LLC; 2010.

10

inadequate glycemic control with diet and exercise alone (19%), a single OAD agent (47%), or a combination of OAD agents (35%). As shown in **Table 10**.3, the reductions in A1C and FPG were significantly greater with extended-release exenatide compared with regular exenatide. In addition, reductions from mean baseline (97/94 kg) in body weight were observed with both extended-release exenatide (-2.3 kg) and regular exenatide (-1.4 kg). In this study, the most common adverse events were nausea (extended-release exenatide 14.0%; regular exenatide 5.0%), diarrhea (extended-release exenatide 9.3%; regular exenatide 4.1%), and injection site erythema (extended-release exenatide 5.4%; regular exenatide 2.4).

TABLE 10.3 — Glycemic Efficacy of Extended-Release Exenatide and Regular Exenatide in a 24-Week, Randomized, Open-Label Trial

	Bydureon 2 mg (q7d) $n=129$	Byetta 10 mcg (bid) $n=123$
A1C (%)		
Mean baseline	8.5	8.4
Mean change	-1.6	-0.9
Difference from Byetta (%)	-0.7[a]	—
Achieving ≤7% (%)	58[a]	30
FPG (mg/dL)		
Mean baseline	173	168
Mean change	-25	-5
Difference from Byetta (%)	-20[a]	—

[a] $P<0.001$ extended-release exenatide vs regular exenatide.

Bydureon [package insert]. San Diego, CA: Amylin Pharmaceuticals, Inc; 2012.

Prescribing Extended-Release Exenatide

Extended-release exenatide (2 mg per dose) should be administered via subcutaneous injection once every 7 days (weekly). The dose can be administered at any time of day, with or without meals. Prior treatment with regular exenatide is not required when initiating the extended-release formulation. Patients changing from the extended-release to the immediate-release formulation of exenatide may experience transient (approximately 2 weeks) elevations in blood glucose concentrations. Extended-release exenatide should not be used in patients with severe renal impairment (CrCl <30 mL/min) or ESRD.

■ Liraglutide (Victoza)

Liraglutide is an acylated GLP-1 analog that shares 97% amino acid sequence identity with native GLP-1. Liraglutide self-associates into a heptameric structure that delays absorption from the SC injection site and slows its metabolism, thereby resulting in a prolonged elimination half-life compared with native GLP-1. This structural modification also results in resistance to GLP-1 inactivation by DPP-4. This pharmacokinetic profile allows for once-daily administration. Liraglutide reduces both FPG and PPG levels, an effect that lasts throughout a 24-hour dosing interval. It increases insulin secretion, reduces postprandial glucagon secretion, delays gastric emptying, and improved β-cell function. Its use has been associated with reductions in body weight and systolic blood pressure.

Liraglutide is indicated as an adjunct to diet and exercise to improve glycemic control in adults with type 2 diabetes mellitus. The results of phase 3 clinical trials have demonstrated that liraglutide can be used as monotherapy, or in combination with one or two OADs, such as MET, SFUs, or TZDs.

Phase 3 Clinical Trials

The efficacy and safety of liraglutide were assessed in the Liraglutide Effect and Action in Diabetes (LEAD) phase 3 program consisting of six large, multicenter, randomized trials of 26- or 52-weeks in duration that enrolled >4000 adult patients with type 2 diabetes (**Table 10.4**). Three of the trials included both placebo and active control groups, while others were either placebo- or active-controlled. Four of the trials used double-blind, double-dummy methodology; however, LEAD-6 was open-label and the insulin glargine arm in LEAD-5 was open-label since the basal insulin dose was individually titrated. LEAD-3 compared liraglutide monotherapy with

TABLE 10.4 — The LEAD Phase 3 Clinical Trial Program With Liraglutide

Design	Patients	Treatment
LEAD-1: Combined With One OAD 26-week randomized, double-blind, placebo- and active-controlled	1041 previously treated with OAD(s)	LIRA 0.6 mg/d + RSG PBO + GLIM 2-4 mg/d LIRA 1.2 mg/d + RSG PBO + GLIM 2-4 mg/d LIRA 1.8 mg/d + RSG PBO + GLIM 2-4 mg/d LIRA PBO + RSG 4 mg/d + GLIM 2-4 mg/d LIRA PBO + RSG PBO + GLIM 2-4 mg/d
LEAD-2: Combined With One OAD 26-week randomized, double-blind, placebo- and active-controlled	1091 previously treated with OAD(s)	LIRA 0.6 mg/d + GLIM PBO + MET 2 g/d LIRA 1.2 mg/d + GLIM PBO +MET 2 g/d LIRA 1.8 mg/d + GLIM PBO + MET 2 g/d LIRA PBO + GLIM 2-4 mg/d + MET 2 g/d LIRA PBO + GLIM PBO + MET 2 g/d
LEAD-3: Monotherapy 52-week randomized, double-blind, active-controlled	746 previously treated with diet/ exercise and/or OAD at ≤50% of highest approved dose	LIRA 1.2 mg/d + GLIM PBO LIRA 1.8 mg/d + GLIM PBO LIRA PBO + GLIM 8 mg/d

LEAD-4: Combined With Two OADs 26-week randomized, placebo-controlled	533 previously treated with one or two OADs	LIRA 1.2 mg/d + MET 2 g/d + RSG 4 g/d LIRA 1.8 mg/d + MET 2 g/d + RSG 4 g/d LIRA PBO + MET 2 g/d + RSG 4 g/d
LEAD-5: Combined With Two OADs 26-week randomized, placebo-controlled with open-label treat-to-target insulin glargine control arm	581 previously treated with one or two OADs	LIRA 1.8 mg/d + MET 2 g/d + GLIM 8 mg/d INSG (titrated) + MET 2 g/d + GLIM 8 mg/d LIRA PBO + MET 2 g/d + GLIM 8 mg/d
LEAD-6: Combined With Two OADs 26-week, randomized, open-label, active-comparator	464 previously treated with maximally tolerated MET and/or SFU	LIRA 1.8 mg/d + previous OAD(s) EXEN 10 mcg BID + previous OAD(s)

glimepiride monotherapy in patients with early-stage diabetes who had not achieved adequate glycemic control with diet and exercise or a single OAD at up to half the maximum approved dose. Change from baseline in A1C was the primary efficacy end point in all LEAD trials. Secondary end points included change from baseline in FPG, PPG, and body weight.

Monotherapy

In the LEAD-3 trial, both doses of liraglutide as monotherapy demonstrated significant improvements in glycemic control in comparison with glimepiride (**Table 10.5**). In addition, A1C reductions from baseline were significantly greater with liraglutide 1.8 mg than with liraglutide 1.2 mg (between-treatment difference of –0.29%). By week 52, significantly more patients in each of the liraglutide groups achieved the target A1C <7%. A1C levels tended to decrease over the first 8 to 12 weeks of treatment with liraglutide. They then remained stable until 52 weeks in the liraglutide 1.8-mg group but increased slightly between week 12 and week 52 with liraglutide 1.2 mg or glimepiride treatment. Patients previously treated with diet and exercise had greater decreases in A1C than did those who were switched from an OAD to liraglutide. Significantly greater reductions in body weight with both doses of liraglutide were also observed compared an increase with glimepiride.

The LEAD-3 trial was extended for an additional 52 weeks of open-label treatment during which 440 of the original study population entered the extension period of whom 321 completed the full 2 years of monotherapy with liraglutide. Of these patients, 110 received liraglutide 1.2 mg, 114 received liraglutide 1.8 mg, and 97 received glimepiride. After 2 years, the mean reductions in A1C with both doses of liraglutide were significantly greater that those glimepiride (–0.9% and –1.1% vs –0.6, respectively). The proportion of patients achieving A1C <7% were significantly greater with liraglutide 1.2 mg and 1.8 mg than with glimepiride (53% and 58% vs 37%). Reductions in FPG also were significantly greater with both doses of liraglutide than with glimepiride. Whereas there was a mean increase in body weight with glimepiride (+1.1 kg), body weight decreased with both doses of liraglutide (–2.1 and –2.7 kg).

In Combination With One OAD

Liraglutide in combination with either rosiglitazone or glimepiride was evaluated in two 26-week, double-dummy, placebo- and active-controlled studies (**Table 10.4**). In LEAD-1, liraglutide used in combination with glimepiride reduced A1C to a significantly greater degree than placebo plus glimepiride or rosiglitazone plus glimepiride (**Figure 10.7**, *top*). The reductions in A1C were greater for patients previously treated with monotherapy compared with combination therapy. However, because the increase with placebo was higher for individuals entering from combination therapy (0.7% vs 0.23%), the differences between treatment groups in favor of liraglutide were similar irrespective of whether individuals were treated previously with monotherapy or combination therapy. A significantly greater proportion of patients treated with liraglutide 0.6, 1.2, or 1.8 mg (24%, 35%, and 42%, respectively) achieved A1C <7% compared with 8% of those who received placebo with glimepiride. The proportions were also significantly greater with liraglutide 1.2 or 1.8 mg (35% and 42%, respectively) compared with that in the rosiglitazone plus glimepiride group (22%). At week 26, all doses of liraglutide decreased FPG significantly more than did placebo (**Figure 10.7**, *bottom*), while only liraglutide 1.2 or 1.8 mg produced greater reductions than rosiglitazone. Changes in body weight with liraglutide 0.6, 1.2, and 5 mg were significantly less than with rosiglitazone (liraglutide +0.7, +0.3, –0.2 kg vs rosiglitazone +2.1 kg, respectively).

In the LEAD-2 trial, reductions in A1C with all three doses of liraglutide plus MET and glimepiride plus MET were significantly greater than with placebo plus MET (**Table 10.6**). The reductions with liraglutide were similar to that with glimepiride; specifically, they were statistically noninferior to glimepiride. The proportions of patients reaching A1C <7% were significantly greater with all doses of liraglutide plus MET compared with placebo plus MET. The proportion of patients in the lira-

TABLE 10.5 — LEAD-3 Trial: Change From Baseline in Glycemic Parameters After 52 Weeks of Treatment With Liraglutide Monotherapy

Efficacy End Point	LIRA (mg/d) + GLIM PBO		GLIM 8 mg + LIRA PBO
	1.2	1.8	
A1C (%):			
Baseline	8.2	8.2	8.2
Change from baseline	−0.8	−1.1	−0.5
Difference from GLIM	−0.3[a]	−0.6[b]	—
Patients A1C <7% (%)	43[b]	51[b]	28
FPG (mg/dL):			
Baseline	168	172	172
Change from baseline	−15	−26	−5
Difference from GLIM	−10[a]	−20[b]	—

Body weight (kg):			
Baseline	92.1	92.6	93.3
Change from baseline	−2.1	−2.5	+1.1
Difference from GLIM	−3.2[b]	−3.6[b]	—

[a] $P<0.05$ vs GLIM.
[b] $P<0.0001$ vs GLIM.

Modified from Garber A, et al. *Lancet.* 2009;373(9662):473-481.

10

FIGURE 10.7 — Change in Glycemic Parameters After 24 Weeks With Liraglutide Added to Rosiglitazone (LEAD-1 Trial)

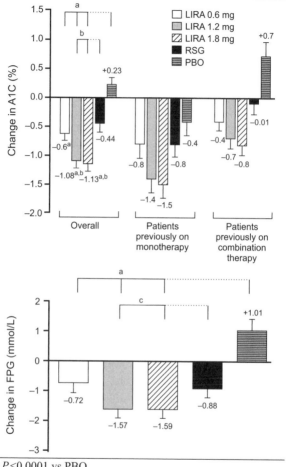

[a] $P<0.0001$ vs PBO.
[b] $P<0.0001$ vs RSG.
[c] $P<0.01$ vs RSG.

Modified from Marre M, et al. *Diabet Med.* 2009;26(3):268-278.

glutide 1.8 mg plus MET group was significantly greater than in the glimepiride plus MET group. Although the proportion of patients with A1C <7% in the glimepiride plus MET group was similar to those receiving liraglutide, the *P* value compared with placebo plus MET was not reported. FPG levels decreased from baseline in the liraglutide plus MET groups as well as in the glimepiride group, whereas FPG increased with placebo plus MET. While body weight decreased in the liraglutide plus MET and placebo plus MET groups, there was an increase in the glimepiride plus MET group.

In Combination With Two OADs

The LEAD-4 and LEAD-5 trials assessed the efficacy of liraglutide as add-on to two OADs: MET and rosiglitazone or MET and glimepiride, respectively (**Table 10.4**).

In LEAD-4, A1C values decreased significantly more in the liraglutide 1.2 and 1.8 mg plus MET and rosiglitazone groups vs placebo plus MET and rosiglitazone. Mean A1C values with both doses of liraglutide decreased from baseline within the first 12 weeks of the study and thereafter remained steady throughout the rest of the trial (**Figure 10.8**, *top*). By week 26, 57.5% and 53.7% of patients in the 1.2- and 1.8-mg liraglutide groups, respectively, had an A1C of <7% compared with 28.1 % in the placebo group. FPG values decreased within 2 weeks of randomization with liraglutide and remained relatively stable thereafter, while there was a significantly smaller decrease with placebo (**Figure 10.8**, *bottom*). In addition, 90-minute PPG at the end of the study decreased from baseline in all treatment groups by –47 mg/dL for 1.2-mg liraglutide, –49 mg/dL 1.8-mg liraglutide, and –14 mg/dL for placebo. Dose-dependent weight loss was observed with 1.2- and 1.8-mg liraglutide (–1.0 and –2.0 kg, respectively) compared with weight gain with placebo (+0.6 kg). The weight loss with liraglutide 1.8 mg was significantly greater than with liraglutide 1.2 mg.

The LEAD-5 trial compared liraglutide 1.8 mg qd, placebo, or open-label insulin glargine, all as add-on to MET and glimepiride. After 26 weeks, the addition of liraglutide 1.8 mg reduced A1C significantly compared

TABLE 10.6 — LEAD-2 Trial: Change in Glycemic Parameters After 24 Weeks With Liraglutide Added to Metformin

| Efficacy End Point | LIRA (mg/d) + MET 2 g/d | | | GLIM 4 mg/d + MET 2 g/d | PBO + MET 2 g/d |
	0.6	1.2	1.8		
A1C (%):					
Baseline	8.4	8.3	8.4	8.4	8.4
Change from baseline	-0.7[a]	-1.0[a,b]	-1.0[a,b]	-1.0[a]	+0.1
Patients A1C <7% (%)	28[c]	35[c]	42[c,d]	36[e]	11
FPG (mmol/L):					
Baseline	10.2	9.9	10.1	10.0	10.0
Change from baseline	-1.1[a]	-1.6[a]	-1.7[a]	-1.3[e]	+0.4
Body weight (kg):					
Baseline	88.3	88.5	88.0	89.0	91.0
Change from baseline	-1.8[f]	-2.6[f,g]	-2.8[f,g]	+1.0	-1.5

^a $P < 0.0001$ vs PBO.
^b Noninferior to glimepiride (upper limit of two-sided 95% CI for treatment difference was <0.4% but not <0%).
^c $P < 0.05$ vs PBO.
^d $P = 0.01$ vs GLIM.
^e P value vs placebo not reported.
^f $P < 0.0001$ vs GLIM.
^g $P \leq 0.01$ vs PBO.

Nauck M, et al. *Diabetes Care*. 2009;32(1):84-90.

10

FIGURE 10.8 — LEAD-4 Trial: Change in Glycemic Parameters After 24 Weeks With Liraglutide Added to Metformin and Rosiglitazone

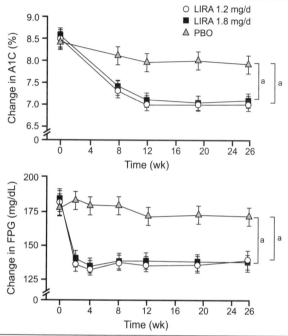

Zinman B, et al. *Diabetes Care.* 2009;32(7):1224-1230.

[a] *P*<0.0001 vs PBO.

with the addition of placebo or insulin glargine (**Table 10.7**). Significantly more patients achieved an A1C <7% with liraglutide than with placebo. FPG levels decreased to a similar degree with liraglutide and insulin glargine, while they increased in the placebo group. There was greater weight loss with liraglutide vs placebo and insulin glargine.

Liraglutide Compared With Exenatide

Liraglutide 1.8 mg qd was compared with exenatide 10 mcg bid, both added to previous treatment with maximally tolerated, but inadequate, doses of MET, an SFU, or both, in a randomized, open-label trial (LEAD-6).

By week 26, liraglutide reduced A1C significantly more than exenatide (1.0% vs 0.79%) (**Figure 10.9**, *top*), and more patients reached A1C <7% with liraglutide than with exenatide (54% vs 43%). Liraglutide treatment also resulted in a greater reduction in FPG than with exenatide (–1.61 mmol/L vs –0.60 mmol/L; *P* <0.0001) (**Figure 10.9**, *bottom*). Weight losses from baseline were similar with both liraglutide and exenatide (–3.24 kg and –2.87 kg).

FIGURE 10.9 — LEAD-6 Trial: Change in Glycemic Parameters After 24 Weeks With Liraglutide or Exenatide Previous Treatment With Metformin, a Sulfonylurea, or Both

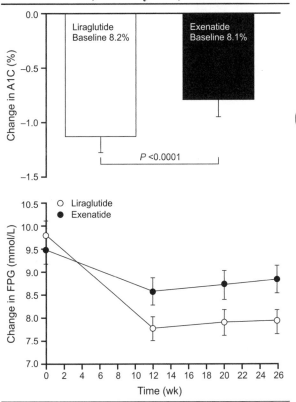

Buse JB, et al. *Lancet*. 2009;374:39-47.

Safety and Tolerability

Throughout the LEAD trials, liraglutide was generally well tolerated, with most adverse events reported to be mild to moderate in severity. GI events (eg, nausea, vomiting, diarrhea) were the most frequently reported adverse events with liraglutide monotherapy and combination therapy and were often dose related. For example, in the LEAD-3 trial with liraglutide monotherapy, 27%, 29%, and 8% of patients who received liraglutide 1.2 mg, 1.8 mg, or glimepiride, respectively, reported treatment-emergent nausea. Nausea generally occurred early during treatment and <10% of patients in the liraglutide 1.8-mg group had experienced nausea by week 4. In the LEAD-4 trial in which liraglutide was added to MET and rosiglitazone, nausea was reported 29% and 40% in the liraglutide 1.2-mg and 1.8-mg groups. However, nausea tended to decrease in frequency over time; for example, there were 216 events during weeks 1 through 4 and 65 events during weeks 4 through 26. In general, serious adverse events were uncommon with liraglutide. In the LEAD-5 trial, patients treated with insulin glargine or placebo reported a 7% frequency of serious adverse events in comparison with a 4% frequency with liraglutide.

Few episodes of minor and major hypoglycemia were reported with liraglutide across the LEAD studies. In the LEAD-3 monotherapy trial, no major hypoglycemic episodes were reported and only 8% of patients treated with liraglutide 1.8 mg reported minor hypoglycemia compared with 24% of glimepiride-treated patients. There were no reports of major hypoglycemia in the LEAD-4 trial. The incidence of minor hypoglycemia also was low (9.0%, 4.9%, and 5.1%) in patients who received liraglutide 1.8 mg, 1.2 mg combined with MET and rosiglitazone, or placebo and MET and rosiglitazone, respectively. Although data are limited, major hypoglycemia with liraglutide seems to occur only when liraglutide is used in combination with an SFU. This may be a result of both agents acting simultaneously to potentiate insulin secretion from β cells, and the fact that insulin secretion stimulated by an SFU is not glucose dependent. This phenomenon of increased hypoglycemic risk in combination with an SFU has also been reported with exenatide.

Dosage and Administration

Liraglutide should be initiated at 0.6 mg qd for 1 week in order to reduce GI symptoms during initiation of treatment. However, this dose is not effective for glycemic control. After 1 week, the dose should be increased 1.2 mg qd. If the 1.2-mg dose does not result in acceptable glycemic control, the dose can be increased to 1.8 mg. Liraglutide can be injected SC in the abdomen, thigh, or upper arm at any time of day, independently of meals. The timing and site of injection can be changed without dosage adjustment. In order to reduce the risk of hypoglycemia, reduction in the dose of a concomitant insulin secretagogue (eg, an SFU) should be considered.

Liraglutide is not recommended as first-line therapy for patients who have inadequate glycemic control on diet and exercise. Since liraglutide is not a substitute for insulin, it should not be used in patients with type 1 diabetes or for the treatment of diabetic ketoacidosis, as it would not be effective in these settings.

It should be noted that since liraglutide causes thyroid C-cell tumors at clinically relevant exposures in rodents, it is contraindicated in patients with a personal or family history of medullary thyroid carcinoma or in patients with Multiple Endocrine Neoplasia syndrome type 2.

■ Summary

The introduction of GLP-1 mimetics inhibitors represents a significant advance in the treatment of type 2 diabetes. Not only are they effective in improving overall glycemic control as indicated by the FBG and PPG values and A1C, but at the same time they are either weight neutral or lead to weight loss. These effects on weight are very important since weight gain associated with intensification of therapy in an effort to normalize or near normalize A1C is a significant challenge in clinical practice. The combination of GLP-1 mimetics with MET appears to be not only effective in terms of metabolic outcomes but also safe in terms of a lower risk of hypoglycemia. It also appears that the weight gain seen with SFUs and TZDs is blunted when these agents are combined with these new classes of antidiabetic agents. Finally, activation of the GLP-1 receptors by these agents may also present the potential to improve β-cell function and, therefore, result in slowing down or halting the natural history of type 2 diabetes. Thus these novel medications may eventually have an important role in the prevention of type 2 diabetes if used early in the course of glucose intolerance.

Amylin Analogue

- **Pramlintide (Symlin)**

Pramlintide is a synthetic analog of human amylin, a naturally occurring neuroendocrine hormone synthesized by pancreatic beta cells that contributes to glucose control during the postprandial period. In healthy individuals, amylin secretion follows the same pattern as insulin, whereby it surges into the bloodstream in response to nutrient uptake (**Figure 10.10-A**). Amylin modulates the rate of gastric emptying, most likely via the vagus nerve, to regulate the inflow of nutrients into the small intestine and thereby reduce the postprandial rise in glucose. Like insulin, amylin secretion is abnormal in patients with type 2 diabetes and is deficient in patients with type 1 diabetes (**Figure 10.10-B**). The rate of gastric emptying is frequently accelerated in people with diabetes with early increases in PPG directly proportional to the rate of gastric emptying. Studies in patients with type 1 diabetes utilizing both solid and liquid meals, showed that amylin prolonged the half-gastric emptying time by 60 to 90 minutes, and did not influence gastric emptying rates of subsequent meals.

Pramlintide slows the rate at which food is released from the stomach to the small intestine following a meal and, thus, it reduces the initial postprandial increase in plasma glucose. This effect lasts for approximately 3 hours following pramlintide. Pramlintide does not alter the net absorption of ingested carbohydrate or other nutrients.

In patients with diabetes, glucagon concentrations are abnormally elevated during the postprandial period, contributing to hyperglycemia. Pramlintide has been shown to decrease postprandial glucagon concentrations in insulin-using patients with diabetes.

FIGURE 10.10 — Amylin: Cosecreted With Insulin and Deficient in Diabetes

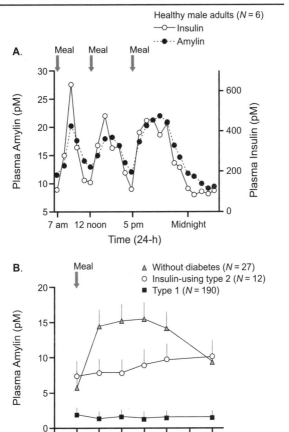

Data from: Kruger DF, et al. *Diabetes Educ.* 1999;25:389-397.

When administered prior to a meal, pramlintide has been shown to reduce total caloric intake. This effect appears to be independent of the nausea that can accompany pramlintide.

■ Clinical Efficacy

Postprandial Glucose

The effect of pramlintide on PPG excursions was assessed in a five-way crossover study in patients with type 2 diabetes using the rapid-acting insulin analog, insulin lispro. Following four separate standardized meals, each subject received pramlintide at different times relative to the meal (−15, 0, +15, and +30 minutes) and, on one occasion, they received placebo 15 minutes before the meal. Insulin lispro was administered immediately before meals. Administration of pramlintide either at or just prior to a meal caused a greater reduction in PPG than either placebo or postmeal pramlintide. Results from this study confirmed that pramlintide, as an adjunct to mealtime insulin therapy, significantly reduced PPG excursions compared with insulin therapy alone. Pramlintide achieved its effects with an average reduction in mealtime insulin dose of approximately 30%.

Long-Term Glycemic Control With Pramlintide

Several long-term clinical trials have shown the benefit of adding pramlintide to an existing regimen of insulin therapy to improve glycemic control in insulin-using patients with type 2 diabetes. A 52-week, randomized, placebo-controlled, double-blind, dose-ranging study in 538 insulin-treated patients compared the efficacy and safety of 30-, 75-, or 150-mcg subcutaneous (SC) doses of pramlintide tid with placebo. Compared with placebo, at week 13 there were significant reductions in A1C in patients receiving the 75-mcg and 150-mcg pramlintide doses. (The 30-mcg dose was subtherapeutic.) The mean A1C reduction from baseline to week 52 of 0.6% in the 150-mcg–dose group was also significantly greater than in the placebo group ($P=0.0068$). The greater reduction in A1C with pramlintide was achieved without increases in insulin use or severe hypoglycemia. Moreover, the proportion of patients who were able to achieve reductions in both A1C and body weight was 3-fold greater with the 150-mcg dose compared with placebo (48% vs 16%). In addition, there was a significant reduction in body weight in all pramlintide-dose groups compared with placebo. It is important to note that due to pH differences between formulations, the 75- and 150-mcg pramlintide doses used in this study were bioequivalent to the 60- and 120-mcg doses used in other studies.

Another 52-week, randomized, placebo-controlled, double-blind, dose-ranging study in 656 insulin-treated patients with type 2 diabetes compared the efficacy and safety of 60-, 90-, or 120-mcg doses of SC pramlintide tid to placebo. Treatment with pramlintide 120 mcg resulted in a sustained reduction from baseline in A1C (–0.68% and –0.62% at weeks 26 and 52, respectively), which was significantly greater than seen with placebo (**Figure 10.11-A**). The proportion of patients who achieved an A1C <8% was approximately 2-fold greater in patients receiving the 120-mcg dose compared with those receiving placebo (48% vs 28%). Once again, the glycemic improvement with pramlintide 120 mcg was accompanied by a reduction in body weight (–1.4 kg) while the placebo group experienced weight gain (+0.7 kg) (**Figure 10.11-B**).

Clinical Practice Study

In order to assess efficacy and safety of pramlintide in a typical clinical practice setting, an open-label study was performed in 166 insulin-using patients with type 2 diabetes who were not able to achieve glycemic control using insulin alone. In this study, pramlintide was initiated at a dose of 120 mcg at major meals. Patients were instructed to reduce their mealtime insulin dose by 30% to 50% upon initiation of pramlintide, then they subsequently adjusted their insulin regimen according to premeal and postmeal glucose monitoring once pramlintide therapy was established. At 6 months, there was a baseline-subtracted A1C reduction of –0.56% from baseline and a body weight reduction of –2.76 kg from baseline. Pramlintide significantly reduced both fasting and PPG (**Figure 10.12**). These changes were achieved with dose reductions of total, short-acting, and long-acting insulin (–6.4%, –10.3%, and –4.20%, respectively).

■ Weight-Loss Effects of Pramlintide

Several long-term, placebo-controlled studies have shown that improved glycemic control in pramlintide-treated patients was not accompanied by increased body

FIGURE 10.11 — Change in A1C and Body Weight Over 52 Weeks in 656 Patients With Type 2 Diabetes Treated With Insulin Plus Various Doses of Pramlintide

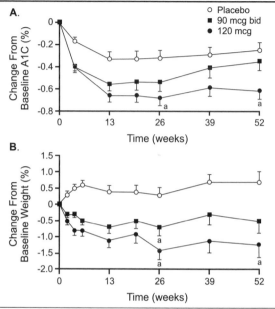

Change from baseline in mean A1C *(A)* and body weight (kg) *(B)*.

[a] *P* = 0.01 compared with placebo.

Adapted from Hollander PA, et al. *Diabetes Care*. 2003;26:784-790.

weight. The greater reduction in A1C with pramlintide compared with placebo has been associated with a sustained and statistically significant reduction in body weight. These findings are further supported by the results of a pooled post hoc analysis of data from 498 overweight/obese (BMI <25 kg/m2) pramlintide- or placebo-treated type 2 diabetic patients who participated in two placebo-controlled long-term trials. At week 26, pramlintide treatment resulted in significant reductions compared with placebo in A1C and body weight (placebo-corrected −0.41% and −1.8 kg, respectively). The greatest reductions in body weight were seen in

FIGURE 10.12 — 7-pt Glucose Profile in Patients With Type 2 Diabetes

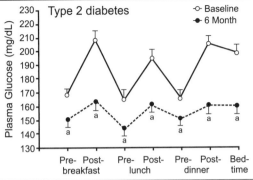

After 6 months of pramlintide therapy as an adjunct to mealtime insulin, postprandial glucose excursions and glucose fluctuations througout the day were reduced in patients with type 2 diabetes.

[a] $P<0.05$.

Karl D, et al. *Diabetes Technol Ther*. 2007;9:191-199.

pramlintide-treated patients with a BMI >40 kg/m2 and in those treated with MET.

■ Tolerability

Pramlintide treatment has been generally well tolerated in patients with diabetes. No evidence of cardiac, hepatic, or renal toxicity, changes in serum lipids, or clinically relevant changes in laboratory parameters, vital signs, electrocardiograms, or abnormal findings upon physical examinations have been observed.

In patients with type 2 diabetes, the most common adverse events, other than hypoglycemia, were GI, including nausea (30%) and vomiting (7%). These symptoms, particularly nausea, appeared early after initiation of therapy, were mostly of mild-to-moderate intensity, were dose dependent, and resolved over time. Slow titration of pramlintide has been shown to significantly reduce the incidence of nausea.

■ Hypoglycemia

The use of pramlintide with insulin has been associated with an increased risk of insulin-induced severe hypoglycemia in both type 1 and type 2 diabetes. When severe hypoglycemia associated with pramlintide occurs, it is usually seen within the first 3 hours after pramlintide injection. Pramlintide alone (without concomitant insulin use) does not cause hypoglycemia.

It should be emphasized that the addition of any anti-hyperglycemic agent to a patient's current insulin therapy has the potential to increase the risk of insulin-induced hypoglycemia, particularly at the start of therapy. In one of the initial long-term pivotal studies of patients with type 1 and insulin-requiring type 2 diabetes where full-dose pramlintide was added to existing insulin regimens in double-blind fashion without titration, it was observed that the severe hypoglycemia event rate during the first 4 weeks of therapy was higher in the pramlintide group compared with the placebo group. In another study in patients with type 1 diabetes, it was shown that this risk was short-term and manageable with adequate glucose monitoring, a 30% to 50% reduction of premeal insulin doses at initiation of pramlintide, and gradual upward titration of the pramlintide dose during its initiation. In the previously discussed clinical practice study, in patients with type 2 diabetes, proactive reduction in premeal insulin doses at initiation of pramlintide was also shown to reduce the incidence of hypoglycemia.

■ Dosing of Pramlintide

Pramlintide is available in a 60 mcg or 120 mcg pen. Patients with type 2 diabetes generally use the 120 mcg pen which delivers doses of either 60 or 120 mcg. Pramlintide should always be administered at a distinct injection site >2 inches away from concomitant insulin injections. All patients should reduce premeal insulin by 50% to lessen the risk of insulin-induced hypoglycemia, monitor blood glucose frequently, and contact their health care provider if symptoms of nausea and/or hypogly-cemia are severe or unusually persistent and when the dosage of pramlintide or insulin is changed. General guidelines and dosing for patients with type 2 diabetes:

- Initiate pramlintide at the 60 mcg dose taken immediately prior to major meals
- Titrate pramlintide to 120 mcg dose after 3 or more days with no clinically significant nausea

- Optimize insulin to achieve glycemic targets once the maintenance dose of pramlintide is reached and blood glucose concentrations are stable

■ Practical Tips for Patients On Pramlintide

Start With a Low Dose and Titrate Slowly

Pramlintide can cause nausea, anorexia, and vomiting, especially in type 1 diabetes where a more gradual titration is required. It is extremely important not to rush the dose titration. Patients with type 2 diabetes generally experience fewer GI side effects. In patients with type 2 diabetes, start with a dose of 60 mcg, followed by escalation to the final dose of 120 mcg if the patient is asymptomatic. If the patient experiences nausea or other GI side effects, do not increase the dose of pramlintide until the GI side effects dissipate.

Take Pramlintide Just Prior to the Meal

In a dose-timing study of pramlintide, PPG concentrations were lowered most effectively when pramlintide was administered just before the meal (Figure 11.3). This reduction of PPG occurred whether the patient was using insulin lispro or regular insulin.

10

When Initiating Pramlintide, Decrease Dose of Mealtime Insulin by 50%

Pramlintide not only works to reduce glucose appearance via the mechanisms previously described but it may also lead to a reduction in food intake greater than anticipated by a patient newly starting pramlintide. Further adjustments of the insulin dose either up or down should be based on home glucose monitoring results and experience with pramlintide.

Timing of the Insulin Dose May Be Important

Many patients who have experience with pramlintide take a fast-acting insulin analog as they approach the end of a meal. The reason is because they will know how much and what types of food they have eaten, so the insulin-dose calculation using carbohydrate counting or other means will be more accurate. Pramlintide delays gastric emptying, and thus the peak in PPG may overlap with the peak action of the fast-acting analogs when given a little later than the beginning of the meal.

SUGGESTED READING

Buse JB, Henry RR, Han J, Kim DD, Fineman MS, Baron AD; Exenatide-113 Clinical Study Group. Effects of exenatide (exendin-4) on glycemic control over 30 weeks in sulfonylurea-treated patients with type 2 diabetes. *Diabetes Care*. 2004;27:2628-2635.

Buse JB, Rosenstock J, Sesti G et al. A study of two glucagon-like peptide-1 receptor agonists for the treatment of type 2 diabetes: liraglutide once daily compared with exenatide twice daily in a randomized, 26-week, open-label trial (LEAD-6). *Lancet*. 2009;374:39-47.

Buse JB, Weyer C, Maggs DG. Amylin replacement with pramlintide in type 1 and type 2 diabetes: a physiological approach to overcome barriers with insulin therapy. *Clin Diabetes*. 2002;20:137-144.

Chapman I, Parker B, Doran S, et al. Effect of pramlintide on satiety and food intake in obese subjects and subjects with type 2 diabetes. *Diabetologia*. 2005;48:838-848.

Croom KF, McCormack PL. Liraglutide. A review of its use in type 2 diabetes mellitus. *Drugs*. 2009;69:1985-2004.

DeFronzo RA, Ratner RE, Han J, et al. Effects of exenatide (exendin-4) on glycemic control and weight over 30 weeks in metformin-treated patients with type 2 diabetes. *Diabetes Care*. 2005;28:1092-1100.

Edelman SV, Weyer C. Unresolved challenges with insulin therapy in type 1 and type 2 diabetes: potential benefit of replacing amylin, a second beta-cell hormone. *Diabetes Technol Ther*. 2002;4:175-189.

Garber A, Henry R, Ratner R et al. Liraglutide versus glimepiride monotherapy for type 2 diabetes (LEAD-3 Mono): randomized, 52-week, phase III, double-blind, parallel-treatment trial. *Lancet*. 2009; 373:473-481.

Heine RJ, Van Gaal LF, Johns D, et al. Exenatide versus insulin glargine in patients with suboptimally controlled type 2 diabetes: a randomized trial. *Ann Intern Med*. 2005;143:559-569.

Henry RR, Ratner RE, Stonehouse AH, et al. Exenatide maintained glycemic control with associated weight reduction over 2 years in patients with type 2 diabetes. Presented at: 66th Scientific Sessions of the American Diabetes Association; June 9-13, 2006; Washington, DC. Poster 485-P.

Hollander PA, Levy P, Fineman MS, et al. Pramlintide as an adjunct to insulin therapy improves long-term glycemic and weight control in patients with type 2 diabetes: a 1-year randomized controlled trial. *Diabetes Care*. 2003;26:784-790.

Hollander P, Maggs DG, Ruggles JA, et al. Effect of pramlintide on weight in overweight and obese insulin-treated type 2 diabetes patients. *Obes Res*. 2004;12:661-668.

Karl D, Philis-Tsimikas A, Darsow T, et al. Pramlintide as an adjunct to insulin in patients with type 2 diabetes in a clinical practice setting reduced A1C, postprandial glucose excursions, and weight. *Diabetes Technol Ther*. 2007;9:191-199.

Kendall DM, Riddle MC, Rosenstock J, et al. Effects of exenatide (exendin-4) on glycemic control over 30 weeks in patients with type 2 diabetes treated with metformin and a sulfonylurea. *Diabetes Care*. 2005;28:1083-1091.

Maggs DG, Fineman M, Kornstein J, et al. Pramlintide reduces postprandial glucose excursions when added to insulin lispro in subjects with type 2 diabetes: a dose-timing study. *Diabetes Metab Res Rev*. 2004;20:55-60.

Marre M, Shaw J, Brändle M, et al. Liraglutide, a once daily human GLP-1 analogue, added to a sulphonylurea over 26 weeks produces greater improvements in glycemic and weight control compared with adding rosiglitazone or placebo in subjects with type 2 diabetes (LEAD-1 SU). *Diabet Med*. 2009;26(3):268-278.

Matthews DR, Marre M, Le-Thi TD, et al. Liraglutide, a human GLP-1 analogue, significantly improves beta cell function in subjects with type 2 diabetes. *Diabetologia*. 2008;51(suppl 1):S356.

Nauck MA, Frid A, Hermansen K, et al. Efficacy and safety comparison of liraglutide, glimepiride, and placebo, all in combination with metformin in type 2 diabetes. *Diabetes Care*. 2009;32:84-90.

Ratner RE, Maggs D, Nielsen LL, et al. Long-term effects of exenatide therapy over 82 weeks on glycemic control and weight in over-weight metformin-treated patients with type 2 diabetes mellitus. *Diabetes Obes Metab*. 2006;8:419-428.

Ratner RE, Want LL, Fineman MS, et al. Adjunctive therapy with the amylin analogue pramlintide leads to a combined improvement in glycemic and weight control in insulin-treated subjects with type 2 diabetes. *Diabetes Technol Ther*. 2002;4:51-61.

Riddle MC, Henry RR, Poon TH, et al. Exenatide elicits sustained glycemic control and progressive reduction of body weight in patients with type 2 diabetes inadequately controlled by sulphonylureas with or without metformin. *Diabetes Metab Res Rev*. 2006;22:483-491.

Russell-Jones D, Vaag A, Schmitz O, et al. Liraglutide vs insulin glargine and placebo in combination with metformin and sulphonylurea therapy in type 2 diabetes mellitus: a randomized controlled trial (LEAD-5 met þ SU). *Diabetologia*. 2009;52:4026-4055.

Schmitz O, Russell-Jones D, Shaw J, et al. Liraglutide, a human GLP-1 analogue, reduces bodyweight in subjects with type 1 diabetes, irrespective of body mass index at baseline. *Diabetologia*. 2008;51(suppl 1):S354.

10

Seino Y, Rasmussen MF, Zdravkovic M, et al. Dose-dependent improvement in glycemia with once-daily liraglutide without hypoglycemia or weight gain: a double-blind, randomized, controlled trial in Japanese patients with type 2 diabetes. *Diabetes Res Clin Pract*. 2008:81:161-168.

Vilsbøll T, Zdravkovic M, Le-Thi T, et al. Liraglutide, a long-acting human glucagon-like peptide-1 analog, given as monotherapy significantly improves glycemic control and lowers body weight without risk of hypoglycemia in patients with type 2 diabetes. *Diabetes Care*. 2007;30:1608-1610.

Weyer C, Gottlieb A, Kim DD, et al. Pramlintide reduces postprandial glucose excursions when added to regular insulin or insulin lispro in subjects with type 1 diabetes: a dose-timing study. *Diabetes Care*. 2003;26:3074-3079.

Whitehouse F, Kruger DF, Fineman M, et al. A randomized study and open-label extension evaluating the long-term efficacy of pramlintide as an adjunct to insulin therapy in type 1 diabetes. *Diabetes Care*. 2002;25:724-730.

Zander M, Madsbad S, Madsen JL, Holst JJ. Effect of 6-week course of glucagon-like peptide 1 on glycemic control, insulin sensitivity, and beta-cell function in type 2 diabetes: a parallel-group study. *Lancet*. 2002;359:824-830.

Zinman B, Hoogwerf B, Durant Garcia S, et al. The effect of adding exenatide to a thiazolidinedione in suboptimally controlled type 2 diabetes: a randomized trial. *Ann Intern Med*. 2007;146:477-485.

Zinman B, Gerich J, Buse J, et al. Efficacy and safety of the human GLP-1 analog liraglutide in combination with metformin and TZD in patients with type 2 diabetes mellitus (LEAD-4 Met+TZD). *Diabetes Care*. 2009;32:1224-1230.

11 Treatment Algorithm

The primary treatment goals of managing type 2 diabetes are to:

- Eliminate symptoms of hyperglycemia
- Recognize the symptoms of hypoglycemia
- Achieve and maintain normal or near-normal metabolic and biochemical parameters (both fasting and postprandial blood glucose levels, A1C [**Table 11.1**], LDL and HDL cholesterol, and fasting triglycerides)
- Achieve normal blood pressure and address pro-coagulant state
- Reduce insulin resistance and its adverse metabolic consequences
- Assist the patient in achieving and maintaining a reasonable body weight
- Prevent or delay the development and progression of microvascular and macrovascular complications

Therapeutic efforts to achieve these goals involve using a variety of treatment modalities:

- Dietary modifications
- Regular physical activity
- Aspirin therapy
- Antidiabetic agents
- Insulin injections.

An individualized approach is recommended based on the following:

- Patient age
- The presence of coexisting illnesses and/or diabetes-related complications
- Lifestyle, including:
  - Attitude
  - Habits
  - Cultural/ethnic status
- Financial considerations

TABLE 11.1 — Glycemic Control for People With Diabetes[a]

	Normal	Goal[b]	Additional Action Suggested
Whole blood values:			
Average preprandial glucose[c]	<100 mg/dL	80-120 mg/dL	<80 mg/dL or >140 mg/dL
Average bedtime glucose[c]	<110 mg/dL	100-140 mg/dL	<100 mg/dL or >160 mg/dL
Plasma values:			
Average preprandial glucose[d]	<110 mg/dL	90-130 mg/dL	<90 mg/dL/>150 mg/dL
Average bedtime glucose[d]	<120 mg/dL	110-150 mg/dL	<110 mg/dL/>180 mg/dL
A1C	<6%	7%	>8%

[a] The values shown in this table are by necessity generalized to the entire population of individuals with diabetes. Patients with comorbid diseases, the very young, older adults, and others with unusual conditions or circumstances may warrant different treatment goals. These values are for nonpregnant adults. Additional action suggested depends on individual patient circumstances. Such actions may include enhanced diabetes self-management education, comanagement with a diabetes team, referral to an endocrinologist, change in pharmacologic therapy, initiation of or increase in self-monitoring of blood glucose, or more frequent contact with the patient. Glycosylated hemoglobin (A1C) is referenced to a nondiabetic range of 4.0% to 6.0% (mean 5.0%, SD 0.5%).

[b] Recommended target glycemic goals for A1C and blood and plasma glucose values vary somewhat between management algorithms proposed by the American Diabetes Association, the American Association of Clinical Endocrinologists, and the Texas Diabetes Council.

[c] Measurement of capillary blood glucose.

[d] Values calibrated to plasma glucose.

12 Assessment of the Treatment Regimen

Certain key clinical and metabolic parameters should be monitored during office visits:
- To assess glycemic control:
  - A1C level
  - Plasma glucose values
- To assess CV risk:
  - Lipoprotein analysis
  - Blood pressure
  - Body weight
- To assess for evidence of diabetic complications
  - Kidney test
  - Dilated eye examination
  - Foot examination.

The metabolic goals for these parameters are shown in **Table 12.1**.

Glycemic control is assessed during office visits with determinations of plasma glucose levels and assays for glycated hemoglobin. Patients can evaluate the effects of their treatment regimen on a day-to-day basis between office visits by using SMBG at home. A combination of physician and patient assessment methods are used to obtain the most accurate information about the degree of metabolic control.

Measuring Plasma Glucose Concentrations

Day-to-day glycemic control is reflected in measurements of plasma glucose concentrations. However, because this measurement is an isolated finding at a single point in time, it may not represent a patient's usual metabolic state. Some limitations of plasma glucose measurements include the following:
- It is difficult to know the meaning of a single random or fasting plasma glucose determination.

TABLE 12.1 — Metabolic Goals of Effective Management

- Glycosylated hemoglobin:
  - Within 1% point above the upper range of normal (7%)
  - Within 3 SD from the mean
- FPG level between 80 mg/dL and 120 mg/dL
- 2-hour postprandial plasma glucose level <160 mg/dL
- Systolic/diastolic blood pressure <130/85 mm Hg if no evidence of proteinuria (<120/80 mm Hg with evidence of proteinuria)
- Approach or maintain ideal body weight
- Lipoprotein goals:
  - Triglyceride level <150 mg/dL
  - HDL cholesterol level >45 mg/dL (>55 in women)
  - LDL cholesterol level <100 mg/dL

- Random determinations may reflect peak, trough, or values in between because of the wide daily variations in glucose levels.
- The stress of an office visit may result in higher than usual glucose values.
- Some patients may become atypically adherent to their treatment regimen or use extra insulin before an office visit, resulting in an uncharacteristically low glucose level.
- The presence of an intercurrent illness at the time of an office visit can alter blood glucose levels.

Home glucose monitoring data are appropriate for assessing glycemic control and making changes in the therapeutic regimen of patients being treated with diet, oral agents, and insulin therapy. Inaccurate or suspicious results would be revealed by a glycated hemoglobin assay, which reflects the level of glucose control for the preceding 2 to 3 months. Because a single plasma glucose measurement does not provide an adequate assessment of any type of therapy, other corroborating data, such as symptoms of hypoglycemia or uncontrolled diabetes, a glycated hemoglobin value, and repeated plasma glucose measurements, are needed.

The timing of plasma glucose measurements has an impact on the significance of the findings:

- A postprandial sample obtained 1 to 2 hours after a patient has eaten is the most sensitive measurement because glucose levels are the highest during this time; total carbohydrate content of the meal will be reflected in this glucose value.
- A preprandial or fasting plasma glucose level reflects how efficiently carbohydrates from a meal have been cleared from the plasma.

Measuring Glycated Hemoglobin

Assays of HbA_1, A1C, and glycated hemoglobin are used extensively to provide an accurate time-integrated measure of average glycemic control over the previous 2 to 3 months and to correlate plasma glucose measurements and patients' SMBG results. Because these assays do not reflect the glucose level at the time a blood sample is tested, measurements of glycated hemoglobin are not useful for making day-to-day adjustments in the treatment regimen.

Glycation refers to a carbohydrate-protein linkage. This irreversible process occurs as glucose in the plasma attaches itself to the hemoglobin component of red blood cells. Because the life span of red blood cells is 120 days, glycated hemoglobin assays reflect average blood glucose concentration over that time.

The amount of circulating glucose concentration to which the red cell is exposed influences the amount of glycated hemoglobin. Therefore, the hyperglycemia of diabetes causes an increase in the percentage of glycated hemoglobin in patients with diabetes; A1C shows the greatest change, whereas the remaining glycated hemoglobins are relatively stable.

Levels of A1C and HbA_1 correlate best with the degree of diabetic control obtained several months earlier. Regardless of which assay is used, however, certain conditions can interfere with obtaining accurate results:
- False low concentrations are likely in the presence of conditions that decrease the life of the red blood cell, such as:
  - Hemolytic anemia
  - Bleeding
  - Sickle cell trait

12

- False high concentrations are likely in the presence of conditions that increase the life span of the red blood cell, eg, patients without a spleen. Other conditions that produce falsely elevated glycated hemoglobins include:
  - Uremia
  - High concentrations of fetal hemoglobin
  - High aspirin doses (>10 g/day)
  - High concentrations of ethanol.

Regular monitoring of glycated hemoglobin (eg, every 3 to 6 months) is essential for all patients with diabetes, regardless of their type of therapy. On a daily basis, patients typically measure capillary blood glucose levels before meals, postprandially, and at bedtime, particularly with intensive insulin regimens in which near-normal glycemia is being actively pursued. Even when preprandial levels seem satisfactory, patients' glycated hemoglobin results often are higher than expected. This finding would not have been evident through glucose measurements alone, and the need for further efforts to control blood glucose would not have been apparent without obtaining a glycated hemoglobin measurement. Home A1C testing is now available (Becton-Dickinson). The patient applies a drop of blood to a reagent card, which is mailed to a central laboratory. The results are then mailed back to the patient.

A disposable test kit for glycosylated A1C is now available for home testing by patients with diabetes.

Measuring Other Glycated Proteins

Enhanced glycation of other proteins occurs in diabetes and has been proposed as another method of assessing average glucose control. Because of the shorter half-life of serum proteins (17 to 20 days) compared with hemoglobin (56 days), measurement of serum fructosamine reflects a shorter period of average glucose control (2 to 3 weeks) (**Figure 12.1**). Traditionally, fructosamine measurements are particularly useful for following patients with GDM.

FIGURE 12.1 — Cooperative Relationship Between Fructosamine and A1C Values

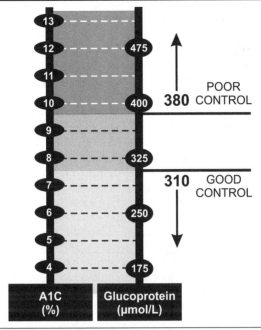

This figure shows the equivalent relationship between fructosamine (glucoprotein) values, which reflect the prior 2 to 3 *weeks* of control, compared with the more commonly used glycosylated hemoglobin (A1C) values, which reflect the prior 2 to 3 *months* of control.

New devices that are available or soon to be released will have the capabilities of measuring serum ketones, lipoproteins, microalbumin, and other important clinical measurements that traditionally could only be obtained by venipuncture or urine collection and measured in a laboratory.

Self-Monitoring of Blood Glucose

This method of self-evaluation using capillary blood samples has become one of the more important tools for monitoring and improving glycemic control and making adjustments in the diabetes therapeutic regimen. SMBG is a relatively painless procedure that involves pricking the fingertip with a lancet to obtain a drop of blood that is placed on a test strip. Reagents on the test strip contain an enzyme that causes glucose to react with a dye to produce a color change. The color intensity is proportional to the amount of glucose present. The test strip is placed in a small, hand-held meter that quantifies the glucose concentration using reflectance spectrometry. Some test strips can be read visually; other systems measure the electrical current produced by the glucose oxidation reaction to quantify the glucose concentration. Results obtained by SMBG tend to have good agreement with plasma glucose concentrations obtained by clinical laboratory procedures if done properly. Patient technique tends to be the source of most discrepancies. Typically, plasma venous glucose measurements are within 15% of the results of whole blood capillary glucose determinations.

SMBG is not a goal in itself but rather a means of achieving the goal of normal or near-normal glycemic control. It should be considered an important part of a comprehensive treatment regimen that includes:

- Diabetes education
- Counseling
- Management by a multidisciplinary team of health care providers.

Goals of treatment and thus the reason for performing SMBG must be clearly defined for the patient. Patients must be motivated and capable of learning the proper technique of SMBG and committed to applying the results to modify their treatment. Health care providers must be able to discuss SMBG results in a nonderogatory, helpful way that provides encouragement through open, honest communication and an atmosphere of support.

Reasons for Performing SMBG

The following reasons for performing SMBG have been outlined in a consensus statement by the ADA:

1. *To achieve or maintain a specific level of glycemic control*—As evidenced by results of the DCCT and

UKPDS, intensive therapy that is closely monitored using SMBG can help patients achieve near-normoglycemia and delay the onset and slow the progression of diabetic complications in type 1 diabetes and type 2 diabetes. Therefore, SMBG at least four times daily is essential for evaluating and adjusting insulin doses in patients on intensive insulin regimens and, with lesser frequency, for patients on less-complex insulin or combination regimens or those using oral agents and diet, directed toward achieving near-normoglycemia.

2. *To prevent and detect hypoglycemia*—Hypoglycemia is a major complication of treatment regimens, particularly those involving intensive application of pharmacologic therapy to achieve near-normoglycemia. The elderly are particularly susceptible to hypoglycemia, and certain oral antidiabetic agents, such as the SFUs, can produce hypoglycemia. Therefore, appropriately timed SMBG is the only way to detect asymptomatic hypoglycemia so that appropriate action (adjusting insulin/oral agents, modifying diet/exercise) can be taken to prevent it from becoming severe.

3. *To avoid severe hyperglycemia*—Illness and certain drugs that alter insulin secretion (eg, phenytoin, thiazide diuretics) or insulin action (eg, prednisone) can increase the risk of severe hyperglycemia and/or ketoacidosis. SMBG should be initiated or used more frequently in all of these situations to detect hyperglycemia before it becomes severe. In addition, patients on insulin therapy can use SMBG data to adjust their insulin doses to avoid severe hyperglycemia.

4. *To adjust care in response to lifestyle changes in patients on pharmacologic therapy*—Glucose levels change in response to variations in diet, exercise, and stressful situations. SMBG can help identify patterns of response to planned exercise and daily activity and help modify pharmacologic therapy during times of increased or decreased caloric consumption.

12

Advantages and Disadvantages of SMBG

SMBG enables the patient to be involved in self-management and provides immediate feedback regarding the impact of diet, exercise, and pharmacologic therapy on blood glucose levels. Patients who are educated about SMBG, how to use the results, and how to make self-adjustments of insulin doses using algorithms (for insulin-requiring type 2 patients and type 1 patients) can achieve better daily glycemic control and have a better sense of self-control and participation in their own care. SMBG also provides worthwhile feedback that the physician and other members of the diabetes health care team can incorporate into ongoing evaluation of the treatment regimen. However, health care professionals need to make a point of requesting and reviewing a patient's SMBG data to provide helpful guidance and encouragement.

Advantages of SMBG include:
- Accurate, immediate results for detecting hypoglycemia and hyperglycemia
- Day-to-day assessment of glycemic control
- Follow-up information after changes in treatment to enhance accurate adjustments in pharmacologic therapy
- Enhanced patient independence, self-confidence, and participation in their treatment
- Storage of test results.

Disadvantages of SMBG include:
- Discomfort of lancing the finger to obtain blood (many meters today allow alternate-site testing)
- Complexity of some testing procedures, requiring mental acuity and dexterity
- Potential malfunction of equipment that could lead to inaccurate results that may affect treatment decisions
- False results because of inaccurate technique that may affect treatment decisions.

SMBG Systems

A combination of factors affect the overall performance of SMBG systems:
- The analytic performance of the meter
- The ability of the user
- The quality of the test strips
- The downloading capacity of home and office computers.

Analytic error can range from 4% to 33%; a goal of future SMBG systems is an analytic error of ± 5%. User performance is most affected by the quality and extent of training, which currently is hindered by reimbursement policies for diabetes education. Initial and regular assessments of a patient's SMBG technique are necessary to assure accurate results. Patients need to be advised that test strips can be adversely affected by environmental factors. In addition, cautious use of generic test strips is warranted because of the complex process of calibrating test strips to specific meters.

A listing of available blood glucose meters, along with their features and capabilities, are compared in the annual *Diabetes Forecast Consumer Guide* and can be found at www.forecast.diabetes.org/consumerguide. The ADA Consensus Panel advises periodic comparisons **12** between a patient's SMBG system and a sample obtained simultaneously and measured by a referenced laboratory. Remember that whole blood glucose values are generally 15% lower than plasma values.

Who Should Perform SMBG?

Virtually all patients with diabetes should perform SMBG because of the value of this evaluation tool in promoting improved glycemic control and reinforcing adherence to therapy. The frequency of SMBG is dictated by the complexity of the therapeutic regimen. For example, insulin-using type 2 diabetics (particularly those on an intensive regimen) would need to perform more daily SMBG evaluations than patients who are achieving acceptable glycemic control with diet, exercise, and oral agents.

Recommended Frequency of SMBG

The frequency of SMBG varies considerably based on the complexity of the therapeutic regimen and the clinical situation of the individual. In addition to guiding therapy, SMBG also has educational and motivational advantages. For example, intermittent measurements 1 to 2 hours after meals can provide an assessment of glycemic response to various types of foods, thus helping patients learn which foods have the greatest and least impact on blood glucose, as well as how the size of a meal affects glucose levels. SMBG also can help motivate patients (especially obese patients trying to lose weight), because they can observe immediate decreases in their blood glucose levels in response to dietary modifications, exercise, and oral therapy.

Patients who demonstrate consistent, acceptable glucose results may require fewer tests (ie, one to three tests per week). However, testing requirements may increase when metabolic control worsens.

SMBG for Patients Who Do Not Take Insulin

Traditionally, SMBG was viewed as not necessary for type 2 patients on diet therapy or oral agents because glucose levels remained relatively stable on these treatment regimens. For these patients, SMBG was recommended only for monitoring short-term adjustments in therapy or for patients at risk for hypoglycemia. Because better glycemic control has been shown to be associated with a greater frequency of SMBG, this evaluation measure now is recommended for all patients, including those not taking insulin. The frequency of testing depends on how stable the patient is. Patients with less than optimal control should monitor their levels more frequently.

SMBG recommendations for patients on diet therapy:

- Prebreakfast—two to three tests per week
- 1 to 2 hours postdinner—two to three tests per week.

Monitoring glucose values from these two important time points, in addition to an A1C or fructosamine value every 3 to 6 months, is an efficient way to follow patients on diet and oral agents.

SMBG recommendations for patients using oral agents alone or combination therapy (daytime oral agents, evening insulin):

- Prebreakfast—four to seven tests per week
- Prelunch—two to three tests per week
- 2 hours postdinner—two to three tests per week.

Patients in this category generally require one to three tests per day when SMBG values are consistent. Patients can make nonpharmacologic changes in their diabetic regimen depending on the results (**Table 12.2**).

TABLE 12.2 — Techniques Used to Adjust for Premeal Hyperglycemia

Nonpharmacologic
- Increase the time interval between insulin injection and consumption of the meal.
- Consume less than the usual amount of calories.
- Eliminate or replace foods containing refined carbohydrates or that have a high glycemic index, such as fruit exchanges.
- Spread the calories over an extended period of time.
- Exercise lightly after a meal.

Pharmacologic
- Increase the amount of fast-acting insulin via an algorithm.
- Make the appropriate long-term adjustment in preceding insulin dose to prevent hyperglycemia at a particular time if a consistent trend is identified.

Edelman SV, Henry RR. *Diabetes Reviews*. 1994;3:310.

12

SMBG is critical for all patients who take exogenous insulin, particularly those on intensive insulin regimens or on combination therapy. The type of insulin regimen used should dictate the frequency of SMBG, with attention to insulin pharmacokinetics and the timing of insulin injections. The best time to evaluate the effectiveness of a dose is at the peak time of action of a particular type of insulin (**Table 9.1**).

Frequent SMBG is necessary to fine-tune an insulin regimen to the needs and responses of a given patient. Ideally, SMBG should be performed four to six times per day (before each meal, at bedtime, and occasionally after meals and at 3 AM, which is the approximate time of early morning glucose nadir). A more intensive SMBG schedule would be a preprandial and 2-hour postprandial measurement and at bedtime, depending on the frequency of insulin doses.

SMBG recommendations for patients on insulin therapy include:

- One injection per day—two tests per day; no less than one to three depending on metabolic control.
- Two injections per day—four tests per day (before each meal and at bedtime)
- Intensive regimen (multiple injections, external pump)—four to seven tests per day.

Results should be recorded in a logbook that is brought to each office visit so the physician can evaluate the effectiveness of the insulin regimen and determine the most appropriate insulin dosage adjustments (**Figure 12.2**). Selected patients should be instructed to apply their SMBG results as the data become available. Making immediate dosage adjustments based on SMBG feedback is evidence of the true benefit of this self-assessment tool. Additionally, most meter logs can be downloaded directly to a personal computer.

When SMBG reveals premeal hyperglycemia, a number of different methods can be used in addition to adjusting the dose of insulin to reduce daily glycemic excursions (**Table 12.2**).

Applying SMBG Results to Adjust Insulin Doses

Patients can be taught how to analyze and use SMBG data to effectively make adjustments in their insulin doses so that they can maintain and improve glycemic control. Insulin algorithms can be used with SMBG to make appropriate day-to-day changes in insulin dosing and to guide long-term treatment. The insulin algorithm shown in **Figure 12.3** is used for patients receiving intensive insulin therapy. Self-adjustment guidelines for patients on a split-mixed regimen are shown in **Table 12.3**; insulin unit changes are provided by the physician on an individualized basis.

Advances in Glucose Monitoring

Over the past several years, home glucose monitoring devices have become smaller, faster, and easier to operate with data analysis capabilities. Computer-generated data analysis can assist the caregiver and the patient in many different areas, including data collection from blood glucose meters, certain insulin pumps, and other new devices. Computer software programs can also create charts and graphs that reveal trends and patterns in blood glucose values for easier evaluation by the patient and the caregiver. There are many software programs that are not only user-friendly for the patient, but are easy to read and analyze by the caregiver. Several programs can generate one-page summaries of a person's diabetes monitoring data intended for optimal presentation of information. Information typically provided includes the standard day plot, before and after meals, pie graphs, the preceding 14 days in a combination graph format (where diet, exercise, and medication are shown with blood glucose levels) and a glucose line plot. The goal ranges and usual insulin doses are usually printed on the bottom of the page if applicable for that patient.

■ Advances in Devices for Bloodletting

The fingerstick devices used to get a drop of blood for testing from the patient have improved with depth-

FIGURE 12.2 — Weekly Self-Monitoring Blood Glucose Record Sheet

Name _____

Address _____

City _____

State _____ Zip _____ – _____

SS #: _____ – _____ – _____

Home PH#: (___) ___ – ___

Work PH#: (___) ___ – ___

Fax #: (___) ___ – ___

Pager #: (___) ___ – ___

INSTRUCTIONS: Record time of day in upper box and glucose readings in lower box.

Day/Date (mm/dd/yy)	AM Breakfast Before	AM Breakfast After	AM INSULIN	Noon	PM Dinner Before	PM Dinner After	PM INSULIN	Comments
SUNDAY ___/___/___								
MONDAY ___/___/___								
TUESDAY ___/___/___								

274

WEDNESDAY							
/ /							
THURSDAY							
/ /							
FRIDAY							
/ /							
SATURDAY							
/ /							

Daily Averages   **Weekly Averages**

	SUNDAY	MONDAY	TUESDAY	WEDNESDAY	THURSDAY	FRIDAY	SATURDAY	
Times of Day								
Glucose Readings								
Weight								

Total Units for the Week: AM _____ + PM _____ = _____

12

275

FIGURE 12.3 — Algorithm Form Used for Patients on Intensive Insulin Therapy

Name _____ Date _____

Provider _____ Phone (____) _____

Time Between Injection/Meal (min)		Blood Glucose Value (mg/dL)	Breakfast	Lunch	Dinner	Bedtime	Bedtime Snack Size
Humalog	Regular						
0	5-15	<80	_____	_____	_____	_____	Large
5	30	81-150	_____	_____	_____	_____	Medium
5-15	30-45	151-200	_____	_____	_____	_____	Small
15-30	45-60	201-250	_____	_____	_____	_____	None
30	60	251-300	_____	_____	_____	_____	None
30+	60+	301-350	_____	_____	_____	_____	None
30+	60+	351-400	_____	_____	_____	_____	None
30+	60+	401-450	_____	_____	_____	_____	None
30+	60+	451+	_____	_____	_____	_____	None

AM long-acting insulin dose _____

PM long-acting insulin dose _____   ☐ Take before dinner   ☐ Take at bedtime

As the premeal blood glucose value increases, the amount of regular insulin recommended also increases and is adjusted based on postprandial glucose values. The time between the insulin injection and the meal also should be increased as the premeal blood glucose values increase, thus improving postprandial glucose values. If the patient consistently requires higher regular insulin doses at a particular time (3 consecutive days), appropriate long-term adjustments should be made.

Diabetes Clinic, VA San Diego Healthcare System, San Diego, California.

12

TABLE 12.3 — Patient Self-Adjustment of Insulin Dosage, Split-Mixed Regimen

High Glucose Values

1. If the prebreakfast blood sugar is >140 mg/dL for 3 days in a row, increase the evening NPH dose by _____ units.
2. If the prelunch blood sugar is >150 mg/dL for 3 days in a row, increase the morning regular insulin dose by _____ units.
3. If the predinner blood sugar is >150 mg/dL for 3 days in a row, increase the morning NPH insulin dose by _____ units.
4. If the bedtime blood sugar is >180 mg/dL for 3 days in a row, increase the predinner regular insulin dose by _____ units.

Low Glucose Values

1. If the prebreakfast blood sugar is <100 mg/dL for 3 days in a row, decrease the evening NPH insulin dose by _____ units.
2. If the prelunch blood sugar is <100 mg/dL for 3 days in a row, decrease the morning regular insulin dose by _____ units.
3. If the predinner blood sugar is <100 mg/dL for 3 days in a row, decrease the morning NPH insulin dose by _____ units.
4. If the bedtime blood sugar is <100 mg/dL for 3 days in a row, decrease the predinner regular insulin dose by _____ units.

General Considerations

1. If more than one change in insulin dose is needed, adjust the NPH dose first before making any changes in the regular dose.
2. Remember not to make changes in the insulin dose more frequently than every 3 days, and do not hesitate to call me for any questions at (____)____-_____.

_____

Physician/Caregiver

Diabetes Clinic, VA San Diego Healthcare System, San Diego, California.

adjustable and sharp, thin lancets. There is a meter that has the capability of getting blood from areas other than the fingertips, such as the forearm, for patient comfort and convenience. Other companies have developed bloodletting devices that can be used on the fingertips and other areas with special attachments to the "finger sticker." Laser technology has also been designed to facilitate the bloodletting for these home devices.

■ Advances in Continuous Glucose Monitoring

SMBG is a fundamental part of diabetes management. It is mandatory for tight glucose control. Intermittent measurement of capillary blood glucose via fingersticks has long been the method of choice for self-monitoring. However, such measurements provide isolated glucose values which do not reflect variations occurring throughout the day and night. In addition, this approach is dependent on patient education, diligence, and consistency. Hence systems monitoring blood glucose concentrations on a continuous basis have been developed. These devices allow for frequent and automatic glucose measurements, and thus can detect and track changes in glucose levels over time. This has tremendous implications for achieving near normalization of glucose control while avoiding the most serious complication of intensive glucose management, hypoglycemia. Several such devices are currently available.

12

The Dexcom Seven Plus, the Dexcom G4 Platium, and the Medtronic Guardian Real-Time are currently available and are composed of three basic parts: a sensor, a transmitter, and a receiver or monitor. The sensor, like a patch, is worn for up to 5 days and then replaced. It is placed just under the skin and is attached to a plastic sensor mount with adhesive to adhere to the skin. The small, unobtrusive transmitter snaps into the sensor mount and sends glucose information wirelessly to the pager-sized receiver, which can be worn on the belt or carried in a handbag. The sensor measures glucose every 1 to 5 minutes (frequency varies according to the device). The receiver displays the readings over time and provides high and low glucose level alarms that warn in advance when levels are trending toward hypoglycemic or hyperglycemic levels as determined the physician.

These systems also store up to 60 days of data, which can be analyzed by the patient or physician.

It is important to note that these systems measure interstitial glucose, a distinct physiologic space when compared with blood glucose. However, clinical trials with the various devices have shown there is an adequate correlation between interstitial and capillary blood glucose measurements. Nevertheless, the use of such systems adds information on PPG excursions, nocturnal hypoglycemia or hyperglycemia not previously detected by fingerstick monitoring, thereby facilitating the tailoring of treatment regimens for the individual patient.

SUGGESTED READING

American Diabetes Association. Standards of medical care in diabetes—2013. *Diabetes Care*. 2013;36(suppl 1):S11-S66.

American Diabetes Association. *Medical Management of Non–insulin-dependent (Type II) Diabetes*. 3rd ed. Alexandria, VA: American Diabetes Association; 1994:52-54.

Buckingham B, Caswell K, Wilson DM. Real-time continuous glucose monitoring. *Curr Opin Endocrinol Diabetes Obes*. 2007;14:288-295.

Fleming DR. Accuracy of blood glucose monitoring for patients: what it is and how to achieve it. *Diabetes Educ*. 1994;20:495-500.

Fonda SJ, Salkind SJ, Walker MS, Chellappa M, Ehrhardt N, Vigersky RA. Heterogeneity of responses to real-time continuous glucose monitoring (RT-CGM) in patients with type 2 diabetes and its implications for application. *Diabetes Care*. 2013;36(4):786-792.

Fox L, Beck R, Weinzimer S, et al. Accuracy of the FreeStyle Navigator Continuous Glucose Monitoring System in children with T2DM. Presented at: 66th Scientific Sessions of the American Diabetes Association; June 9-13, 2006; Washington, DC. Poster 391-P.

Greyson J. Quality control in patient self-monitoring of blood glucose. *Diabetes Care*. 1993;16:1306-1308.

Harman-Boehm I. Continuous glucose monitoring in type 2 diabetes. *Diabetes Res Clin Pract*. 2008;82(suppl 2):S118-S121.

Harris MI, Cowie CC, Howie LJ. Self-monitoring of blood glucose by adults with diabetes in the Unites States population. *Diabetes Care*. 1993;16:1116-1123.

Mazze RS, Strock E, Borgman S, Wesley D, Stout P, Racchini J. Evaluating the accuracy, reliability, and clinical applicability of continuous glucose monitoring (CGM): is CGM ready for real time? *Diabetes Technol Ther*. 2009;11:11-18.

Nettles A. User error in blood glucose monitoring. The National Steering Committee for Quality Assurance Report. *Diabetes Care*. 1993;16:946-948.

Peragallo-Dittko V, ed. *A Core Curriculum for Diabetes Education*. 2nd ed. Chicago, IL: American Association of Diabetes Educators; 1993:259-279.

Sola-Gazagnes A, Vigeral C. Emergent technologies applied to diabetes: what do we need to integrate continuous glucose monitoring into daily practice? Where the long-term use of continuous glucose monitoring stands in 2011. *Diabetes Metab*. 2011;37(suppl 4):S65-S70.

12

Yeh HC, Brown TT, Maruthur N, et al. Comparative effectiveness and safety of methods of insulin delivery and glucose monitoring for diabetes mellitus: a systemic review and meta-analysis. *Ann Intern Med.* 2012;157:336-347.

13   Acute Complications

Patients with type 2 diabetes are prone to developing acute complications such as:

- Metabolic:
  - DKA
  - Hyperosmolar hyperglycemic nonketotic syndrome (HHNS)
  - Hypoglycemia
- Infection (poor wound healing)
- Quality of life:
  - Nocturia
  - Poor sleep
  - Daytime tiredness
  - Tooth and gum disease
  - Cognitive impairment.

The most common acute complications of diabetes are metabolic problems (DKA, HHNS, hypoglycemia) and infection. In addition, the quality of life of patients with chronic and severe hypoglycemia is adversely affected. Characteristic symptoms of tiredness and lethargy can become severe and lead to increased falls in the elderly, decreased school performance in children, and decreased work performance in adults.

Metabolic

■ Diabetic Ketoacidosis

This acute metabolic complication typically results from a profound insulin deficiency (absolute or relative) associated with uncontrolled type 1 diabetes mellitus and less commonly in severely decompensated type 2 diabetes.

Individuals with type 2 diabetes may develop DKA under certain conditions:

- Poor nutrition that contributes to dehydration and catabolism of fat to provide necessary calories
- Severe physiologic stress (eg, infection, myo-

cardial infarction) that leads to increased levels of counterregulatory hormones (eg, epinephrine, cortisol, and glucagon), which stimulate lipolysis, elevate free fatty acids, and stimulate hepatic ketogenesis
- Chronic poor metabolic control that leads to decreased insulin secretion and decreased glucose uptake (glucose toxicity)
- Dehydration that leads to decreased excretion of ketones in urine and a buildup of ketone bodies in the blood.

Key characteristics include:
- Hyperglycemia (300 to 800 mg/dL although usually <600 mg/dL; the glucose concentration is not related to severity of DKA)
- Ketosis: serum ketones usually 10 to 20 mM and acidosis (pH 6.8-7.3, HCO_3 <15 mEq/L)
- Dehydration caused by:
  – Nausea
  – Vomiting
  – Inadequate oral intake
- Electrolyte depletion (eg, potassium, magnesium, etc).

Precipitating factors vary from individual to individual and may include the following (approximately 50% of which are preventable):
- Illness and infection; increased production of glucagon and glucocorticoids by adrenal gland promotes gluconeogenesis; increased production of epinephrine and norepinephrine increases glycogenolysis
- Inadequate insulin dosage due to omission or reduction of doses by patient, physician, or clinic; patients with GI distress often decrease or eliminate their insulin doses thinking that less insulin is needed when food intake is decreased; this practice can be dangerous because GI symptoms are key features of DKA
- Initial manifestation of type 1 diabetes in the elderly misdiagnosed as type 2 diabetes

- Chronic untreated hyperglycemia (glucose toxicity) and hyperinsulinemia.

Pathophysiology of DKA

DKA is a metabolic acidosis caused by a significant insulin deficiency. The following physiologic abnormalities are characteristic of DKA and require prompt correction:

- Chronic hyperglycemia and glucose toxicity
- Acidosis caused by catabolism of fat and the buildup of ketone bodies
- Low blood volume because of dehydration (loss of fluid and electrolytes)
- Hyperosmolality because of renal water loss and water depletion from sweating, nausea, and vomiting; and associated potassium loss.

Symptoms and Signs of DKA

The symptoms and signs of DKA are shown in **Table 13**.**1**. These are classic for DKA in type 1 diabetes, although they are not as severe in patients with type 2 diabetes because some insulin secretion is maintained. Polyuria and polydipsia are symptoms of osmotic diuresis secondary to hyperglycemia. Nonspecific symptoms include weakness, lethargy, headache, and myalgia; specific symptoms of DKA are GI and respiratory. The GI symptoms probably are related to the ketosis and/or acidosis. The chief respiratory complaint of dyspnea actually is an inability to catch one's breath. This type of hyperventilation unrelated to exertion is the ventilatory response to metabolic acidosis termed Kussmaul's respiration.

13

Because the signs are not specific to DKA, physicians should be alert to a constellation of evidence that points to the possibility of DKA.

Because other diseases and conditions may mimic DKA and precipitate and/or coexist with DKA, the following differential diagnoses (and representative DKA symptoms) should be considered:

- Cerebrovascular accident (altered mental status)
- Brainstem hemorrhage (hyperventilation, glucosuria)
- Hypoglycemia (altered mental status, tachycardia)

TABLE 13.1 — Symptoms and Signs of Classic Diabetic Ketoacidosis

Symptoms of DKA
- Nausea
- Vomiting
- Abdominal pain
- Dyspnea
- Myalgia
- Headache
- Anorexia
- Characteristic symptoms of hyperglycemia

Signs of DKA
- Hypothermia
- Hyperpnea (Kussmaul's respiration)
- Acetone breath
- Dehydration (intravascular volume depletion, hypotension)
- Hyporeflexia
- Acute abdomen (tenderness to palpation, muscle guarding, diminished bowel sounds)
- Stupor (mild to frank coma)
- Hypotonia
- Uncoordinated ocular movements

Davidson MB. *Diabetes Mellitus: Diagnosis and Treatment.* 3rd ed. New York, NY: Churchill Livingstone; 1991.

- Metabolic acidosis (hyperventilation, anion-gap acidosis):
  - Uremia
  - Salicylates
  - Methanol
  - Ethylene glycol
- Gastroenteritis (nausea, vomiting, abdominal pain)
- Pneumonia (hyperventilation).

Laboratory Evaluation

Initial laboratory values are shown in **Table 13.2**.

Treatment

Although aggressive therapy is not usually necessary in type 2 diabetes, the following treatment strategies are for severe cases and for true type 1 diabetes misdiagnosed as type 2 diabetes because of the patient's age at presentation. The goals of treatment are to:

TABLE 13.2 — Initial Laboratory Values for Patients Experiencing Diabetic Ketoacidosis

Test	Result	Remarks
Glucose	300-800 mg/dL	Concentrations not related to severity of DKA
Ketone bodies	Strong, at least in undiluted plasma	Measures only acetoacetate, not β-hydroxybutyrate
HCO_3	0-15 mEq/L	Concentrations related to severity of DKA
pH	6.8-7.3	Concentrations related to severity of DKA
K	Low, normal, or high	Total-body depletion; heart responsive to extracellular concentration
Phosphate	Usually normal or slightly elevated	Associated with phosphaturia; marked decrease with occasionally slightly low treatment in levels of both serum and urine phosphates
Creatitine/BUN	Usually mildly increased	May be prerenal; spurious increases in creatinine by acetoacetate in some automated methods
WBC count	Usually increased	Possibility of leukemoid reaction (even in absence of infection)
Amylase	Often increased	Predominant form of salivary gland origin
Hemoglobin, hematocrit, total protein	Often increased	Secondary to contracted plasma volume
AST, ALT, LDH	Can be mildly elevated	Spurious increases in transaminases due to acetoacetate interference in older colorimetric methods

Davidson MB. *Diabetes Mellitus: Diagnosis and Treatment*. 3rd ed. New York, NY: Churchill Livingstone; 1991:183.

13

- Correct fluid and electrolyte disturbances
- Correct acidosis and ketogenesis
- Restore and maintain normal glucose metabolism.

The cornerstones of DKA therapy are administering fluids and insulin immediately. Potassium and phosphate replacement and bicarbonate therapy also may be necessary for certain patients, depending on the severity of the DKA. This is rarely the case in patients with type 2 diabetes. The following treatment guidelines provide an overview for managing DKA. It is not unusual that patients with type 2 diabetes can be treated adequately in a general hospital ward and not in an intensive care unit.

Fluid and Electrolyte Replacement

- This is based on the degree of dehydration and the patient's CV status.
- It also plays a critical role in lowering glucose concentrations; hyperglycemia will continue despite appropriate insulin therapy if hydration is not adequate.
- Oral hydration with a sodium-containing fluid is appropriate for a patient with mild DKA who is not vomiting.
- Most adults require IV fluid administration with normal (0.9%) or half-normal (0.45%) saline (normal saline should be used when intravascular volume depletion is extreme, and half-normal saline, when plasma volume contraction is more moderate).
- One liter of fluid should be given per hour for the first 2 hours; the rate can be decreased to 500 mL per hour when signs of intravascular volume depletion have subsided.
- IV fluids are continued until intravascular volume has been fully restored, as indicated by normal filling of neck veins or when the patient can tolerate fluids.

Insulin Therapy

- Most patients with type 2 diabetes can be treated successfully with frequent (every 2 to 3 hours) injections of Humalog or Novolog insulin subcutaneously (5 to 15 units).

- A low dose of regular insulin can be administered via IV infusion at a rate of approximately 5 units per hour.
- If a 10% decrease in glucose concentration from the initial level is not observed after 2 hours, the infusion rate should be doubled to 10 units per hour.
- The insulin infusion can be discontinued and intermediate-acting NPH insulin can be started when HCO_3 is >15 mEq/L and the patient can drink and eat light foods.
- The major mistake with severe DKA is premature discontinuation of aggressive fluid and insulin therapy. Ketogenesis must be curtailed and requires insulin therapy. Serum glucose levels are not reflective of ketone body generation.

Potassium Replacement

- Not usually necessary in patients with type 2 diabetes
- May be necessary after fluid and insulin therapy has been started because all modes of therapy reduce the serum [K].
- The goal is to maintain the serum [K] within the normal range.
- An electrocardiogram (ECG) should be done as soon as possible. Potassium replacement is withheld if the patient is anuric or if the T waves are abnormally tall and peaked or have a high-normal configuration. If the T waves are normal, 20 mEq of potassium (with appropriate anion) is added to the first liter of replacement fluid. Low or flat T waves require the addition of 40 mEq of potassium.
- An ECG should be done every 1 to 2 hours to evaluate treatment and adjust the potassium replacement regimen. Patients who are able to eat can receive potassium orally via food intake or potassium supplementation (12 to 15 mEq three times daily with meals).

13

Phosphate Replacement

- Phosphate levels should be measured initially; some physicians use potassium phosphate for replacement if PO_4 is in the low or low-normal range.

Bicarbonate Therapy

- This is not necessary in most patients but may be considered under certain circumstances, such as in patients with life-threatening hyperkalemia, lactic acidosis, or severe acidosis (pH <7.0) with shock that does not respond to fluid replacement.
- When necessary, bicarbonate should be added to 0.45% saline and infused slowly over at least 1 hour; it should never be given in an IV bolus because of the risk of death secondary to hypokalemia.

Glucose concentrations should be decreased by about 75 to 100 mg/dL/h with low-dose insulin infusion, reaching levels of 200 to 300 mg/dL within 4 to 5 hours. Dextrose generally is added to the infusion at this point in therapy to avoid hypoglycemia from continued insulin administration, which still is necessary to treat ketosis and acidosis. Approximately 12 to 24 hours of treatment is necessary to reverse ketosis for most patients; some patients may have ketone bodies for several days.

■ Hyperosmolar Hyperglycemic Nonketotic Syndrome

This acute metabolic complication is a life-threatening crisis with a high mortality rate that usually is seen in:

- Elderly patients with type 2 diabetes (particularly those in nursing homes without access to free water)
- People with undiagnosed diabetes
- Those with diabetes that is diagnosed after a long period of uncontrolled hyperglycemia.

Pathophysiology of HHNS

Hyperosmolar hyperglycemic nonketotic syndrome has four key clinical features:

- Severe hyperglycemia—blood glucose usually >600 mg/dL (>33.3 mM) and generally 1000 mg/dL to 2000 mg/dL (55.5 mM to 111.1 mM)
- Absence of or slight ketosis
- Plasma or serum hyperosmolality (>340 mOsm)
- Profound dehydration.

In clinical practice, patients often are seen who have these characteristics but also have mild ketosis and acidosis. Although HHNS and DKA represent opposite ends of a continuum, many patients have some aspects of each syndrome. The two conditions have some similarity in pathophysiology, clinical signs and symptoms, and treatments, with certain important exceptions.

Symptoms and Signs of HHNS

Patients typically develop excessive thirst, confusion, and physical signs of severe dehydration. A comparison of the key features of HHNS and DKA is shown in **Table 13.3**; several important differences exist in the symptoms and signs:

- GI symptoms usually are milder in HHNS than in DKA in the absence of ketosis and acidosis. Because of a lack of severe GI problems (which prompt patients with DKA to seek medical attention within 1 to 2 days), patients with HHNS may tolerate polyuria and polydipsia for weeks and consequently lose significant quantities of fluids and electrolytes before seeking help. Average fluid loss in HHNS is 9 L vs 6.5 L in DKA.
- Kussmaul's respiration is rarely observed because of a lack of severe acidosis.
- Decreased mentation (mild confusion, lethargy) and lack of normal responsiveness are common and correlate best with serum osmolality. These are the usual reasons that patients with HHNS seek medical attention.
- Focal neurologic signs may be present and may mimic a cerebrovascular event (hemisensory deficits, hemiparesis, aphasia, seizures); these signs decline as biochemical status returns to normal.

13

TABLE 13.3 — Diabetic Ketoacidosis and Hyperglycemic Hyperosmolar Nonketotic Syndrome: Comparison of Some Salient Features

Feature	DKA	HHNS
Age of patient	Usually <40 years	Usually >60 years
Duration of symptoms	Usually <2 days	Usually >5 days
Glucose level	Usually <600 mg/dL (<33.3 mmol/L)	Usually >800 mg/dL (>44.4 mmol/L)
Sodium concentration	More likely to be normal or low	More likely to be normal or high
Potassium concentration	High, normal, or low	High, normal, or low
Bicarbonate concentration	Low	Normal
Ketone bodies	At least 4+ in 1:1 dilution	<2+ in 1:1 dilution
pH	Low	Low
Serum osmolality	Usually <350 mOsm/kg (<350 mmol/kg)	Usually >350 mOsm/kg (>350 mmol/kg)
Cerebral edema	Often subclinical; occasionally clinical	Subclinical has not been evaluated; rarely clinical
Prognosis	3% to 10% mortality	10% to 20% mortality
Subsequent course	Insulin therapy required in virtually all cases	Insulin therapy not required in many cases

Peragallo-Dittko V, ed *A Core Curriculum for Diabetes Education.* 2nd ed. Chicago, IL: American Association of Diabetes Educators; 1993:326.

A diagnosis of HHNS usually is easily made if one has a high index of suspicion. Patients may be admitted to the neurology or neurosurgical service because only neurologic conditions are considered initially. Routine urine and blood tests can help clarify the diagnosis of HHNS. Health care professionals need to be alert for signs of HHNS in patients at chronic-care facilities because this diagnosis tends to be overlooked in such settings.

Laboratory Evaluation

Typical laboratory values in HHNS are shown in **Table 13.3**.

Treatment

Lifesaving measures may be needed immediately. The primary treatment goal is rehydration to restore circulating plasma volume and correct electrolyte deficits. In addition, the precipitating event should be identified and corrected, and other goals similar to those described for treatment of DKA should be instituted, including providing adequate insulin to restore and maintain normal glucose metabolism. Glucose concentration is the major biochemical end point because patients with HHNS do not have ketosis or acidosis.

- CV status should be monitored closely and frequently during fluid replacement to avoid precipitating CHF, given the fact that most patients with HHNS are older and have preexisting heart disease.
- Insulin is administered in the same manner as in patients with DKA. At glucose concentrations of 250 mg/dL, the rate of insulin infusion should be decreased to 2 to 3 U/h and dextrose should be added to the IV fluid because oral intake will not be possible for many hours to a few days.
- Dextrose (50 g) should be given intravenously every 8 hours and insulin dose adjusted accordingly (decreased 1 to 3 U/h) based on plasma glucose measurements every 4 hours.
- Potassium replacement follows the same guidelines as for DKA, with consideration of the special conditions of patients with HHNS (under-

13

lying renal disease is associated with lower urinary potassium losses; preexisting heart disease is associated with greater susceptibility to the effects of potassium).

- Bicarbonate therapy is contraindicated in absence of acidosis.
- Phosphate replacement follows the same guidelines as for DKA, with consideration of the effect of phosphate on underlying renal disease.

■ Hypoglycemia

This metabolic problem occurs in both type 1 and less commonly in type 2 diabetes when there is an imbalance between food intake and the appropriate dosage and timing of drug therapy (oral agents, insulin). Other factors that contribute to hypoglycemia are:

- Exercise
- Alcohol intake
- Other drugs
- Decreased liver or kidney function.

Signs of Hypoglycemia

The incidence of hypoglycemia in patients with type 2 diabetes is several orders of magnitude lower than in type 1 diabetes. Nonetheless, patients taking insulin, SFUs, and/or glinides are prone to hypoglycemia.

Hypoglycemia should be suspected in patients who demonstrate the following clinical signs; a diagnosis of hypoglycemia is confirmed in a symptomatic patient if a plasma glucose level <60 mg/dL (<3.3 mM) is found:

- Mild hypoglycemia is associated with adrenergic or cholinergic symptoms such as:
  - Pallor
  - Diaphoresis
  - Tachycardia
  - Palpitations
  - Hunger
  - Paresthesias
  - Shakiness
- Moderate hypoglycemia (<40 mg/dL) is associated with neuroglycopenic symptoms of altered mental and/or neurologic functioning such as:
  - Inability to concentrate
  - Confusion

- Slurred speech
- Irrational or uncontrolled behavior
- Slowed reaction time
- Blurred vision
- Somnolence
- Extreme fatigue
- Severe hypoglycemia (<20 mg/dL) is associated with extreme impairment of neurologic function to the extent that the assistance of another person is needed to obtain treatment; symptoms include:
  - Completely automatic/disoriented behavior
  - Loss of consciousness
  - Inability to arouse from sleep
  - Seizures
- Nocturnal hypoglycemia is associated with over 50% of cases of severe hypoglycemia; early symptoms do not awaken patients and the predinner intermediate-acting insulins may cause hyperinsulinemia and hypoglycemia in the early morning hours.

It is important to understand that hypoglycemia does not necessarily progress in a linear fashion from mild to severe. For example, some patients might develop neuroglycopenic symptoms before adrenergic or cholinergic symptoms, and other patients may overlook or ignore adrenergic or cholinergic symptoms and progress to neuroglycopenia.

Treatment

The goal of treatment is to normalize the plasma glucose level as quickly as possible:
- Mild hypoglycemia is treated most effectively by having the patient ingest approximately 15 g of readily available carbohydrate by mouth. Sources of carbohydrate (15 g) include:
  - Three glucose tablets (5 g each)
  - ½ cup fruit juice
  - 2 tablespoons raisins
  - Five Lifesavers candy
  - ½ to ¾ cup regular soda (not diet)
  - 1 cup milk

13

If symptoms continue, treatment may need to be repeated in 15 minutes. Most patients can resume normal activity following treatment.

- For moderate hypoglycemia, larger amounts of carbohydrate (15 to 30 g) that are rapidly absorbed may be needed. Patients usually are instructed to consume additional food after the initial treatment and wait approximately 30 minutes before resuming activity. Measuring blood glucose levels during treatment and the recovery periods can help determine the effectiveness of treatment. Some patients, however, may continue to have neuroglycopenic symptoms for an hour or longer after blood glucose levels have increased to above 100 mg/dL.

- Severe hypoglycemia requires rapid treatment. IV glucose (50 cc 50% dextrose or glucose followed by 10% dextrose drip) is the most effective route; however, glucagon (1 mg for adults) can be administered intramuscularly at home with positive results. Several emergency kits for intramuscular administration of glucagon by a family member or friend are available from Lilly (glucagon for injection vials and emergency kit) and Novo Nordisk (BlucaGen HypoKit). Individuals who are unable to swallow should be given glucose gel, honey, syrup, or jelly on the inside of the cheek. After the initial response, a rapid-acting, carbohydrate-containing liquid should be given until nausea subsides; then a small snack or meal can be consumed. Blood glucose levels should be monitored frequently for several hours to assure that the levels remain normal and to avoid overtreatment. The individual's health care team should be informed of any severe hypoglycemic episodes.

Prevention of Hypoglycemia

Patients can take certain measures to avoid hypoglycemia:

- Know the signs and symptoms of hypoglycemia.
- Try to eat meals on a regular schedule.
- Carry a source of carbohydrate (at least 10 to 15 g).

- Perform SMBG regularly for early detection of low blood glucose levels; initiate treatment at the first signs of hypoglycemia.
- Take regular insulin at least 30 minutes before eating. (Patients who take their regular insulin immediately before or after a meal will be prone to delayed hypoglycemia.) A fast-acting insulin analogue should be taken 5 minutes before consumption of meal.
- Schedule exercise appropriately; adjust meal times, caloric intake, or insulin dosing to accommodate physical activity; use SMBG (before, during, after strenuous activity) to determine the effect of exercise on blood glucose levels and to detect low blood glucose levels.
- Check blood glucose level before going to sleep to avoid nocturnal hypoglycemia; perform nocturnal (3 AM) monitoring:
  - If hypoglycemia has occurred during the night
  - When evening insulin has been adjusted
  - When strenuous activity has occurred the previous day
  - During times of irregular eating schedules or erratic glucose control
- Several nutrition bars that are low in fat have been developed to help prevent hypoglycemia (eg, Extend Bar).

Infection

Infection is the primary cause of metabolic abnormalities leading to diabetic coma in patients with diabetes. Because of the potentially severe consequences of untreated infections, prompt diagnosis and treatment are essential. Infections are often occult in diabetic patients and require a high index of suspicion. Common infections in patients with diabetes are shown in **Table 13.4**.

Quality of Life

Patients with blood glucose values consistently >200 mg/dL will have a reduced quality of life. Poorly controlled

TABLE 13.4 — Infections Common or Special to Patients With Diabetes Mellitus

Type of Infection	Comments
Cutaneous: furunculosis, carbuncles	For reasons not clear, patients with diabetes mellitus may be prone to recurrent furunculosis and carbuncles. Unless vascular insufficiency is present, warm compresses may be used for treatment. Antibiotics are sometimes needed with and without drainage.
Vulvovaginitis (less frequently, scrotal infections)	*Candida* skin infection commonly occurs in warm, moist areas, particularly in the region of the genitalia (also on the inner thighs and under the breasts). This is particularly common in people with type 2 diabetes who are overweight, have poor metabolic control, or who have been taking antibiotics. These infections can cause extreme discomfort to the patient and result in breakdown of skin, which may allow entry of more virulent organisms. Good glycemic control and local supportive antifungal treatment usually will resolve the problem. Occassionally, oral antifungal therapy is needed.
Cellulitis, alone or in combination with lower extremity vascular ulcers	To prevent the spread of infection to bone and the necessity of amputation, treatment of infected ulcers and surrounding cellulitis must be aggressive. Antibiotics effective against bacteria recovered from the site (both aerobes and anaerobes should be expected) should be used, as well as surgical debridement and drainage.
Urinary tract	Asymptomatic bacteriuria occurs in up to 20% of patients with diabetes mellitus; some suggest that it be treated. Certainly, a patient with neurogenic bladder is susceptible to urinary tract infection and sepsis. Treatment is mandatory in patients with pyelonephritis. Patients with serious urinary tract infections should be hospitalized, the offending pathogens identified, and appropriate susceptibility tests performed.

Ear

Malignant external otitis is relatively rare, but when it occurs, it is most often seen in elderly diabetic patients with chronically draining ear and sudden onset of severe pain. *Pseudomonas aeruginosa* is the usual pathogenic organism. This condition is fatal in ~50% of cases. Immediate treatment should include appropriate antibiotic therapy and surgical debridement when indicated.

American Diabetes Association. *Medical Management of Type 2 Diabetes*. 6th ed. Alexandria, VA: American Diabetes Association; 2008.

13

blood glucose values will lead to excessive thirst and urination, causing nocturia and poor sleep. Poor sleep will lead to daytime tiredness and poor work performance in adults. Patients will have frequent urinary tract infections, tooth and gum disease, and blurry vision. It has also been shown that the elderly experience cognitive impairment and a higher incidence of falls.

SUGGESTED READING

Peragallo-Dittko V, ed. *A Core Curriculum for Diabetes Education*. 2nd ed. Chicago, IL: American Association of Diabetes Educators; 1993.

Porte D, Sherwin RS. *Ellenburg and Rifkin's Diabetes Mellitus*. 5th ed. Stamford, CT: Appleton and Lange; 1997.

14   Long-Term Complications

The long-term complications that may co-exist with or develop in patients with type 2 diabetes include:

- Macrovascular disease
- Microvascular disease:
  - Diabetic retinopathy
  - Diabetic nephropathy
  - Diabetic neuropathy:
    - Symmetric distal neuropathy
    - Mononeuropathy
    - Diabetic amyotrophy
    - Gastroparesis
    - Diabetic diarrhea
    - Neurogenic bladder
    - Impaired CV reflexes (sudden death)
    - Sexual dysfunction
- Diabetic foot disorders
- Obesity.

The long-term, chronic complications of diabetes have the greatest impact on the health of individuals with diabetes as well as on the health care system. Diabetes and its associated vascular complications are the fourth leading cause of death in the United States. Consequently, early detection and aggressive treatment of these complications are essential to reduce associated morbidity and mortality. Striving for tight metabolic control also has been proven to help delay the onset and prevent the development of microvascular complications (diabetic retinopathy, nephropathy, and neuropathy).

The DCCT, a multicenter, randomized clinical trial, investigated the effects of intensive therapy vs traditional therapy on the development and progression of microvascular complications of type 1 diabetes mellitus. The aim of intensive therapy was to achieve and maintain near-normal blood glucose values following a regimen of three or more daily insulin injections or treatment with an insulin pump. In contrast, only one or two insulin injections were used in conventional therapy. Patients were assessed for the presence or progression of retinopathy, nephropathy, and neuropathy. Intensive therapy was highly effective in delaying the onset and slowing the progression of these complications in patients with type 1 diabetes. Similar benefits were observed in the UKPDS in type 2 diabetes. Given to these findings, the ADA recommended striving for the best possible glycemic control in patients with type 1 and type 2 diabetes, with the following goals:

- Fasting and preprandial blood glucose level 80 mg/dL to 120 mg/dL
- PPG level <160 mg/dL
- A1C 7% (normal reference range=4% to 6%) or three standard deviations from the mean of the normal range.

Obesity presents a major management challenge since it increases insulin resistance and glucose intolerance as well as contributing to the risk of cardiovascular complications. Therefore, two recently FDA-approved pharmacologic options for weight management in overweight or obese adults are discussed in this chapter.

Macrovascular Disease

The incidence of the three major macrovascular diseases (coronary artery, cerebrovascular, and peripheral vascular) is greater in individuals with diabetes than in nondiabetic individuals, accounting for up to 80% of mortality in adults with diabetes. Atherosclerosis develops at an earlier age, accelerates more rapidly, and is more extensive in patients with diabetes than in nondiabetics matched by age, weight, and sex.

Type 2 diabetes is a risk factor for macrovascular disease, as are conditions that commonly coexist in patients with diabetes (hypertension, dyslipidemia, and central obesity). Smoking and lack of exercise contribute to an increased risk in both those with type 2 diabetes and the nondiabetic population. In addition, renal insufficiency can increase the risk of and accelerate macrovascular disease in diabetic individuals with microalbuminuria or gross proteinuria.

Weight control and exercise are safe and effective methods for modifying macrovascular risk and should form the basis to which all other treatments are added. The following treatments for hypertension and dyslipidemia should be applied when appropriate.

■ Hypertension

Hypertension should be treated vigorously in all patients with diabetes to limit and/or prevent the development and progression of atherosclerosis, nephropathy, and retinopathy. Lowering elevated blood pressure is the most important and immediate consideration, with a therapeutic goal of <130/80 mm Hg if there is no evidence of protein in the urine. The goal for patients with isolated systolic hypertension (180 mm Hg) is 160 mm Hg; further reductions to 140 mm Hg are suggested if the treatment is well tolerated. The goal for patients with renal insufficiency should be <120/80 mm Hg with a mean blood pressure <93 mm Hg.

Treatment should be initiated with a no-salt added diet and weight loss (for obese patients) combined with appropriate aerobic exercise. Because patients with diabetes can be uniquely impacted by certain side effects of antihypertensives, physicians must be familiar with the potential complications with the various classes of antihypertensive drugs (**Table 14.1**).

In general, reductions in systolic or diastolic blood pressure of 5% to 10% occur with most antihypertensives. The potential benefits of the commonly prescribed antihypertensives are shown in **Table 14.2**. Treatment guidelines include:

- One or more antihypertensive medications may be necessary to achieve satisfactory blood pressure control.
- Adding a second drug to small or moderate doses of the first drug often results in better control with fewer side effects than using full doses of the first agent.

Angiotensin-Converting Enzyme Inhibitors and Angiotensin II Receptor Blockers

ACE inhibitors and now the ARBs commonly are the first choices for therapy because they are effective and have a low incidence of side effects. They are useful in diabetic patients with and without nephropathy. In the UKPDS, the ACE inhibitor captopril was equally effica-

14

TABLE 14.1 — Potential Complications of Common Antihypertensive Agents in the Patient With Diabetes

Drug	Potential Complications
Angiotensin-converting enzyme (ACE) inhibitors	Proteinuria (can occur in patients with severe bilateral renal artery stenosis), reduced renal function, hyperkalemia, cough, leukopenia/agranulocytosis (rare)
Angiotensin receptor blockers	Have the same renal-protective effects as ACE inhibitors; they do not cause cough but can cause hyperkalemia
β-Adrenergic Blockers:	
Nonselective β₁- and β₂-blockers	Cardiac failure, impaired insulin release with hyperglycemia, hypoglycemia unawareness, delayed recovery from hyperglycemia, impotence
Cardioselective (cardioselectivity may be lost with high doses) β₁-blockers	Blunted symptoms of hypoglycemia, hypertension associated with hypoglycemia, hyperlipidemia, impotence
α-Blockers	Orthostatic hypotension
Calcium channel blockers	Pedal edema, constipation, heart block, negative inotropic effect (depending on agent selected)
Thiazide and loop diuretics	Hypokalemia, hyperglycemia, dyslipidemia, impotence

TABLE 14.2 — Potential Benefits of Common Antihypertensive Agents

Class	Effects on Coronary Events Rates	Effects on Progression of Renal Disease	Effects on Stroke
ACE inhibitors	Beneficial	Beneficial	Beneficial
ARBs	Beneficial	Beneficial	Beneficial
β-Blockers	Beneficial	Beneficial	Beneficial
α-Blockers	Controversial	Unknown	Unknown
CCBs	Controversial	Controversial	Beneficial
NDCCBs	Unknown	Beneficial	Unknown
Thiazide diuretics	Beneficial	Probably beneficial	Beneficial
Loop diuretics	Unknown	Unknown	Unknown

Adapted from American Diabetes Association. *Diabetes Care.* 2002;25:137.

14

cious as the β-blocker atenolol in reducing microvascular and CV complications of type 2 diabetes. They have no negative impact on carbohydrate or lipid metabolism, can slow the rate of progression of proteinuria in diabetic nephropathy, reduce the decline in renal function, and prevent progression of retinopathy. Caution should be used in patients with peripheral occlusive disease because renal artery stenosis may be present, which could lead to renal decline with ACE inhibitors.

ACE inhibitors have now been shown to be cardioprotective in addition to having beneficial effects on the diabetic kidney. The Heart Outcomes Prevention Evaluation (HOPE) trial studied >3500 subjects with diabetes who had documentation of previous CV events and were >55 years of age. Subjects were randomized to either ramipril (10 mg/day) or placebo and vitamin E or placebo. Within 4.5 years, the ramipril-treated group experienced a 22% reduction in MI, a 33% reduction in stroke, a 37% reduction in any CV event, and a 24% reduction in the development of overt nephropathy when compared with the placebo group.

These benefits occurred despite minor reductions in blood pressure, raising the possibility that ACE inhibitors have benefits for diabetic patients independent of blood pressure lowering. As with the ACE inhibitors, ARBs have been shown to slow the progression of albuminuria and are protective in diabetic nephropathy. Based on the results of these studies, ACE inhibitors and ARBs should be considered as first-line therapy in people with diabetes with mild-to-moderate hypertension and/or microalbuminuria or macroalbuminuria.

Serum potassium should be monitored during therapy with ACE inhibitors in patients with suspected hyporeninemic hypoaldosteronism (type IV renal tubular acidosis) to prevent severe hyperkalemia.

More than a decade ago, the results from the Candesartan and Lisinopril Microalbuminuria (CALM) study suggested that combining an ACE inhibitor and an ARB reduces blood pressure and urinary albumin levels more than either agent alone. More recently, the ONTARGET trial randomized 25,620 patients with CHD or diabetes plus other CV risk factors who were >55 years of age and free of heart failure to receive the ACE inhibitor ramipril, the ARB telmisartan, or a combination of the two and followed them for a mean of 55 months.

Although the monotherapies were noninferior to each other in terms of the primary end point of CV death, MI, stroke, or heart failure hospitalization, combination therapy was associated with more renal dysfunction, hypotension, and GI upset compared with the ACE inhibitor alone. Furthermore, a population-based longitudinal analysis using linked administrative and laboratory data for 32,312 elderly patients (mean age 76.1 years, median creatinine level 92 μmol/L), seen in clinical practice who were new users of an ACE inhibitor, an ARB, or a combination of both medications ($n = 1750$). Renal dysfunction was more common among patients given combination therapy (adjusted hazard ratio [HR] 2.36). Hyperkalemia was also more common among patients given combination therapy (adjusted HR 2.42). Most patients took combination therapy for only a short time (median 3 months) before at least one agent was stopped.

β-*Blockers*

β-Blockers are being used more frequently as antihypertensive agents following the beneficial effects reported with atenolol in the UKPDS. Besides equal efficacy to the ACE inhibitor captopril, atenolol did not cause an increased incidence of hypoglycemic episodes. However, it is probably prudent to avoid β-blockers in patients with a history of severe hypoglycemia or hypoglycemic unawareness. The potential to blunt counterregulatory responses or prolong hypoglycemia needs to be weighed against the clear-cut benefits of β-blockers to reduce mortality in diabetic patients with recent MI. Selective β-blockers may be more beneficial than the nonselective β-blockers and have a lower incidence of side effects.

14

α-*Blockers*

α-Adrenergic blockers have been associated with improved insulin sensitivity and modest decreases in LDL cholesterol, but no long-term randomized studies have been conducted examining renal or CV outcomes. Orthostatic hypotension can occur, so caution should be used in patients with diabetic autonomic neuropathy.

Calcium Channel Blockers

There are three subclasses of CCBs: the dihydropyridine group (DCCBs) and the benzothiazepines and phenylalkylamines (NDCCBs). The DCCBs are a heterogenous class of compounds with significant pharmacologic differences and a primary vasodilatory effect. Due to conflicting evidence, it is unclear whether the DCCBs reduce CV events or progression of nephropathy. They may protect against stroke but appear to be less effective than ACE inhibitors in reducing CV events. An increase in CV mortality has been reported with the short-acting DCCB nifedipine. Short-acting DCCBs are not approved for and should not be used to treat hypertension in diabetic patients.

Use of the NDCCBs has been associated with decreased proteinuria in short-term studies of patients with overt diabetic nephropathy.

Direct Renin Inhibitors

The benefits of inhibition of the renin-angiotensin-aldosterone system (RAAS) stimulated a search for alternate inhibitory mechanisms of action. This resulted in development of direct renin inhibitors of which aliskiren (Tekturna) currently is the only available agent of this class. Aliskiren is approved for the treatment of hypertension. The efficacy and safety of aliskerin in diabetic patients with renal disease (either the presence of albuminuria or reduced GFR) were assessed in the ALTITUDE study in which 8570 patients who were receiving an ARB or ACEI were randomized to aliskiren 300 mg once daily or placebo. After a median follow-up of about 27 months, the trial was terminated early for lack of efficacy. In addition, there was a higher risk of renal impairment, hypotension, and hyperkalemia with aliskiren compared with placebo-treated patients. Consequently, aliskiren is specifically contraindicated for use with an ACEI or ARB in patients with diabetes.

Diuretics

Low-dose thiazide diuretic use has been associated with reduced risk of CHF and stroke in large randomized trials. Treatment of systolic hypertension with low-dose thiazides in older diabetic subjects significantly reduced

CV events. Their effects on progression of renal impairment have not been studied in large randomized clinical trials. Low-dose thiazides probably do not impair insulin sensitivity or worsen the lipid profile as high doses have been reported to do. Low-dose thiazide diuretics may be particularly useful in combination with other antihypertensive agents. The loop diuretics have been used in combination therapy, particularly in diabetic patients with decreased renal function.

■ Dyslipidemia

Lipid abnormalities that accelerate atherosclerosis and increase the risk of CV disease are significantly more common in patients with type 2 diabetes than in nondiabetic individuals. In addition, central obesity associated with type 2 diabetes is also a risk factor for CV disease. These combined factors have resulted in CV disease becoming a major cause of morbidity and mortality in type 2 diabetes.

The characteristic lipid abnormalities in type 2 diabetes are:

- Hypertriglyceridemia usually due to elevated triglyceride-rich, very low-density lipoprotein (VLDL) levels and sometimes increased chylomicrons as well
- Decreased HDL levels
- Phenotype B pattern (excessive amounts of small, dense LDL and intermediate-density lipoprotein particles), which contributes to an increased CV risk.

Given this higher risk of premature CV disease in type 2 diabetes, all patients should be screened for lipid abnormalities at the initial evaluation using a fasting lipid profile to determine serum triglycerides, total cholesterol, HDL cholesterol, and LDL cholesterol levels. Shown in **Table 14.3** are acceptable, borderline, and high-risk lipid levels for adults. LDL cholesterol is calculated from the formula:

LDL = total cholesterol − HDL − (triglycerides ÷ 5)

This calculation is not accurate if the triglycerides are >400 mg/dL, and LDL should be measured directly by

TABLE 14.3 — Lipid Levels for Adults

Risk for Adult Diabetic Patients	Cholesterol (mg/dL)	HDL Cholesterol[a] (mg/dL)	LDL Cholesterol (mg/dL)	Triglycerides (mg/dL)
Low	<200	>45	<100	<200
Borderline	200–239	35–45	100–129	200–399
High	≥240	<35	≥130	≥400

[a] For women, the HDL cholesterol values should be increased by 10 mg/dL.

American Diabetes Association. *Diabetes Care.* 2002;25(suppl 1):S74-S77.

ultracentrifugation. The recommendations for treatment decisions based on elevated LDL are shown in **Table 14.4**. Pharmacologic therapy should be initiated after nutrition and behavioral interventions. However, when clinical CV disease is present or LDL is very high ($\geq$200 mg/dL), pharmacologic therapy should be initiated at the same time.

Because lipid abnormalities often reflect poor glycemic control, the first treatment approach to dyslipidemia in type 2 diabetes should be optimizing diabetes control with diet, exercise, and pharmacologic therapy as needed. As glycemic control improves, lipid levels also usually improve, particularly when insulin resistance is the underlying metabolic abnormality responsible for the lipid disorder.

Limiting calories and saturated fat intake has proved to be highly effective in improving, but not usually normalizing, the dyslipidemia of type 2 diabetes. Increased intake of soluble fiber, particularly from oat and bean products, has been shown to reduce LDL cholesterol levels. The NCEP has designed a stepped approach for restricting dietary fat and cholesterol that can be modified to incorporate specific requirements for diabetic nutrition. The following guidelines should be implemented with the assistance of a registered dietitian:

- Step 1 diet guidelines: limit saturated fat intake to 8% to 10% of daily calories, with 30% of calories from total fat; limit cholesterol to <300 mg cholesterol per day. If this approach is not adequate for meeting lipid goals, initiate Step 2.
- Step 2 diet guidelines: limit saturated fat intake to <7% of daily calories; limit cholesterol intake to <200 mg/day.
- If triglycerides are >1000 mg/dL, all dietary fats should be reduced to lower circulating chylomicrons.

Recommendations for effective diet therapy for the treatment of lipid disorders in diabetes are shown in **Table 14.5**.

Lipid-lowering pharmacologic agents are usually necessary when the lipid profile does not normalize in response to diet, exercise, and other efforts to improve

TABLE 14.4 — Treatment Decisions Based on LDL Cholesterol Level in Adults With Diabetes

Risk Factors	Medical Nutrition Therapy		Drug Therapy	
	Initiation Level (mg/dL)	LDL Goal (mg/dL)	Initiation Level (mg/dL)	LDL Goal (mg/dL)
With CHD, PVD, or CVD	≥100	<100	≥100	<100
Without CHD, PVD, or CVD	≥100	<100	≥130[a]	<100

[a] For patients with LDL between 100 and 129 mg/dL, a variety of treatment strategies are available, including more aggressive nutrition therapy and pharmacologic treatment with a statin; in addition, if the HDL is <40 mg/dL, a fibric acid such as fenofibrate may be used in these patients. Nutrition therapy should be attempted before starting pharmacologic therapy.

American Diabetes Association. *Diabetes Care.* 2002;25(suppl 1):S75.

TABLE 14.5 — Diet Recommendations for the Treatment of Lipid Disorders in Diabetes

- Calorie restriction and increased physical activity for weight loss as indicated
- Saturated and transunsaturated fat intake <10% and preferably <7% of total energy intake
- Total dietary cholesterol intake <200 mg/day
- Emphasis on complex carbohydrates (at least five portions per day of fruits/vegetables); soluble fibers (legumes, oats, certain fruits/vegetables) have additional benefits on total cholesterol, LDL cholesterol level, and glycemic control
- Replacing saturated fat with carbohydrate or monounsaturated fats (eg, canola oil, olive oil)

glycemic control. The ADA follows an order of priority for the treatment of diabetic dyslipidemia (**Table 14.6**). LDL cholesterol is considered the first priority, followed by HDL cholesterol raising, triglyceride lowering, and treatment of combined hyperlipidemia. Commonly used pharmacologic agents for the treatment of dyslipidemia are listed in **Table 14.7**:

- When elevated LDL cholesterol is the primary lipoprotein abnormality: HMG-CoA reductase inhibitors (atorvastatin, fluvastatin, lovastatin, pitavastatin, pravastatin, rosuvastatin, simvastatin) are indicated. These agents reduce cholesterol synthesis and are useful as monotherapy for the familial forms of hypercholesterolemia, or in combination with BASs. Most HMG-CoA reductase inhibitors are indicated for the reduction of both LDL cholesterol and triglyceride levels. When serum triglycerides are consistently elevated >200 mg/dL, with or without low HDL levels, medication is warranted in addition to a low-fat diet.

- BASs (Colestid, Questran, Welchol) have several disadvantages in patients with diabetes. The older bile binders, in particular, must be taken 1 hour before or 4 hours after other oral medications so there is no interference with absorption. Bile binders also cause fairly significant constipation, and this is especially bothersome in the diabetic population because it exacerbates the constipation of

14

TABLE 14.6 — Order of Priorities for Treatment of Diabetic Dyslipidemia in Adults

- LDL cholesterol lowering:
  - Lifestyle interventions
  - Preferred: HMG CoA reductase inhibitor (statin)
  - Others: bile-acid binding resin, cholesterol absorption inhibitor, fenofibrate, or niacin
- HDL cholesterol raising:
  - Lifestyle interventions
  - Nicotinic acid or fibrates
- Triglyceride lowering:
  - Lifestyle interventions
  - Glycemic control
  - Fibric acid derivative (gemfibrozil, fenofibrate), niacin, high-dose statins (in those who also have high LDL cholesterol)
- Combined hyperlipidemia:
  - First choice: improved glycemic control plus high-dose statin
  - Second choice: improved glycemic control plus statin plus fibric acid derivative
  - Third choice: improved glycemic control plus statin plus nicotinic acid

Decision for treatment of high LDL cholesterol before elevated triglycerides is based on clinical trial data indicating safety as well as efficacy of the available agents. The combination of statins with nicotinic acid, fenofibrate, or especially gemfibrozil may carry an increased risk of myositis. Patients with triglyceride levels >400 mg/dL require special consideration.

Adapted from ADA. *Diabetes Care*. 2004;27(suppl 1):S69.

diabetic gastroparesis. Bile binders also can worsen hypertriglyceridemia in patients with diabetes.

The newest BAS, colesevelam (Welchol) may provide an additional benefit in patients with type 2 diabetes with dyslipidemia since it is not only indicated for the treatment of primary dyslipidemia as monotherapy or in combination with a HMG-CoA reductase inhibitor, but was recently approved to improve glycemic control in adults with type 2 diabetes (see *Chapter 8*) and appears to be better tolerated, in terms of GI adverse events (eg, constipation), than the older BASs. A

TABLE 14.7 — Pharmacologic Agents for Treatment of Dyslipidemia in Adults

Agent	Effect on Lipoprotein			Clinical Trials in Diabetic Subjects
	LDL	HDL	Triglyceride	
First-Line Agents for Lowering LDL, Raising HDL, and Decreasing Triglycerides				
LDL-lowering HMG-CoA reductase inhibitor	↓↓	↔↑	↔↓	4S (simvastatin) CARE (pravastatin) CARDS (atorvastatin) HPS (simvastatin)
Fibric acid derivatives	↓↔↑	↑	↓↓	Helsinki (gemfibrozil) DAIS (fenofibrate) VA-HIT (gemfibrozil)
Second-Line Agents				
LDL-lowering bile acid-binding resins	↓	↔	↑	None
LDL- and triglyceride-lowering nicotinic acid[a]	↓	↑↑	↓↓	None

[a] In diabetic patients, nicotinic acid should be restricted to ≤2 g/d; short-acting nicotinic acid is preferred.

14

315

recently approved oral-suspension formulation for once or twice daily administration may be more convenient and easier to take than multiple tablets for some patients.

- Nicotinic acid is highly effective at improving all lipoprotein parameters, although it significantly worsens glucose intolerance and is contraindicated in most patients with type 2 diabetes. Niaspan is a new slow-release niacin preparation that may be tolerated in a subset of severe dyslipidemic individuals with diabetes.

- Despite earlier warnings that HMG-CoA reductase inhibitors should not be used with gemfibrozil (Lopid) or fenofibrate (Tricor) in patients with mixed disorders, they offer a safe and effective approach to diabetic patients with elevated triglycerides and LDL cholesterol values. When adding one medication to the other, creatinine phosphokinase (CPK) should be measured and LFTs should be performed in 3 weeks and again in 6 weeks, along with a lipoprotein profile. Once a stable dose is maintained and the CPK and LFTs are below three times the upper limit of normal, monitoring these values frequently becomes unnecessary. Caution should be used if the patient is on other medications that could cause hepatitis or myositis. Last, this combination should only be used in compliant patients who will not get lost to medical follow-up.

- When hypertriglyceridemia is the primary lipid abnormality (triglyceride levels consistently >200 mg/dL with or without low HDL levels), a fibric acid derivative is the drug of choice; gemfibrozil reduces triglyceride levels usually with small decreases in LDL cholesterol and small increases in HDL cholesterol. Fenofibrate is a fenofibric acid derivative that may lower LDL cholesterol in addition to reducing triglyceride values and increasing HDL levels. These agents are particularly effective at decreasing hepatic VLDL production and enhancing the clearance of VLDL triglycerides by stimulating lipoprotein lipase, and they are well tolerated.

- Low HDL levels are extremely difficult to treat. Nicotinic acid can be of benefit but often leads to deterioration in glucose control. Fibrates also improve HDL modestly. Perhaps the best medications to increase HDL in type 2 diabetic subjects are the glitazones, which can increase HDL up to 20%.
- An effective therapeutic option for combined dyslipidemia is the use of an HMG-CoA reductase inhibitor that is indicated for the treatment of elevated LDL cholesterol and triglyceride levels. LDL cholesterol can be reduced up to 60% and triglycerides up to 40% with an HMG-CoA reductase inhibitor.

Microvascular Complications

Retinopathy, nephropathy, and neuropathy are the major microvascular complications of type 2 diabetes. Prevention, early detection, and aggressive treatment are essential to reduce associated morbidity and mortality. Good metabolic control has been clearly shown to prevent the development and delay the progression of these complications in both types of diabetes.

■ Diabetic Retinopathy

The development and progression of retinopathy depend on the duration of diabetes and the duration and severity of hyperglycemia. Because diabetic retinopathy does not cause symptoms until it has reached an advanced stage, early and frequent evaluation for vision problems is critical for patients with diabetes. The following findings also support the importance of early detection:

- Diabetes is the leading cause of all new cases of blindness (13%).
- Loss of vision associated with diabetic retinopathy and macular edema can be reduced by at least 50% with laser photocoagulation if identified in a timely manner.

Patients must be completely informed about the possible relationship between hyperglycemia and retinopathy, stressing the importance of promptly reporting any visual symptoms. They should be aware that hypertension can worsen retinopathy and therefore be encouraged to take any antihypertensive medications that have been prescribed. Most important, patients should understand the potential visual complications associated with diabetic retinopathy and how to prevent or reduce the severity of these problems.

The three categories of diabetic retinopathy that are part of a continuum are:

- Nonproliferative or background
- Preproliferative
- Proliferative.

Nonproliferative

Background changes are the earliest stage of retinopathy and are characterized by microaneurysms and intraretinal "dot and blot" hemorrhages (**Figure 14.1**). If serous fluid leaks into the area of the maculae (where central vision originates), macular edema can occur and cause disruption in light transmission and visual acuity.

FIGURE 14.1 — Background Diabetic Retinopathy

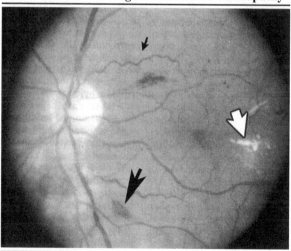

Note microaneurysm *(small black arrow)*, hard exudate *(white arrow)*, and hemorrhage *(large black arrow)*.

Courtesy of Albert Sheffer, MD.

Macular edema cannot be observed directly but is suggested by the presence of hard exudates close to the maculae. Any of these findings should prompt immediate referral to an ophthalmologist.

Preproliferative

Advanced background retinopathy with certain lesions is considered the preproliferative stage and indicates an increased risk of progression to proliferative retinopathy. This stage is characterized by "beading" of the retinal veins; soft exudates (also called "cotton-wool" spots that are ischemic infarcts of the inner retinal layers) (**Figure 14.2**); and irregular, dilated, and tortuous retinal capillaries or occasionally newly formed intraretinal vessels. Any one of these signs suggests the need for further evaluation by an ophthalmologist.

Proliferative

Proliferative retinopathy is the final stage of this degenerative condition and imparts the most serious

FIGURE 14.2 — Preproliferative Retinopathy

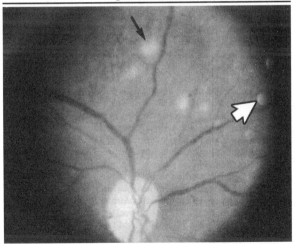

The soft or cotton-wool exudate *(black arrow)* has indistinct margins in contrast to the hard exudate in **Figure 14.1**, which has sharp margins and is brighter. The round structures with distinct margins *(white arrow)* are artifacts.

Courtesy of Albert Sheffer, MD.

threat to vision. Neovascularization typically covers more than one third of the optic disk and may extend into the posterior vitreous. These fragile new vessels, which are prone to bleeding, probably develop in response to ischemia. Bleeding that occurs in the vitreous or preretinal space can cause visual symptoms such as "floaters" or "cobwebs" or retinal detachment that results from contraction of fibrous tissue. Sudden and painless vision loss usually is related to a major retinal hemorrhage.

Evaluation and Referral

Because visual acuity frequently changes in response to fluctuations in glycemic control (particularly extreme variations, eg, low-to-high and high-to-low), the reason for any vision changes should be thoroughly investigated. All patients with diabetes should have annual eye examinations with complete visual history, visual acuity examinations, and careful ophthalmoscopic examinations with dilated pupils. High-quality fundus photographs can detect most clinically significant diabetic retinopathy. Indications for referral to an ophthalmologist are shown in **Table 14**.**8**. Patients with type 1 diabetes should begin having annual eye examinations after 5 years of diabetes. Patients with type 2 diabetes should have annual eye examinations starting at the time of diagnosis because of the probability that glucose intolerance was present for up to 4 to 7 years before the diagnosis of diabetes.

Treatment

Treatment of nonproliferative and preproliferative retinopathy typically involves blood glucose control and blood pressure control. The only standard treatment for background retinopathy, in addition to optimizing metabolic control and blood pressure, is photocoagulation treatment. Results of the Early Treatment Diabetic Retinopathy Study revealed the effectiveness of argon laser photocoagulation applied focally (eg, spot-welding the leaking microaneurysms) in treating macular edema and stabilizing vision. Photocoagulation can slow the progression of vision loss in cases of macular edema and reduce visual loss by >50% when used as a preventive measure to limit neovascularization and vitreous hemorrhages. Panretinal laser treatment

TABLE 14.8 — Reasons to Refer Patients With Type 2 Diabetes Mellitus to an Ophthalmologist

Asymptomatic Patients (annual examinations are imperative)
- Hard exudates near macula
- Any preproliferative or proliferative characteristics
- Pregnancy (prior to conception and during first trimester)

Symptomatic Patients (annual examinations)
- Blurry vision persisting for >1 to 2 days when not associated with a change in blood glucose
- Sudden loss of vision in one or both eyes
- Black spots, cobwebs, or flashing lights in field of vision

High-Risk Patients (annual examinations)
- Neovascularization covering more than one third of optic disk
- Vitreous or preretinal hemorrhage with any neovascularization, particularly on optic disk
- Macular edema

American Diabetes Association. *Diabetes Care*. 2002;25(suppl 1):S90.

has been proven effective and is the treatment of choice for patients with proliferative retinopathy and high-risk characteristics. A scatter pattern of 1200 to 1600 burns is applied throughout the periphery of the retina, avoiding the macular area.

Vitrectomy may be required to treat retinal detachment and large vitreous hemorrhages. This procedure generally is reserved for patients with poor vision in whom the benefits outweigh the risks.

■ Diabetic Nephropathy

Over 20% of adults who have had diabetes for ≥20 years have clinically apparent nephropathy. This disease is progressive, takes years to develop, and requires laboratory evaluation for early detection because it generally is asymptomatic in the early stages.

Structural and functional changes in the kidneys occur early in the course of poorly controlled diabetes but do not produce clinical symptoms. The first sign of nephropathy is microalbuminuria (30 to 300 mg albumin/24 hours), which may be apparent at the time of diagnosis in patients with type 2 diabetes. The presence of microalbuminuria is not only a predictable marker of early diabetic nephropathy, but is also very strongly associated with coronary artery disease in patients with type 2 diabetes. In addition, hyperfiltration, indicated by an elevated CrCl, is also a finding in early diabetic nephropathy. The important clinical point is that in this early stage of nephropathy, aggressive management may reverse or completely stabilize any abnormalities. Overt nephropathy is defined as urinary protein excretion >0.5 g/24 hours and clinical proteinuria characterized by albumin excretion rates >300 mg (0.3 g)/24 hours, typically accompanied by hypertension. The following conditions play a role in the development and acceleration of renal insufficiency:

- Chronic uncontrolled hyperglycemia
- Hypertension (virtually all patients who develop nephropathy also have hypertension [systolic blood pressure >135 mm Hg, diastolic blood pressure >85 mm Hg])
- Neurogenic bladder leading to hydronephrosis and infections
- Urinary tract infection (UTI) and obstruction
- Nephrotoxic drugs (nonsteroidal anti-inflammatory drugs, chronic analgesic abuse, radiocontrast dyes [should be performed only when adequate hydration and diuresis can be assured and if no other diagnostic alternatives are available]).

Patients with diabetes often develop uremia at lower creatinine levels than patients with renal insufficiency resulting from other causes. Second, even with dialysis, the prognosis for patients with diabetes is worse than that for nondiabetic patients. Patients with diabetes tend to start dialysis earlier because they develop symptoms sooner than other patients with renal disease. Therefore, a renal transplant is the preferred method of treatment, if possible, at this stage.

Evaluation

A routine urinalysis should be done at the time of diagnosis and then yearly. If the urinalysis is positive for protein (>300 mg of albumin or macroalbuminuria), then a 24-hour quantitative measure along with a CrCl is important to obtain. If the urinalysis is negative, a test for microalbuminuria is indicated. The easiest method is the albumin-to-creatinine ratio in a random spot collection. The gold standard is a 24-hour collection and can be used to accurately follow the patient over time and assess the success of therapy. If a UTI is present, it should be treated promptly before determining the significance of proteinuria. A positive result (>30 mg protein/24 hour) indicates the need for pharmacologic therapy with an ACE inhibitor or an ARB.

Annual screening is important for patients who have negative results (particularly those without microalbuminuria and hypertension), given that certain factors can interfere transiently with this evaluation (eg, exercise, infections, fever, uncontrolled diabetes, hypertension). The mean albumin excretion of three timed urine collections can be used to establish a diagnosis of microalbuminuria if the values are equivocal.

It is important for physicians to inform patients with diabetes about the relationship between high blood pressure and renal disease, and the benefits of maintaining glycemic control. Patients should be encouraged to have their blood pressure checked regularly (in addition to obtaining their own blood pressure cuff to measure blood pressure at home), take antihypertensive medications that have been prescribed, decrease their protein intake to approximately 10% of daily calories, and monitor glucose levels frequently with SMBG and take any other measures to improve glycemia. The importance of reporting symptoms of UTI should be emphasized, along with following proper treatment for this infection and avoiding nephrotoxic drugs.

Treatment

Treatment is aimed at early detection and prevention, focusing specifically on improving glycemic control, aggressively treating hypertension (eg, with ACE inhibitor or ARB therapy and other agents as necessary), and restricting protein intake. If proteinuria is persistent or progressive, hypertension does not respond to treatment, or serum creatinine continues to be elevated, a nephrologist should be consulted. There is also evidence that treating an elevated LDL cholesterol level and taking antioxidants such as vitamin E and C, may be beneficial to the diabetic kidney.

14

Improving Glycemic Control

Considerable evidence supports the importance of optimizing glycemic control in delaying the development and slowing the progression of diabetic nephropathy. In the DCCT and UKPDS, intensive metabolic control was associated with a decrease in the development of microalbuminuria and clinical-grade proteinuria in patients with type 1 and type 2 diabetes. The benefits of improved glycemia appear to be greatest before the onset of macroalbuminuria; once overt diabetic nephropathy has developed, improved glycemia has little beneficial effects on the progression of renal disease.

Research has revealed a glycemic threshhold for developing microalbuminuria, establishing a A1C level of <7% (normal is 4% to 6%) as the new glycemic goal, whereas previously it was <8%. The risk of developing microalbuminuria is substantially reduced at <7%.

Treating Hypertension

Controlling hypertension through aggressive therapeutic intervention can reduce proteinuria and considerably delay the progression of renal insufficiency. ACE inhibitors and ARBs offer effective antihypertensive effects in addition to significant delaying of the progression of diabetic nephropathy to ESRD. ACE inhibitors and ARBs decrease proteinuria by minimizing efferent glomerular vasoconstriction and reducing glomerular hyperfiltration. In cases where the glomerular filtration rate has already declined, ACE inhibitors also can partially reverse or prevent a further decrease. ACE inhibitors and ARBs should be considered as first-line therapy in all normotensive and hypertensive patients with diabetes who have microalbuminuria or macroalbuminuria. ARBs (losartan, valsartan, irbesartan, candesartan) do not cause cough.

When blood pressure cannot be adequately controlled with the maximum dose of an ACE inhibitor or ARB, additional antihypertensive medications may be needed, such as CCBs, α-blockers (indapamide) and centrally acting agents (clonidine patch). Patients with renal insufficiency and hypertension may be given a diuretic as part of the antihypertensive regimen because of related sodium and fluid retention; a loop diuretic usually is necessary if the creatinine level exceeds 2 mg/dL.

Restricting Protein Intake

Protein intake should be limited to 0.8 g/kg/day or approximately 10% of daily calories, derived primarily from lean animal and vegetable or plant sources, in patients with diabetes and evidence of nephropathy. Vegetable proteins appear to have beneficial renal effects compared with animal sources and provide an important protein supplement or substitute in low-protein diets. The value of restricting protein intake in the absence of diabetic renal disease has not been clearly demonstrated. Low-protein diets can be made more palatable with a greater variety of vegetable protein sources and increased consumption of high-fiber complex carbohydrates and monounsaturated fats.

■ Diabetic Neuropathy

The various diabetic neuropathies are one of the more common yet distressing long-term complications of diabetes, affecting 60% to 70% of patients with type 1 and type 2 diabetes. The categories of diabetic neuropathy are shown in **Table 14.9**. As discussed below, there are several approaches to the management of specific types of diabetic neuropathy. However, there are few options for treating the underlying pathophysiology. Therefore, the results of an 8-year observational study in Australia are of some interest. The results showed that treatment of diabetic patients with either a statin or fibrate reduced the risk of developing peripheral neuropathy by 35% and 48%, respectively. Several possible underlying mechanisms for this protective effect were suggested, including the fact that statins are mild anti-inflammatory agents and fibrates, which are peroxisome PPARα agonists, are strong anti-inflammatory agents. Although these results are encouraging, this was an observational study and not an intervention trial. Therefore, the results need to be confirmed in controlled trials and should be interpreted with some caution.

Symmetric Distal Neuropathy

These neuropathies develop most often in the lower extremities, causing numbness and tingling (pins-and-

TABLE 14.9 — Types of Diabetic Neuropathies

Sensorimotor Peripheral Neuropathies
- Symmetric, distal, bilateral of upper/lower extremities
- Mononeuropathies
- Diabetic amyotrophy

Autonomic Neuropathies
- Gastroparesis diabeticorum
- Diabetic diarrhea
- Neurogenic bladder
- Impaired cardiovascular reflex responses
- Impotence

needles paresthesias) usually during the night. Some patients develop painful burning and stabbing symptoms that can interfere with their quality of life and may be associated with neuropathic cachexia syndrome that includes anorexia, depression, and weight loss. Treatments that have varying degrees of effectiveness, particularly for painful neuropathies, include tricyclic antidepressants, carbamazepine, phenytoin, and counter-irritants such as topical capsaicin. Aspirin or propoxyphene should be prescribed as necessary for pain; narcotic analgesics generally should be avoided because of the risk of addiction with chronic use, however, in some cases, these drugs are necessary. Gabapentin (Neurontin) and tramadol (Ultram) are medications that benefit a subset of patients with painful neuropathy.

In general, treatment strategies for painful peripheral neuropathy include initial use of nonsteroidal anti-inflammatory drugs, such as aspirin and Tylenol, which can offer pain relief, especially in patients with musculoskeletal or joint abnormalities secondary to long-standing neuropathy. The tricyclic antidepressants, such as amitriptyline, remain the most commonly used drugs in the treatment of painful neuropathy. After 6 weeks of treatment, many patients report significant pain relief, independent of mood but correlating with increasing drug dosage. The topical cream capsaicin may be added to the patient's therapeutic regimen if neuropathic pain persists in spite of treatment with maximally tolerated doses of antidepressant medication.

In an outpatient setting, approximately two thirds of diabetic patients treated with a combination of antidepressant medication and capsaicin cream experience substantial relief of neuropathic pain. In patients who experience continued pain on combination therapy, an anticonvulsant (eg, gabapentin) or tramadol can be added as a third drug. If neuropathic pain persists despite the outlined treatment regimen, referral to a specialist, addition of a transcutaneous nerve stimulation (TENS) unit, acupuncture, or a series of local nerve blocks may be helpful, although the prognosis for pain relief in these patients is poor. A treatment flowchart for managing painful diabetic neuropathy is shown in **Figure 14**.**3**.

Mononeuropathy

These neuropathies can occur in virtually any cranial or peripheral nerve, are asymmetric, and have an abrupt onset. Cranial mononeuropathies are the most common, particularly those involving the third and sixth cranial nerves, causing extraocular muscle motor paralysis and peripheral palsies. Patients can develop palsies involving the peroneal (foot drop), median, and ulnar nerves. Spontaneous recovery over 3 to 6 months is typical. Patients with diabetes are more prone to developing compression neuropathies such as carpal tunnel syndrome.

Diabetic Amyotrophy

This neuropathy often is asymmetric, is more common in men, and is often characterized by severe pain, muscle wasting in the pelvic girdle and quadricep muscles, and mild sensory involvement. This condition usually is self-limiting, with complete recovery typically occurring in 6 to 12 months. Treatment is focused on maintaining glycemic control and symptomatic relief using physical therapy and analgesics.

14

Gastroparesis

This neuropathy should be suspected in patients with nausea, vomiting, early satiety, abdominal distention, and bloating following a meal, and is secondary to delayed emptying and retention of gastric contents. The delay in gastric emptying usually is asymptomatic, although glycemic control can be affected. Postprandial hypoglycemia and delayed hyperglycemia develop when

FIGURE 14.3 — Managing Painful Diabetic Neuropathy

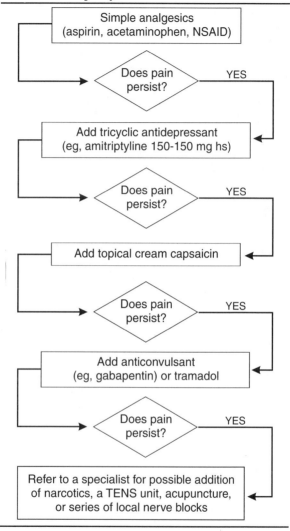

Simple analgesics (aspirin, acetaminophen, NSAID)

Does pain persist? — YES

Add tricyclic antidepressant (eg, amitriptyline 150-150 mg hs)

Does pain persist? — YES

Add topical cream capsaicin

Does pain persist? — YES

Add anticonvulsant (eg, gabapentin) or tramadol

Does pain persist? — YES

Refer to a specialist for possible addition of narcotics, a TENS unit, acupuncture, or series of local nerve blocks the balance between exogenous insulin administration and nutrient absorption is disrupted because of gastric stasis. Therefore, gastroparesis should be considered even in the absence of GI symptoms in a patient who suddenly develops unexplainable poor glycemic control after having had satisfactory control.

Primary treatment is focused on optimizing glucose control with insulin; secondary treatment involves dietary modifications in the form of a low-fat, low-residue diet. When patients remain symptomatic despite these measures, treatment with the following prokinetic agents is recommended:

- Erythromycin lactobionate 1.5 to 3.0 mg/kg body weight intravenously every 6 to 8 hours (acute treatment, effective in eliminating residue from stomach); common side effects are nausea and vomiting.
- Oral treatment with cisapride (only obtained by special request because of cardiac side effects), 10 to 20 mg before meals and at bedtime (enhances gastric emptying through serotoninergic mechanisms, effective in acute conditions); minimal side effects (abdominal cramping, frequent bowel movements); long-term use may cause hyperprolactinemia, galactorrhea, menstrual irregularities.
- Oral metoclopramide HCl is generally used with caution because of adverse reactions (nervousness, anxiety, dystonic effects, and the potential for irreversible tardive dyskinesia).
- Oral treatment with domperidone, a peripheral dopamine antagonist (FDA approval pending), 10 to 20 mg 3 to 4 times daily (accelerates gastric emptying); minimal side effects (abdominal cramping, frequent bowel movements) and rare adverse reactions (hyperprolactinemia, galactorrhea).

Diabetic Diarrhea

Intermittent diarrhea may alternate with constipation and can be difficult to treat. Diabetic diarrhea is a diagnosis of exclusion. High-fiber intake can be helpful, along with diphenoxylate (Lomotil), loperamide (Imodium), or clonidine. Small-intestine stasis contributes to bacterial overgrowth, causing diarrhea. Treatment with one of the following antibiotics for 10 to 14 days is recommended:

- Doxycycline hyclate, 100 mg every 12 hours
- Amoxicillin trihydrate, 250 mg every 6 hours
- Metronidazole, 250 mg every 6 hours
- Ciprofloxacin HCl, 250 mg every 12 hours.

A trial of pancreatic enzymes is also recommended to rule out exocrine pancreatic insufficiency. In many instances, tincture of opium is the only medication that can help the patient live a nearly normal daily life.

Neurogenic Bladder

Frequent small voidings and incontinence that may progress to urinary retention characterize this neuropathy. Confirmation of this diagnosis requires demonstration of cystometric abnormalities and large residual urine volume. Most medical treatment is inadequate, although scheduling frequent voidings every 3 to 4 hours combined with bethanechol 10 to 50 mg 3 to 4 times daily supplemented by small doses of phenoxybenzamine may be helpful. Surgical intervention may be necessary if patients do not respond to pharmacologic therapy because chronic urinary retention can lead to UTI.

Impaired Cardiovascular Reflexes

Orthostatic hypotension and fixed tachycardia are the most disturbing and disabling autonomic symptoms. Typical treatment of orthostatic hypotension includes elevating the head of the bed, compression stockings for lower limbs and torso, supplementary salt intake, and the use of fludrocortisone (0.05 mg initially with gradual increases of 0.1 mg up to 0.5 to 1 mg). This pharmacologic therapy should be used cautiously in patients with cardiac disease because it causes sodium and water retention and may precipitate CHF.

Sexual Dysfunction

Erectile dysfunction, or impotence, is defined as the consistent inability of a man to attain or keep an erection for satisfactory sexual intercourse. It is a couples' disorder, as both patient and partner suffer. Diabetic impotence is usually caused by circulatory and nervous system abnormalities and is a very common complaint in the male diabetic population. The classic clinical picture includes a patient with normal sexual desire but the inability to physically act on that desire. If a patient says that he has morning erections, he can masturbate without problems, or his libido is abnormally low, look for other causes of impotence such as psychological problems or a low androgen state. Orgasm and ejaculation are usually normal. Even if the patient does not have any psychological problems that could cause the impotence, he may develop a secondary psychological fear of failure that could complicate the clinical picture. A woman may experience lack of lubrication and painful intercourse.

The diagnosis can be made in most cases by a good sexual, psychosocial, and medical history, a physical examination, and laboratory tests. A testosterone level should be drawn to rule out a low androgen state, which is rarely a cause for impotence.

Hyperprolactinemia is also an uncommon cause of impotence. Hemochromatosis is a condition that is underdiagnosed and is associated with impotence and glucose intolerance. Serum iron stores, including ferritin levels, are abnormally high in this disorder. If the patient has femoral bruits and/or peripheral occlusive disease, a vascular workup may help identify the cause of impotence.

It is important to be sure the patient is not taking any medications that can cause impotence such as β-blockers and thiazide diuretics. ACE inhibitors, ARBs, CCBs, and α-blockers do not generally cause impotence.

Despite the prevalence of this disorder, nearly all **14** patients can be successfully treated with either nonsurgical or surgical means. Yohimbine HCl, an α_2-adrenergic blocking agent, has been widely used as a nonhormonal medication for the treatment of impotence. However, there has been a consistent lack of data to show that it is more effective than placebo.

Testosterone given by injection or via a scrotal or skin patch is only indicated when the serum testosterone levels are low on several occasions. If there might be binding protein abnormalities, a free testosterone level is indicated. As mentioned above, a low testosterone state is rarely a cause of impotence.

Until the late 1990s, there were no truly effective oral medications for erectile dysfunction (ED). Since then, the convenience and outcomes of the treatment of ED have improved considerably as a result of the availability of the class of drugs called phosphodiesterase-type 5 (PDE-5) inhibitors, which include sildenafil (Viagra), vardenafil (Levitra), and tadalafil (Cialis). All improve erectile function in the same basic way, by inactivating cyclic GMP thereby resulting in an increase in nitric oxide levels leading to relaxation of the vessels that supply blood to the erectile tissue in the penis. The PDE-5 inhibitors do not automatically trigger erections; sexual stimulation also is needed to start the process.

Many clinical trials have shown sildenafil, vardenafil, and tadalafil improve erectile function regardless of the underlying cause or causes including diabetes. Although all of these PDE-5 inhibitors increase the number and quality of erections and sexual experiences in men with diabetes, they have slightly different chemical structures that affect how quickly they work and how quickly they wear off (**Table 14.10**). Which drug may be best for an individual patient is not known since there have been no studies that compared these medications.

TABLE 14.10 — Dosing of Phosphodiesterase-5 Inhibitors

	Sildenafil	Vardenafil	Tadalafil
Dosage (mg/day without food):			
Usual	50	10	10
Maximum	100	20	20
When to take	30-60 minutes prior to sexual activity		
Duration of effects	Up to 4 hours	Up to 4 hours	24-36 hours
Warning	Should not be taken with nitrates; should be used with caution or not at all with α-blockers		

The side effects of the PDE-5 inhibitors include headaches, lightheadedness, dizziness, flushing, distorted vision, dyspepsia, syncope, and MI. Men at highest risk for syncope are those taking nitrates. They may also have adverse effects in individuals with hypertrophic cardio-myopathy because of a decrease in preload and afterload, which can increase the outflow obstruction, culminating in an unstable hemodynamic state. In 1999, the American College of Cardiology and the AHA published recommendations for the use of sildenafil, which would also apply to vardenafil and tadalafil. The document reiterates caution with respect to the use of sildenafil in the following situations:

- Patients with active coronary ischemia who are not taking nitrates
- CHF and borderline blood pressure or low volume status
- Complicated, multidrug, antihypertensive regimen
- Patients taking drugs that prolong the half-life by blocking enzyme CYP3A4 (eg, erythromycin, cimetidine).

Vacuum constrictor devices are a viable therapeutic option for diabetic patients with impotence. No surgery or injections are required, patient acceptance is excellent, and there are few side effects. The majority of these external penile devices have a vacuum chamber that goes over the penis, a vacuum pump that creates negative pressure within the chamber allowing for engorgement of the penis with blood, and a constrictor band that is placed over the base of the penis when tumescence is achieved. Side effects are minor and include ecchymoses, hematomas, and pain. These devices are effective in men with both total and partial impotence. Many patients discover that they do not need the device after a brief period of time, which indicates that a fear of failure or other psychological problems were the initial cause of impotence.

Intracavernosal injection of vasoactive agents such as papaverine or prostaglandins can be self-administered and work by relaxing corporal smooth muscle. Intracavernosal injections will work best in patients with diabetic impotence whose arterial inflow and corporal veno-occlusion mechanism are normal. Side effects include the formation of painless fibrotic nodules within the corpora cavernosa and priapism. Titration guidelines should be followed when initiating therapy. Despite the route of administration, patient acceptance is also good. The Medical Urethral System for Erection (MUSE) is also available.

Penile prostheses represent an excellent surgical option for the treatment of impotence. The options range from simple malleable or semirigid prostheses to inflatable devices that use hydraulic principles to inflate and deflate the penis when desired. Surgical complications are very low, especially when the patient's glycemic control has been acceptable prior to surgery. With the availability of oral medications, intracavernosal injections, and vacuum devices, surgery is chosen less often.

Diabetic Foot Disorders

More than half of all nontraumatic amputations in the United States occur in individuals with diabetes, and the majority of these could have been prevented with proper foot care. Efforts aimed at prevention, early detection, and treatment of diabetic foot disorders can have a significant impact on the incidence of these problems.

■ Detection and Treatment

The physician and patient must diligently examine the patient's feet on a regular basis for signs of redness or trauma, especially if neuropathy is present. Lack of pain, position, and vibratory sensations caused by neuropathy, associated deformities, and vascular ischemia can facilitate the development of foot lesions. Foot pressure that is abnormally distributed predisposes a neuropathic patient to pressure ischemia and skin breakdown. Autonomic neuropathy causes decreased sweating and dry skin that can result in cracked, thickened skin that is susceptible to infection and ulceration.

Pressure perception can be assessed using the Semmes Weinstein (SW) monofilaments, which are available in three thicknesses: 1-g fiber (SW 4.17 rating), 10-g fiber (SW 5.07 rating), and 75-g fiber (SW 6.10 rating). The following evaluation procedure has been recommended:

Place the monofilament against the skin and apply pressure to different areas of the bottom of the foot until the filament buckles. The patient should be able to feel the monofilament when it buckles and identify the location being tested. The 5.07-thickness monofilament, which is equivalent to 10-g of linear pressure, detects the presence or absence of protective sensation and is useful for identifying a foot at risk for ulceration and in need of special care.

Daily inspection of feet can help detect early skin lesions, and proper footwear can minimize the development of foot problems. Patients should be taught to cut toenails straight across, not trim calluses themselves, regularly wash their feet with warm water and mild soap, and avoid going barefoot or wearing constricting shoes. Minor wounds that are not infected can be treated with mild antiseptic solution, daily dressing changes, and foot rest. Patient guidelines for care of the diabetic foot are shown in **Table 14.11**.

Podiatrists should be consulted for assistance with more serious foot problems and for regular nail and callus care in high-risk individuals. If an ulcer develops, the skin must be debrided and the pressure alleviated; infections should be treated promptly with medications appropriate for the offending organism. Healing is facilitated by bed rest with foot elevation and the use of an orthopedic walking cast to relieve pressure but allow mobility. IV antibiotics, surgical debridement, distal arterial revascularization, and local foot-sparing surgery may help prevent amputation in cases of seriously infected foot ulcers.

14

Obesity

According the CDC National Health and Nutrition Examination Survey III, two thirds of adult men and women in the United States diagnosed with type 2 diabetes have a BMI of ≥ 27. This presents a major challenge since obesity increases insulin resistance and glucose intolerance. Historically, pharmacologic and lifestyle options have been disappointing. Two new pharmacologic options for weight management in overweight or obese adults were recently approved by the FDA.

TABLE 14.11 — Care of the Diabetic Foot

- Wash feet daily and dry carefully, especially between the toes (same after shower, jacuzzi, or swimming)
- Inspect your feet daily for blisters, cuts, scratches, and areas of possible infection. Look between the toes! A mirror can help you see the bottom of your feet and between toes. If it is not possible for you to inspect your feet, seek the help of a family member or friend
- If your feet feel cold at night, wear socks. Do not apply hot water bottles or heating pads
- Avoid extreme temperatures for your feet. Test bath water with your hand to ensure that it is not too hot, and be extremely careful of hot pavement or concrete in the summer
- Inspect your shoes daily for foreign objects, nail points, torn linings, or other problems
- Change socks daily, wear properly fitting socks, and avoid holes or mended socks. "THOR-LO" socks have extra padding in heel and ball of foot for better shock absorption (available in sporting goods stores)
- All shoes should be comfortable at the time of purchase. Do not depend on shoes to break in. Wear them only 1 hour the first day, and only in the house. Check your feet for blisters, and then slowly increase the wearing time
- Do not wear sandals with thongs between the toes, and never wear shoes without socks
- Never walk barefoot, not even in the house, because of danger from stepping on pins, needles, tacks, glass, or other items on the floor
- Do not use chemical agents to remove corns or calluses, and do not cut them yourself; consult your podiatrist and be sure to let him/her know you are diabetic
- Toenails should be cut straight across. If you have trouble or questions about them, see your podiatrist.
- Infections from cuts, scratches, blisters, etc, can cause significant problems in diabetics, and a podiatrist or physician should be seen when infection occurs
- Do not smoke!

Goldman F, et al. *The High Risk Foot in Diabetes Mellitus*. New York, NY: Churchill Livingstone; 1990.

■ Phentermine/Topiramate ER (Qysmia)

This fixed-dose combination of phentermine and topiramate ER was recently approved by the FDA as an adjunct to a reduced-calorie diet and increased physical activity for chronic weight management in adults who are obese (BMI ≥ 30 kg/m^2) or overweight (BMI ≥ 27 kg/m^2) who have at least one weight-related comorbid condition, (eg, hypertension, dyslipidemia, or type 2 diabetes).

Although the exact mechanism of action is not known, the effect of phentermine on body weight is likely mediated by release of catecholamines in the hypothalamus, resulting in reduced appetite and decreased food consumption, but other metabolic effects may also be involved. The precise mechanism of action of topiramate on body weight also is not known, although it may be due to its effects on both appetite suppression and satiety enhancement induced by a combination of pharmacologic effects with various neurotransmitters.

Efficacy

The efficacy of this combination phentermine/topiramate ER on weight loss in conjunction with reduced caloric intake and increased physical activity was studied in two randomized, double-blind, placebo-controlled studies in obese patients (Study 1) and in obese and overweight patients with two or more significant comorbidities (Study 2). Both studies had a 4-week titration period, followed by 52 weeks of treatment. The two co-primary efficacy outcomes after 1 year of treatment were percent weight loss from baseline and treatment response defined as achieving $\geq 5\%$ weight loss from baseline. Patients with type 2 diabetes were excluded from participating in Study 1.

In Study 2, eligible patients were required to have a BMI of ≥ 27 kg/m^2 and ≤ 45 kg/m^2 (no lower limit on BMI for patients with type 2 diabetes) and two or more of the following obesity-related comorbid conditions: elevated blood pressure or requirement for ≥ 2 antihypertensive medications; triglycerides >200-400 mg/dL or treatment with ≥ 2 lipid-lowering agents; impaired FPG, impaired OGTT, or a diagnosis of type 2 diabetes; and/or waist circumference ≥ 102 cm for men or >88 cm for women. During both studies, a well-balanced, reduced-calorie

14

diet to result in an approximate 500 kcal/day decrease in caloric intake was recommended to all patients and patients were offered nutritional and lifestyle modification counseling.

After 1 year of treatment with phentermine/topiramate ER, all dosage levels resulted in statistically significant weight loss compared with placebo (**Table 14.12**) and a statistically significant greater proportion of patients randomized to phentermine/topiramate ER than placebo achieved 5% and 10% weight loss. Secondary end points included changes in cardiovascular, metabolic and anthropometric risk factors associated with obesity. Treatment with phentermine/topiramate ER resulted in small, significant reductions in FPG, blood pressure, and plasma lipids.

Safety

In clinical trials with the fixed-dose, single-capsule formulations of phentermine/topiramate ER, adverse events that occurred at a rate of $\geq 5\%$ and at a rate ≥ 1.5 times placebo included paraesthesia, dizziness, dysgeusia, insomnia, constipation, and dry mouth. In the 1-year placebo-controlled clinical studies, the rates of discontinuations due to adverse events were:

- Phentermine 3.75 mg/topiramate ER 23 mg: 11.6%
- Phentermine 7.5 mg/topiramate ER 46 mg: 11.6%
- Phentermine 15 mg/ topiramate ER 92 mg: 17.4%
- Placebo: 8.4%.

The most common adverse events that led to discontinuation of treatment are shown in **Table 14.13**.

Prescribing Qysmia

This combination of phentermine/topiramate ER should be taken once daily in the morning with or without food. Avoid dosing in the evening due to the possibility of insomnia. Gradual dose titration is recommended as follows:

- Start treatment with phentermine 3.75 mg/topiramate ER 23 mg extended-release daily for 14 days; after 14 days, increase to the recommended dose of phentermine 7.5 mg/topiramate ER 46 mg once daily.

- Evaluate weight loss after 12 weeks of treatment with phentermine/topiramate ER 7.5 mg/46 mg. If the patient has not lost ≥3% of baseline body weight with this dosage, discontinue or escalate the dose, as it is unlikely that the patient will achieve and sustain clinically meaningful weight loss at this dosage.
- Escalate the dose to phentermine/topiramate ER 11.25 mg/69 mg for 14 days; followed by increase to phentermine/topiramate ER 15 mg/92 mg daily.
- Evaluate weight loss following dose escalation to phentermine/topiramate ER 15 mg/92 mg after an additional 12 weeks.
- If a patient has not lost ≥5% of baseline body weight, discontinue treatment (*see below*) as it is unlikely that the patient will achieve and sustain clinically meaningful weight loss with continued treatment.

Discontinuation of phentermine/topiramate ER 15 mg/92 mg should proceed gradually by taking a dose every other day for at least 1 week prior to stopping treatment altogether, due to the possibility of precipitating a seizure.

Phentermine/topiramate ER is contraindicated in pregnancy and in patients with glaucoma, hyperthyroidism, and during or within 14 days following administration of an MAOI.

All dosage formulations of phentermine/topiramate ER are Schedule IV controlled substances.

14

■ Lorcaserin (Belviq)

Lorcaserin is indicated as an adjunct to a reduced-calorie diet and increased physical activity for chronic weight management in adults who are obese (BMI ≥30 kg/m^2) or overweight (BMI ≥27 kg/m^2) who have at least one weight-related comorbid condition, (eg, hypertension, dyslipidemia, type 2 diabetes).

Lorcaserin is a 5-HT2C receptor agonist. Its precise mechanism of action is not known but it is believed to decrease food consumption and promote satiety by selectively activating 5-HT2C receptors on anorexigenic

TABLE 14.12 — Change From Baseline in Body Weight With Combination Phentermine/Topiramate ER After 1 Year in Overweight or Obese People

	Placebo	Phentermine/Topiramate ER	
		3.75 mg/23 mg	15 mg/92 mg
STUDY 1: Obese Patients (BMI ≥35 kg/m²)	$n = 498$	$n = 234$	$n = 498$
Weight loss (kg)			
Baseline	115.7	118.6	115.2
Change from baseline	-1.6	-5.1[a]	-10.9[b]
Difference from placebo		-3.5	-9.4
Patients losing ≥5% body weight (%)	17	45[a]	67[b]
Risk difference from placebo	—	27.6	49.4
Patients losing ≥10% body weight (%)	7	19[a]	47[b]
Risk difference from placebo	—	11.4	39.8

340

STUDY 2: Overweight and Obese Patients ($\leq 27\ kg/m^2$ to $\geq 45\ kg/m^2$)	$n = 979$	$n = 488$	$n = 981$
Weight loss (kg)			
Baseline	103.3	102.8	103.1
Change from baseline	-1.2	-7.8[a]	-9.8[b]
Difference from placebo		-6.6	-8.6
Patients losing $\geq$5% body weight (%)	21	62[a]	70[b]
Risk difference from placebo	—	41.3	53.0
Patients losing $\geq$10% body weight (%)	7	37[a]	48[b]
Risk difference from placebo	—	29.9	40.3

[a] $P < 0.0001$ vs placebo.

[b] $P < 0.01$ vs 3.75 mg/23 mg dose in Study 1 or 7.5 mg/46 mg dose in Study 2.

Allison DB, et al. *Obesity (Silver Spring)*. 2012;20(2):330-342; Gadde KM, et al. *Lancet*. 2011;377(9774):1341-1352.

14

TABLE 14.13 — Adverse Events With Incidence ≥1% Leading to Treatment Discontinuation in 1-Year Clinical Trials

| Adverse Event Leading to Discontinuation | Placebo (%) n = 1561 | Phentermine/Topiramate ER | | |
		3.75 mg/23 mg (%) n = 240	7.5 mg/46 mg (%) n = 498	15 mg/92 mg (%) n = 1580
Blurred vision	0.5	2.1	0.8	0.7
Headache	0.6	1.7	0.2	0.8
Irritability	0.1	0.8	0.8	1.1
Dizziness	0.2	0.4	1.2	0.8
Paresthesia	0.0	0.4	1.0	1.1
Insomnia	0.4	0.0	0.4	1.6
Depression	0.2	0.0	0.8	1.3
Anxiety	0.3	0.0	0.2	1.1

Qsymia [package insert]. Mountain View, CA: Vivus, Inc; 2012.

pro-opiomelanocortin neurons located in the hypo-thalamus. At the recommended daily dose, it selectivity interacts with 5-HT2C receptors compared with 5-HT2A and 5-HT2B receptors, other 5-HT receptor subtypes, the 5-HT receptor transporter, and 5-HT reuptake sites. Lorcaserin is absorbed from the GI tract with peak plasma concentration occurring 1.5 to 2 hours after oral dosing and has a plasma half-life of ~11 hours; steady state is reached within 3 days after twice-daily dosing, and accumulation is estimated to be approximately 70%. Lorcaserin is extensively metabolized by the liver and the metabolites are excreted primarily in the urine (~93%).

Efficacy

The effects of lorcaserin on body weight were evaluated in three randomized, double-blind, placebo-controlled trials of 52 to 104 weeks duration. Two trials enrolled adults without type 2 diabetes while one study was performed in adults with type 2 diabetes. The primary efficacy parameters were weight loss at 1 year assessed as percent of patients achieving ≥5% weight loss, percent of patients achieving ≥10% weight loss, and mean weight change. In all studies, patients were randomized to receive either lorcaserin 10 mg bid or placebo. All patients received one-on-one instruction for a reduced-calorie diet and exercise counseling that began with the first dose of study medication and continued every 4 weeks throughout the trials.

In the two trials in adults without type 2 diabetes, there was statistically significantly greater weight loss with lorcaserin 10 mg bid compared with placebo at week 52 (placebo-adjusted difference −3.3 kg; $P < 0.001$). Significantly more patients treated with lorcaserin 10 mg bid lost ≥5% of body weight compared with placebo (47.2% and 22.6%, respectively; $P < 0.001$).

The patients in the third study were required to have type 2 diabetes with a baseline A1C of 7% to 10%, a BMI of 27-45 kg/m^2, and treatment with MET, an SFU, or both. As shown in **Table 14.14**, by 1 year, weight loss was significantly greater with lorcaserin 10 mg bid compared with placebo, and significantly greater proportions of people treated with lorcaserin experienced ≥5% and ≥10% reductions in body weight than in those who

14

TABLE 14.14 — Changes From Baseline in Body Weight With Lorcaserin After 1 Year in Overweight or Obese People With Type 2 Diabetes

	Lorcaserin 10 mg bid $n = 251$	Placebo $n = 248$
Weight loss (kg)		
Baseline	103.5	102.3
Change from baseline	-4.7	-1.6
Difference from placebo	-3.1[a]	
Patients losing ≥5% body weight (%)	37.5	16.1
Difference from placebo	21.3[a]	
Patients losing ≥10% body weight (%)	16.3	4.4
Difference from placebo	11.9[a]	
Waist circumference (cm)		
Baseline	115.8	113.5
Change from baseline	-5.5	3.3
Difference from placebo	-2.2[a]	

[a] $P < 0.001$ vs placebo.

O'Neil PM, et al. *Obesity (Silver Spring)*. 2012;20(7):1426-1436.

received placebo. Reduction in waist circumference was also significantly greater with lorcaserin treatment. Changes in A1C, FPG, blood pressure, and plasma lipids were secondary end points. Compared with placebo, lorcaserin treatment resulted in statistically significantly greater reductions from baseline in A1C (placebo-subtracted difference −0.5%; $P < 0.001$) and FPG (placebo-subtracted difference −15.1 mg/dL; $P < 0.001$). Changes in blood pressures, heart rate, and plasma lipids with either lorcaserin or placebo were generally small and not clinically or significantly different.

Safety

In placebo-controlled clinical trials of at least 1 year in duration, 8.6% of lorcaserin-treated patients prematurely discontinued treatment due to adverse reactions compared with 6.7% of placebo-treated patients. In patients without type 2 diabetes, the most common adverse events with lorcaserin (>5% and more commonly than with placebo) were headache, dizziness, fatigue, nausea, dry mouth, and constipation. The most common adverse reactions among diabetic patients were hypoglycemia, headache, back pain, nasopharyngitis, cough, and fatigue. Hypoglycemia defined as blood glucose ≤65 mg/dL and, with symptoms, occurred in 7.4% of lorcaserin-treated patients and in 6.3% placebo-treated patients.

Prescribing Belviq

The recommended daily, as well as maximum dose, is one 10-mg tablet twice daily with or without food. Lorcaserin should be discontinued if ≥5% weight loss is not achieved by week 12. Since lorcaserin is a serotonergic agent, coadministration with other serotonergic drugs may lead to the development of a potentially life-threatening serotonin syndrome or neuroleptic malignant syndrome–like reactions.

Lorcaserin is contraindicated in pregnancy.

Lorcaserin is a Schedule IV controlled substance.

14

SUGGESTED READING

Abuaisha BB, Costanzi JB, Boulton AJ. Acupuncture for the treatment of chronic painful peripheral diabetic neuropathy: a long-term study. *Diabetes Res Clin Prac*. 1998;39:115-121.

Allison DB, Gadde KM, Garvey WT, et al. Controlled-release phentermine/topiramate in severely obese adults: a randomized controlled trial (EQUIP). *Obesity (Silver Spring)*. 2012;20:330-342.

American Diabetes Association. Preventive foot care in people with diabetes. *Diabetes Care*. 2004;27(suppl 1):S63-S64.

American Diabetes Association. *Diabetes 2002 Vital Statistics*. Alexandria, VA: American Diabetes Association; 2002.

Backonja M, Beydoun A, Edwards KR, et al. Gabapentin for the symptomatic treatment of painful neuropathy in patients with diabetes mellitus: a randomized controlled trial. *JAMA*. 1998;280:1831-1836.

Bays HF, Goldberg RB, Truitt KE, Jones MR. Colesevelam hydrochloride therapy in patient with type 2 diabetes mellitus treated with metformin: glucose and lipid effects. *Arch Intern Med*. 2008;168:1975-1983.

Belviq [package insert]. Woodcliff Lake, NJ: Eisai Inc; 2012.

Brenner BM, Cooper ME, de Zeeuw D, et al. Effects of losartan on renal and cardiovascular outcomes in patients with type 2 diabetes and nephropathy. *N Engl J Med*. 2001;345:861-869.

Cheitlin MD, Hutter AM, Brindis RG, et al. Use of sildenafil (Viagra) in patients with cardiovascular disease. Technology and Practice Executive Committee. *Circulation*. 1999;99:168-177.

Cohen KL, Harris S. Efficacy and safety of nonsteroidal anti-inflammatory drugs in the therapy of diabetic neuropathy. *Arch Intern Med*. 1987;147:1442-1444.

Diabetes Control and Complications Trial Research Group. The effect of intensive treatment of diabetes on the development and progression of long-term complications in insulin-dependent diabetes mellitus. *N Engl J Med*. 1993;329:977-986.

Diabetic Retinopathy Study Research Group. Indications for photocoagulation treatment of diabetic retinopathy, DRS report no. 14. *Int Ophthalmol Clin*. 1987;27:239-253.

Early Treatment Diabetic Retinopathy Study Research Group. Photocoagulation for diabetic macular edema: ETDRS report no. 1. *Ophthalmology*. 1985;103:1796-1806.

Fidler MC, Sanchez M, Raether B, et al; BLOSSOM Clinical Trial Group. A one-year randomized trial of lorcaserin for weight loss in obese and overweight adults: the BLOSSOM trial. *J Clin Endocrinol Metab*. 2011;96:3067-3077.

Fonseca VA, Rosenstock J, Wang AC, Truitt KE, Jones MR. Cole-sevelem HCl improves glycemic control and reduces LDL cholesterol in patients with inadequately controlled type 2 diabetes on sulfonylurea-based therapy. *Diabetes Care.* 2008;31:1479-1484.

Gadde KM, Allison DB, Ryan DH, et al. Effects of low-dose, controlled-release, phentermine plus topiramate combination on weight and associated comorbidities in overweight and obese adults (CONQUER): a randomised, placebo-controlled, phase 3 trial. *Lancet.* 2011;377:1341-1352.

Garvey WT, Ryan DH, Look M, et al. Two-year sustained weight loss and metabolic benefits with controlled-release phentermine/topiramate in obese and overweight adults (SEQUEL): a randomized, placebo-controlled, phase 3 extension study. *Am J Clin Nutr.* 2012;95:297-308.

Goldman F, Gibbons G, Kruse-Edelmann I. Limb salvage techniques. In: *The High Risk Foot in Diabetes Mellitus.* New York, NY: Churchill Livingstone; 1990.

Gorson KC, Schott C, Herman R, Ropper AH, Rand WM. Gabapentin in the treatment of painful diabetic neuropathy: a placebo controlled, double blind, crossover trial. *J Neurol Neurosurg Psychiatry.* 1999;66: 251-252.

Harati Y, Gooch C, Swenson M, et al. Double-blind randomized trial of tramadol for the treatment of the pain of diabetic neuropathy. *Neurology.* 1998;50:1842-1846.

Heart Outcomes Prevention Evaluation (HOPE) Study Investigators. Effects of ramipril on cardiovascular and microvascular outcomes in people with diabetes mellitus: results of the HOPE study and MICRO-HOPE substudy. *Lancet.* 2000;355:253-259.

Isomaa B, Almgren P, Tuomi T, et al. Cardiovascular morbidity and mortality associated with the metabolic syndrome. *Diabetes Care.* 2001;24:683-689.

Kalin M, Zieve F, Schwartz S, et al. Lipid-lowering effects of co-lesevelam hydrochloride (HCl) in patients with diabetes. *Diabetes.* 2006;55(suppl 1):A119.

Karlsson FO, Garber AJ. Prevention and treatment of diabetic nephropa-thy: role of angiotensin-converting enzyme inhibitors. *Endocr Pract.* 1996;2:215-219.

Krowlewski AS, Laffel LM, Krolewski M, Quinn M, Warram JH. Gly-cosylated hemoglobin and the risk of microalbuminuria in patients with insulin-dependent diabetes mellitus. *N Engl J Med.* 1995;332:1251-1255.

Kumar D, Marshall HJ. Diabetic peripheral neuropathy: amelioration of pain with transcutaneous electrostimulation. *Diabetes Care.* 1997; 20:1702-1705.

14

Labasky RC, Spivack AP. Transurethral alprostadil for treatment of erectile dysfunction: two-year safety update. *J Urol.* 1998;159:907A.

Lakin MM, Montague DK, Vander Brug Medendorp S, Tesar L, Schover LR. Intracavernous injection therapy: analysis of results and complications. *J Urol.* 1990;143:1138-1141.

Leungwattanakij S, Flynn V, Hellstrom WJ. Intracavernosal injection and intraurethral therapy for erectile dysfunction. *Urol Clin North Am.* 2001;28:343-354.

Levine LA, Dimitiou RJ. Vacuum constriction and external erection devices in erectile dysfunction. *Urol Clin North Am.* 2001;28:355-361.

Lewis E, Hunsicker LG, Bain RP, Rohde RD. The effect of angiotensin-converting enzyme inhibition on diabetic nephropathy. *N Engl J Med.* 1993;329:1456-1462.

Lewis EJ, Hunsicker LG, Clarke WR, et al. Renoprotective effect of the angiotensin-receptor antagonist irbesartan in patients with nephropathy due to type 2 diabetes. *N Engl J Med.* 2001;345:851-860.

Mann JF, Anderson C, Gao P, et al; ONTARGET investigators. Dual inhibition of the renin-angiotensin system in high-risk diabetes and risk for stroke and other outcomes: results of the ONTARGET trial. *J Hypertens.* 2013;31:414-421.

Martin CK, Redman LM, Zhang J, et al. Lorcaserin, a 5-HT(2C) receptor agonist, reduces body weight by decreasing energy intake without influencing energy expenditure. *J Clin Endocrinol Metab.* 2011;96:837-845.

Max MB, Culnane M, Schafer SC, et al. Amitriptyline relieves diabetic neuropathy pain in patients with normal or depressed mood. *Neurology.* 1987;37:589-596.

McAlister FA, Zhang J, Tonelli M, Klarenbach S, Manns BJ, Hemmelgarn BR; Alberta Kidney Disease Network. The safety of combining angiotensin-converting-enzyme inhibitors with angiotensin-receptor blockers in elderly patients: a population-based longitudinal analysis. *CMAJ.* 2011;183:655-662.

McQuay HJ, Tramer M, Nye BA, Carroll D, Wiffen PJ, Moore RA. A systematic review of antidepressants in neuropathic pain. *Pain.* 1996;68:217-227.

Mogensen CE, Neldam S, Tikkanen I, et al. Randomised controlled trial of dual blockade of renin-angiotensin system in patients with hypertension, microalbuminuria, and non-insulin dependent diabetes: the candesartan and lisinopril microalbuminuria (CALM) study. *BMJ.* 2000;321:1440-1444.

Montague DK, Angermeier KW. Penile prosthesis implantation. *Urol Clin North Am.* 2001;28:355-361.

Mudaliar SR, Henry RR. Role of glycemic control and protein restriction in clinical management of diabetic kidney disease. *Endocrinol Pract.* 1996;2:220-226.

O'Neil PM, Smith SR, Weissman NJ, et al. Randomized placebo-controlled clinical trial of lorcaserin for weight loss in type 2 diabetes mellitus: the BLOOM-DM study. *Obesity (Silver Spring).* 2012;20:1426-1436.

Padma-Nathan H, Giuliano F. Oral drug therapy for erectile dysfunction. *Urol Clin North Am.* 2001;28:321-334.

Parving HH, Brenner BM, McMurray JJ, et al; ALTITUDE Investigators. Cardiorenal end points in a trial of aliskiren for type 2 diabetes. *N Engl J Med.* 2012;367:2204-2213.

Parving HH, Lehnert H, Brochner-Mortensen J, Gomis R, Andersen S, Arner P. The effect of irbesartan on the development of diabetic nephropathy in patients with type 2 diabetes. *N Engl J Med.* 2001;345:870-878.

Prather CM. Evaluating and managing GI dysfunction in diabetes. *Contemp Intern Med.* 1996;8:47-54.

Qsymia [package insert]. Mountain View, CA: Vivus, Inc; 2012.

Reichard P, Nilsson BY, Rosenqvist U. The effect of long-term intensified insulin treatment on the development of microvascular complications of diabetes mellitus. *N Engl J Med.* 1993;329:304-309.

Rendell MS, Rajfer J, Wicker PA, Smith MD. Sildenafil for the treatment of erectile dysfunction in men with diabetes: randomized controlled trial. Sildenafil Diabetes Study Group. *JAMA.* 1999;281:421-426.

Smith SR, Weissman NJ, Anderson CM, et al; Behavioral Modification and Lorcaserin for Overweight and Obesity Management (BLOOM) Study Group. Multicenter, placebo-controlled trial of lorcaserin for weight management. *N Engl J Med.* 2010;363:245-256.

United Kingdom Prospective Diabetes Study Group. Efficacy of atenolol and captopril in reducing risk of macrovascular and microvascular complications in type 2 diabetes: UKPDS 39. *BMJ.* 1998;317:713-720.

14

15

Prevention of Type 2 Diabetes

According to estimates provided by the CDC, about 35% of adults ages ≥20 years of age had "prediabetes"—based on fasting glucose or A1C levels—in 2010. Data suggest that 79 million US adults had prediabetes in 2010, and the prevalence is still increasing. Unfortunately, recent estimates also indicate that <10% of patients with prediabetes are aware of their diagnosis, indicating a need for wider screening. Our knowledge of the early stages of hyperglycemia that presage the diagnosis of diabetes and the encouraging results of major intervention trials clearly show that individuals at high risk can be identified and diabetes delayed, if not prevented. Recent data indicate that screening and early intervention, reducing the huge burden resulting from the complications of diabetes and the potential ancillary benefits of some of the intervention strategies, strongly suggest that an effort to delay or prevent diabetes is worthwhile.

Diabetes Primary Prevention Trials

Several studies have demonstrated that type 2 diabetes can be delayed and perhaps prevented (**Table 15.1**). These studies used several different interventions, including lifestyle modification, oral antidiabetic agents, and basal insulin, in nondiabetic study subjects at high risk for developing type 2 diabetes.

■ Da Qing IGT and Diabetes Study

In this small, early study, 577 individuals with IGT from the city of Da Qing, China, were randomized either to a control group or to one of three active treatment groups: diet only, exercise only, or diet plus exercise. Follow-up evaluation examinations were conducted at 2-year intervals over a 6-year period to identify subjects who developed type 2 diabetes. The cumulative incidence of diabetes at 6 years was 67.7% in the control group compared with 43.8% in the diet group,

15

TABLE 15.1 — Primary Prevention Trials of Type 2 Diabetes

Study	Intervention	Sample Size	Reduction in Diabetes Risk (%)
ACT-NOW	Pioglitazone	602	81
Da Qing	Diet and/or exercise	577	32-39
DPP	Diet and exercise	3234	58
	Metformin	3234	31
	Troglitazone	585	23
DREAM	Rosiglitazone	5269	62
	Ramipril	5269	9
FDPS	Diet and exercise	522	58
Indian DPP	Diet and exercise	269	29
	Metformin	269	26
STOP-NIDDM	Acarbose	1429	25
TRIPOD	Troglitazone	236	56
XENDOS	Xenical	3305	37

Adapted from Gerstein HC. *Diabetes Care.* 2007;30:432-434.

352

41.1% in the exercise group, and 46.0% in the diet-plus-exercise group. In a proportional hazards analysis, the diet, exercise, and diet-plus-exercise interventions were associated with 31% ($P<0.03$), 46% ($P<0.0005$), and 42% ($P<0.005$) reductions in risk of developing diabetes, respectively.

■ The Finnish Diabetes Prevention Study (FDPS)

The FDPS randomized 522 middle-aged, overweight subjects (mean BMI, 31 kg/m^2) with IGT to either an intensive lifestyle intervention group or a control group. Each subject in the intervention group received individualized counseling aimed at reducing weight, total intake of fat, intake of saturated fat, and increasing intake of fiber and physical activity. The mean duration of follow-up was 3.2 years. The cumulative incidence of diabetes after 4 years was 11% in the intervention group and 23% in the control group. During the trial, the risk of diabetes was reduced by 58% ($P<0.001$) in the intervention group.

■ Diabetes Prevention Program (DPP)

The long-term, National Institutes of Health–funded DPP study was designed to determine whether diabetes could be prevented or delayed in people who had risk factors for developing type 2 diabetes, namely:

- A family history of type 2 diabetes
- Having prediabetes (FPG concentration between 100 and 126 mg/dL or a 2-hour OGTT value between 140 and 200 mg/dL)
- Being overweight
- Hypertension or abnormal cholesterol levels
- History of GDM and/or having given birth to a baby weighing >9 lb
- A member of an ethnic group who has a high incidence of diabetes (American Indians, Latinos, Pacific Islanders, Asian Indians, and African Americans).

The 3234, mostly obese (BMI >31 kg/m^2), participants in the 3½-year DPP study were randomized into one of four treatment groups. The first group was the intensive lifestyle-change group (goals: exercise at least 150 minutes per week and 7% loss of baseline body weight).

15

The other three groups received MET (Glucophage), troglitazone (Rezulin), or placebo, with only minimal lifestyle changes. The DPP is the only study to date that compared lifestyle modifications and pharmacologic interventions.

The DPP ended 1 year early because of the remarkable results gathered from 25 research institutions around the United States that included >4000 subjects. Compared with the placebo group, the subjects randomized to the intensive lifestyle-change group reduced their chances of developing type 2 diabetes by an impressive 58%. In addition, intensive lifestyle changes were effective in all age groups and in both obese and nonobese subjects. Individuals who were given MET with minimal lifestyle changes showed a reduction of 31% in the development of diabetes over the course of study compared with the placebo group. Subanalysis of the results revealed that MET was most effective in younger (<45 years old), heavier (BMI >30 kg/m^2) subjects compared with the older, nonobese subjects. There was also a highly significant (approximately 75%) early reduction in the conversion to type 2 diabetes in the troglitazone group near the end of the first year of the study, although this group was only on medication for an average of 10 months because troglitazone was withdrawn from the study due to liver toxicity. All interventions were more effective in subjects who were randomized earlier in the natural history of their disease (ie, a 2-hour OGTT value between 140 and 160 mg/dL) compared with the subjects whose initial 2-hour OGTT value was between 180 and 200 mg/dL.

During 10-year follow-up since randomization in the original DPP study, the original lifestyle group lost and then partly regained weight. The modest weight loss with MET was maintained. In the 10-year follow-up study, diabetes incidence rates were similar between treatment groups: 5.9, 4.9, 5.6 per 100 person-years for lifestyle, for MET, and for placebo, respectively. The diabetes incidence rates in the 10 years since DPP randomization were reduced by 34% in the lifestyle group and 18% in the MET group compared with placebo. These results indicate that prevention or delay of diabetes with lifestyle intervention or MET can persist for at least 10 years.

■ Troglitazone in the Prevention of Diabetes (TRIPOD) Study

The TRIPOD study provided several important findings. The first important result was that diabetes could be prevented and delayed with troglitazone (400 mg/day) by 56% compared with the placebo group in a cohort of high-risk, nonpregnant, nondiabetic Hispanic women who had a recent history of GDM. In addition, metabolic studies performed during and after the study demonstrated prolonged preservation of pancreatic or β-cell function in the troglitazone-treated group even after the drug was discontinued. Although troglitazone is no longer on the market, this study suggested that similar benefits may be achieved with the other insulin sensitizers that are available (rosiglitazone [Avandia] and pioglitazone [Actos]).

■ Study to Prevent Non–Insulin-Dependent Diabetes Mellitus (STOP-NIDDM)

In the 3-year STOP-NIDDM, patients with IGT were randomized to receive either the carbohydrate-absorption inhibitor acarbose 100 mg tid or placebo. By the end of the study, 32% of patients in the acarbose group and 42% of those in the placebo group developed diabetes, corresponding to a risk reduction of ~25% ($P = 0.0015$). In addition, there was a reduction in CV risk in the acarbose-treated group. The results of this study raised some controversy since 4% of patients were excluded from the intention-to-treat analysis because they did not have IGT at screening or had no postrandomization data. Furthermore, 9.3% of the study population had a fasting plasma glucose value at screening that, according to more recent criteria, could be considered diagnostic of diabetes. However, subsequent analysis in which these patients were excluded still found a significant ($P = 0.0027$) risk reduction with acarbose treatment.

■ Xenical in the Prevention of Diabetes Mellitus in Obese Subjects (XENDOS) Trial

This double-blind trial randomized 3305 patients to lifestyle changes plus either the weight-loss agent orlistat 120 mg or placebo three times daily. Participants had a BMI ≥30 kg/m^2 and normoglycemia (79%) or IGT

15

(21%). After 4 years' treatment, the cumulative incidence of diabetes was 9.0% with placebo and 6.2% with orlistat, corresponding to a risk reduction of 37% ($P = 0.0032$). However, subsequent analyses indicated that the difference in diabetes incidence was detectable only in the subgroup of patients with IGT.

■ Diabetes Reduction Assessment With Ramipril and Rosiglitazone Medication (DREAM) Trial

In the DREAM trial, 5269 people with IFG or IGT, or both, and no previous CV disease were randomized to receive ramipril (15 mg/day) or placebo, or rosiglitazone (8 mg/day) or placebo, using a 2×2 factorial design and were followed for a median of 3 years. The primary outcome was a composite of incident diabetes or death (included because undiagnosed diabetes may be more frequent in those who die than in those who do not).

Ramipril modestly improved glycemic status, including a 9% nonsignificant reduction in the incidence of diabetes and a significant 16% increase in regression to normal glucose levels. In addition, ramipril significantly reduced blood pressure and had a small, favorable effect on liver function. A significantly smaller proportion of patients in the rosiglitazone group than in the placebo group developed the composite primary outcome (11.6% vs 26.0%, respectively, $P < 0.0001$).

Similarly, 10.6% of rosiglitazone-treated patients developed diabetes vs 25% of those that received placebo ($P < 0.0001$), a risk reduction of 62%. Furthermore, the proportion of patients who became normoglycemic by at least 2 years was significantly greater with rosiglitazone than with placebo (50.5% vs 30.3%, respectively; $P < 0.0001$).

While mean body weight increased by ~3% (2.2 kg) with rosiglitazone more than with placebo, there was a favorable effect on the waist/hip ratio with rosiglitazone. In addition, decreases in systolic and diastolic blood pressure with rosiglitazone (1.7 mmHg and 1.4 mmHg, respectively) were greater than the decreases with placebo ($P < 0.0001$). CV event rates were similar in both groups, although 14 (0.5%) patients in the rosiglitazone group and two (0.1%) in the placebo group developed heart failure ($P = 0.01$). However, there were no cases of fatal heart failure. At the final visit, 6.8% of subjects in the rosiglitazone group reported peripheral edema vs 4.9% in the placebo group ($P = 0.003$).

■ Actos Now for Prevention of Diabetes (ACT-NOW) Trial

The double-blind, placebo-controlled ACT-NOW trial assessed whether pioglitazone can reduce the risk of type 2 diabetes in adult patients with IGT. A total of 602 patients were enrolled and the median follow-up period was 2.4 years. Conversion to diabetes was confirmed on the basis of the results of repeat testing of fasting glucose and oral glucose tolerance. Annual incidence rates for type 2 diabetes mellitus were 2.1% in the pioglitazone group and 7.6% in the placebo group, resulting in a relative risk reduction of 72% for conversion to diabetes in the pioglitazone group ($P <0.001$) (**Figure 15.1**). In addition, 48% of the patients in the pioglitazone group converted to normal glucose tolerance compared with 28% of those in the placebo group ($P <0.001$). A1C decreased by 0.04% with pioglitazone treatment while it increased by 0.20% with placebo ($P <0.001$). Compared with placebo, there also were significantly greater reductions in fasting glucose with pioglitazone compared with placebo (11.7 mg/dL and 8.1 mg/dL, respectively,

FIGURE 15.1 — ACT-NOW: Kaplan-Meier Plot of HRs for Time to Development of Diabetes

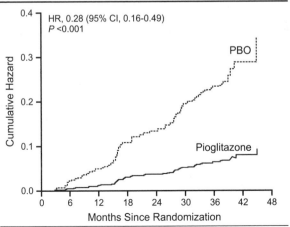

HR, 0.28 (95% CI, 0.16-0.49)
$P <0.001$

DeFronzo RA, et al. *N Engl J Med*. 2011;364:1104-1115.

P <0.001), as well as 2-hour postprandial glucose (30.5 mg/dL vs 15.6 mg/dL, pioglitazone and placebo, respectively, P <0.001). Other findings included a significantly greater decrease in diastolic BP with pioglitazone vs placebo (2.0 mmHg vs 0.0 mmHg, P = 0.03), a reduced rate of carotid intima-media thickening (31.5%, P = 0.047), and a greater increase in the level of HDL-c (7.35 mg/dL vs 4.5 mg/dL, P = 0.008). However, weight gain was greater with pioglitazone than with placebo (3.9 kg vs 0.77 kg, P <0.001), and edema was more frequent (12.9% vs 6.4%, P = 0.007).

■ Nateglinide and Valsartan in Impaired Glucose Tolerance Outcomes Research (NAVIGATOR) Trial

This randomized, double-blind, clinical trial in a total of 9306 subjects with impaired glucose tolerance and either CV disease or CV risk factors used a 2 × 2 factorial design to assign individuals to treatment with nateglinide vs placebo, or valsartan vs placebo, in addition to participation in a lifestyle-modification program. Participants were followed for a median of 5 years. Treatment with nateglinide did not reduce the incidence of diabetes or the co-primary composite CV outcomes. Although treatment with valsartan resulted in a relative reduction of 14% in the incidence of diabetes, it did not reduce the rate of CV events.

Reduced Diabetes Risk in Other Trials

The recently completed ORIGIN trial enrolled over 12,000 subjects over the age of 50 with at least one CV risk factor and either prediabetes (IFG and/or IGT) or early type 2 diabetes. The primary objective was to determine if insulin replacement therapy targeting normal fasting glucose (<95 mg/dL) with insulin glargine reduces the risk of CV events more than standard-care approaches to glycemic control and, in a factorial design, the impact of omega-3 fatty acids. After a median follow-up of 6.2 years, insulin glargine had a neutral effect on cardiovascular outcomes and cancers. However, this study also assessed the progression to type 2 diabetes in subjects with prediabetes (n=752). In this population, insulin glargine resulted in a 28% relative reduction in the development of diabetes, although it also increased hypoglycemia and modestly increased weight.

Several other large-scale clinical trials (**Table 15.2**) reported a remarkably consistent reduction in the incidence of type 2 diabetes in patients with hypertension and/or other CV risk factors treated with either ACE inhibitors (including ramipril) or ARBs for 3 to 6 years. However, unlike the DREAM trial, the effect on the incidence of new-onset diabetes was either a secondary end point or a post hoc analysis.

Taken together, the results of these trials add further evidence that the development of diabetes can be delayed and possibly prevented.

Who Should Be Screened

According to the American Diabetes Association's Standards of Care, screening for prediabetes and diabetes should be conducted with a fasting plasma glucose, A1C, or 75-g 2-hour OGTT in individuals >45 years of age.. Screening should also be considered for people who are <45 years of age and are overweight (BMI >25 kg/m^2) if they have another risk factor, such as a first-degree relative with diabetes or previous GDM, or if they are of an ethnicity other than Caucasian or have hypertension or dyslipidemia. Asian-Americans should be considered for screening at lower levels of BMI (eg, 23 kg/m^2).

Although the results of the trials discussed above are encouraging, broader implementation of screening has been slowed by concern over the cost effectiveness of early interventions in high-risk patients. This concern was addressed in the analysis of the 10-year cost-effectiveness data from the DPP/DPPOS studies which demonstrates that intensive lifestyle intervention is indeed cost effective, and MET is marginally cost-saving, or at least cost-neutral, compared with placebo. Even when the direct nonmedical costs of the interventions are considered, the interventions are cost effective.

Since the natural history of prediabetes is variable, with some patients progressing to type 2 diabetes, some remaining in the prediabetes state, and other regressing

15

TABLE 15.2 — Reduction of Diabetes Risk in Trials With Other Primary End Points

Study	Intervention	Sample Size	Reduction in Diabetes Risk (%)
ALLHAT	Lisinopril	1399[a]	30
CAPPP	Captopril	10,413[b]	14
HOPE	Ramipril	5270[b]	34
LIFE	Losartan	7998[b]	25
ORIGIN	Insulin glargine	1452[a]	28
VALUE	Valsartan	9995[b]	23
WOSCOPS	Pravastatin	5974[b]	30

[a] Cohort with impaired glucose tolerance/prediabetes.
[b] Nondiabetic subjects at increased risk for cardiovascular events.

Adapted from Scheen AJ. *Drugs*. 2004;64:2537-2565; Skyler JS. *Clin Diabetes*. 2004;22:162-166.

to normal glucose regulation, there has been a heightened recent interest in more specific tests that may identify individuals with prediabetes with the greatest risk of type 2 diabetes. The PreDx test (Tethys Bioscience, Inc, Emeryville, CA) is a multianalyte blood test that measures seven biomarkers: fasting glucose, A1C, insulin, hs-CRP, ferritin, interleukin 2 receptor-α, and adiponectin. A validated algorithm is applied to these markers, along with age and gender, and a score between 1 and 10 is generated that estimates the 5-year likelihood of progression from prediabetes to type 2 diabetes. The test is used in clinical practice to help health care providers tailor diabetes prevention interventions in high-risk patients.

Summary

A substantial and growing body of evidence suggests that the onset of type 2 diabetes in patients with prediabetes can be delayed or prevented by several interventions, including intensive lifestyle modification and pharmacologic strategies such as MET, TZDs, and acarbose. Although the long-term efficacy, safety, and durability of the benefits of pharmacologic interventions need further study, they may offer a new strategy for reducing the ongoing epidemic and burden of type 2 diabetes.

15

Abuissa H, Jones PG, Marso SP, O'Keefe JH Jr. Angiotensin-converting enzyme inhibitors or angiotensin receptor blockers for prevention of type 2 diabetes: a meta-analysis of randomized clinical trials. *J Am Coll Cardiol*. 2005;46:821-826.

American Diabetes Association and National Institute of Diabetes, Digestive and Kidney Diseases. The prevention or delay of type 2 diabetes. *Diabetes Care*. 2002;25:742-749.

Buchanan TA, Xiang AH, Peters RK, et al. Preservation of pancreatic beta-cell function and prevention of type 2 diabetes by pharmacological treatment of insulin resistance in high-risk hispanic women. *Diabetes*. 2002;51:2796-2803.

Burnet DL, Elliott LD, Quinn MT, Plaut AJ, Schwartz MA, Chin MH. Preventing diabetes in the clinical setting. *J Gen Intern Med*. 2006;21: 84-93.

Centers for Disease Control and Prevention. National diabetes fact sheet: national estimates and general information on diabetes and prediabetes in the United States, 2011. Atlanta, GA: U.S. Department of Health and Human Services, Centers for Disease Control and Prevention, 2011. CDC Web site. http://www.cdc.gov/diabetes/pubs/pdf /ndfs_2011.pdf. Accessed June 12, 2013.

Chiasson JL, Brindisi MC, Rabasa-Lhoret R. The prevention of type 2 diabetes: what is the evidence? *Minerva Endocrinol*. 2005;30:179-191.

Chiasson JL, Josse RG, Gomis R, Hanefeld M, Karasik A, Laakso M; STOP-NIDDM Trial Research Group. Acarbose for prevention of type 2 diabetes mellitus: the STOP-NIDDM randomised trial. *Lancet*. 2002;359:2072-2077.

DeFronzo RA, Tripathy D, Schwenke DC, et al; ACT NOW Study. Pioglitazone for diabetes prevention in impaired glucose tolerance. *N Engl J Med*. 2011;364:1104-1115.

Diabetes Prevention Research Group. Reduction in the evidence of type 2 diabetes with life-style intervention or metformin. *N Engl J Med*. 2002;346:393-403.

Diabetes Prevention Program Research Group. The 10-year cost-effectiveness of lifestyle intervention or metformin. an intent-to-treat analysis of the DPP/DPPOS. *Diabetes Care*. 2012;35:723-730.

Diabetes Prevention Program Research Group ; Knowler WC, Fowler SE, Hamman RF, et al: 10-year follow-up of diabetes incidence and weight loss in the Diabetes Prevention Program Outcomes Study. *Lancet*. 2009;374:1677-1686.

DREAM Trial Investigators. Rationale, design and recruitment characteristics of a large, simple international trial of diabetes prevention: the DREAM trial. *Diabetologia*. 2004;47:1519-1527.

DREAM Trial Investigators; Bosch J, Yusuf S, Gerstein HC, et al. Effect of ramipril on the incidence of diabetes. *N Engl J Med*. 2006;355:1551-1562.

DREAM (Diabetes REduction Assessment with ramipril and rosiglitazone Medication) Trial Investigators; Gerstein HC, Yusuf S, Bosch J, et al. Effect of rosiglitazone on the frequency of diabetes in patients with impaired glucose tolerance or impaired fasting glucose: a randomised controlled trial. *Lancet*. 2006;368:1096-1105.

Eriksson KF, Lindgarde F. Prevention of type 2 (non-insulin-dependent) diabetes mellitus by diet and physical exercise. The 6-year Malmo feasibility study. *Diabetologia*. 1991;34:891-898.

Freeman DJ, Norrie J, Sattar N, et al. Pravastatin and the development of diabetes mellitus: evidence for a protective treatment effect in the West of Scotland Coronary Prevention Study. *Circulation*. 2001;103:357-362.

Kjeldsen SE, Julius S, Mancia G, et al; VALUE Trial Investigators. Effects of valsartan compared to amlodipine on preventing type 2 diabetes in high-risk hypertensive patients: the VALUE trial. *J Hypertens*. 2006;24:1405-1412.

Knowler WC, Barrett-Connor E, Fowler SE, et al; Diabetes Prevention Program Research Group. Reduction in the incidence of type 2 diabetes with lifestyle intervention or metformin. *N Engl J Med*. 2002; 346:393-403.

Kolberg J, Gerwien R, Watkins S, Wuestehube LJ, Urdea M. Biomarkers in type 2 diabetes: improving risk stratification with the PreDx diabetes risk score. *Expert Rev Mol Diagn*. 2011;11:775-792.

Lindholm LH, Ibsen H, Borch-Johnsen K, et al; the LIFE study group. Risk of new-onset diabetes in the Losartan Intervention For Endpoint reduction in hypertension study. *J Hypertens*. 2002;20:1879-1886.

McCall KL, Craddock D, Edwards K. Effect of angiotensin-converting enzyme inhibitors and angiotensin II type 1 receptor blockers on the rate of new-onset diabetes mellitus: a review and pooled analysis. *Pharmacotherapy*. 2006;26:1297-1306.

NAVIGATOR Study Group; Holman RR, Haffner SM, McMurray JJ, et al. Effect of nateglinide on the incidence of diabetes and cardiovascular events. *N Engl J Med*. 2010;362:1463-1476.

NAVIGATOR Study Group; McMurray JJ, Holman RR, Haffner SM, et al. Effect of valsartan on the incidence of diabetes and cardiovascular events. *N Engl J Med*. 2010;362:1477-1490.

15

Niklason A, Hedner T, Niskanen L, Lanke J; Captopril Prevention Project Study Group. Development of diabetes is retarded by ACE inhibition in hypertensive patients—a subanalysis of the Captopril Prevention Project (CAPPP). *J Hypertens*. 2004;22:645-652.

ORIGIN Trial Investigators; Gerstein HC, Bosch J, Dagenais GR, et al. Basal insulin and cardiovascular and other outcomes in dysglycemia. *N Engl J Med*. 2012;367:319-328.

Scheen AJ. Prevention of type 2 diabetes mellitus through inhibition of the Renin-Angiotensin system. *Drugs*. 2004;64:2537-2565.

Skyler JS. Effects of glycemic control on diabetes complications and on the prevention of diabetes. *Clin Diabetes*. 2004;22:162-166.

Sjostrom L. Analysis of the XENDOS study (Xenical in the Prevention of Diabetes in Obese Subjects). *Endocr Pract*. 2006;12(suppl 1):31-33.

Torgerson JS, Hauptman J, Boldrin MN, Sjostrom L. XENical in the prevention of diabetes in obese subjects (XENDOS) study: a randomized study of orlistat as an adjunct to lifestyle changes for the prevention of type 2 diabetes in obese patients. *Diabetes Care*. 2004:155-161.

Tuomilehto J, Lindstrom J, Eriksson JG, et al; Finnish Diabetes Prevention Study Group. Prevention of type 2 diabetes mellitus by changes in lifestyle among subjects with impaired glucose tolerance. *N Engl J Med*. 2001;344:1343-1350.

Urdea M, Kolberg J, Wilber J, et al. Validation of a multimarker model for assessing risk of type 2 diabetes from a five-year prospective study of 6784 Danish people (Inter99). *J Diabetes Sci Technol*. 2009;3:748-755.

Yusuf S, Sleight P, Pogue J, Bosch J, Davies R, Dagenais G. Effects of an angiotensin-converting-enzyme inhibitor, ramipril, on cardiovascular events in high-risk patients. The Heart Outcomes Prevention Evaluation Study Investigators. *N Engl J Med*. 2000;342:145-153.

16 Resources

Academy of Nutrition and Dietetics
(formerly the American Dietetic Association)
120 S. Riverside Plaza, Suite 2000
Chicago, IL 60606-6995
800/877-1600 or 312/899-0040
www.eatright.org

The Academy of Nutrition and Dietetics is the nation's largest organization of food and nutrition professionals. Information on the website includes nutritional information and links to help find a nutritional professional in a given city or state. Fact sheets are available for healthy habits to help manage and prevent type 2 diabetes, as well as general eating tips and recipes.

American Association of Diabetes Educators (AADE)
200 W. Madison, Suite 800
Chicago, IL 60606
312/644-2233 or 800/338-3633
800/TEAMUP4 (800/832-6874) (Diabetes Educator Access Line)
www.aadenet.org

AADE is a multidisciplinary organization, with state and regional chapters, for health professionals involved in diabetes patient education. The organization sponsors a certification program for diabetes educators and provides grants, scholarships, and awards for educational research and teaching activities. AADE's annual meeting features continuing education programs on diabetes treatment and education. The organization also features a Diabetes Educator Access Line to help people with diabetes locate diabetes education services in their area.

Publications: AADE publishes a bimonthly journal, *The Diabetes Educator*; curriculum guides; consensus statements; self-study programs; and other print and nonprint resources for diabetes educators.

American Association of Kidney Patients (AAKP)
2701 N. Rocky Point Drive
Suite 150
Tampa, FL 33607
800/749-2257 or 813/636-8100
www.aakp.org

AAKP exists to serve the needs, interests, and welfare of all kidney patients and their families. It is a national organization consisting of patients, family members, renal professionals, friends, and institutional members. It contains information regarding reduced kidney function or chronic kidney disease, dialysis, and transplants.

American Diabetes Association (ADA)
Attn: Center for Information
1701 North Beauregard Street
Alexandria, VA 22311
800/342-2383
www.diabetes.org

ADA is both a professional association and a private, nonprofit, voluntary organization with state and local affiliates and chapters. It serves people with diabetes and their families and friends, as well as health professionals and research scientists involved in diabetes-related activities. The organization funds diabetes research and education activities; sponsors educational programs, including an annual meeting, postgraduate courses, consensus meetings, and special symposia; administers a recognition program for diabetes outpatient education; develops professional guidelines for diabetes care; and advocates for diabetes issues in the legislative and public health arenas. Local ADA affiliates often sponsor educational programs and support groups for persons with diabetes and their families.

Publications: ADA publishes monthly and quarterly magazines for patients, including *Diabetes Forecast*; professional journals focusing on basic and clinical research, including *Diabetes*, *Diabetes Care*, *Diabetes Spectrum*, and *Diabetes Reviews*; other publications, including cookbooks, meal planing guides, pamphlets, brochures, and books for patients; and clinical manuals, nutritional guides, audiovisuals, statistical reports, and curriculum guides for professionals.

American Heart Association
Diabetes Information
National Center
7272 Greenville Avenue
Dallas, TX 75231
800/AHA-USA1 (800/242-8721)
http://www.heart.org/HEARTORG/Conditions/Diabetes/Diabetes_UCM_001091_SubHomePage.jsp

This website is filled with important information about type 2 diabetes, insulin resistance, and related cardiovascular risks, as well as ways to reduce chances of heart disease and other complications in diabetes. Information for both the patient and the health care professional is available. There are tools for monitoring blood glucose, blood pressure, and cholesterol.

Centers for Disease Control and Prevention (CDC)
National Center for Chronic Disease Prevention
and Health Promotion (NCCDPHP)
4770 Buford Highway NE
MS K-40
Atlanta, GA 30341-3717
800/CDC-INFO (800/232-4636)
www.cdc.gov/diabetes

An agency of the Public Health Service, Department of Health and Human Services, the CDC develops public health approaches to reduce the burden of diabetes in the United States. The agency supports diabetes-control programs in 26 states and one territory; carries out state and national surveillance activities to assess diabetes prevalence, impact, and possible contributing factors; develops consensus guidelines for clinical and public health practice; supports community-based preventive programs for minority populations and the elderly; and coordinates federal activities concerned with translating research findings into clinical practice, including issues related to cost and reimbursement practices, disability, and quality of life.

Publications: The CDC distributes a practice manual for primary care practitioners and a companion guide for patients, surveillance reports, and guidelines on patient education, educational reimbursement, and maternal and child health. State programs have produced patient and professional publications.

Indian Health Service (IHS)
Division of Diabetes Treatment and Prevention
5300 Homestead Road
Albuquerque, NM 87110
505/248-4182
www.ihs.gov/medicalprograms/diabetes

An agency of the Public Health Service, Department of Health and Human Services, IHS supports 17 model Diabetes Health Care Programs serving Native Americans and Alaskans. These programs develop and evaluate effective and culturally accepted prevention and treatment methods for diabetes and its complications. Diabetes-control officers in each IHS region provide surveillance, training, and other services to promote the use of techniques recommended by the program.

16

Publications: The model programs and the IHS produce culturally relevant publications for native populations, including nutrition guides, complication-specific educational materials, and guides for professionals. Publications are available only to persons working with Native Americans or Alaskan populations.

International Diabetes Federation (IDF)
166 Chaussee de La Hulpe
B-1170 Brussels, Belgium
+32-2-538-5511
www.idf.org

IDF collaborates with more than 100 member associations in over 80 countries, the World Health Organization, and other affiliated organizations and individuals to ensure that people with diabetes receive quality treatment and education services.

Publications: IDF publishes a newsletter, a journal entitled *IDF Bulletin, The Directory 1991: A Guide to the Activities of Member Diabetes Associations*, as well as other publications.

InsulinDependence, Inc.
249 S. Highway 101, 8000
Solana Beach, CA 92075
888/912-3837
www.insulindependence.org

The Diabetes Exercise and Sports Association merged with InsulinDependence in 2011. The organization inspires people with diabetes to set personal fitness goals, educates them on adaptive management strategies through hands-on experience, and equips them to explore their individual capacities.

Joslin Diabetes Center
One Joslin Place
Boston, MA 02215
617/309-2400
www.joslin.org

The Joslin Diabetes Center offers inpatient and outpatient treatment, education, and other support services to adults and children with diabetes; provides professional medical education; sponsors camps for children with diabetes; and supports research to improve treatment and find a cure for diabetes and its complications. The center is affiliated with Harvard Medical School and a number of hospitals in the Boston area and operates affiliated clinics in several states. The Joslin Diabetes Center is one of six Diabetes Endocrinology Research Centers supported by the National Institute of Diabetes and Digestive Kidney Diseases.

Publications: Joslin produces a variety of educational materials for patients and professionals, including manuals, nutrition guides, materials for children with diabetes, and films. *The Joslin Magazine* is issued quarterly to members of the Joslin Society.

Juvenile Diabetes Research Foundation (JDRF)
26 Broadway
New York, NY 10004
800/533-CURE (2873)
www.jdrf.org

JDRF is a private, nonprofit, voluntary organization with chapters throughout the world. JDRF raises funds to support research on the cause, cure, treatment, and prevention of diabetes and its complications. The organization awards research grants for laboratory and clinical investigations and sponsors a variety of career development and research training programs for new and established investigators. JDRF also sponsors international workshops and conferences for biomedical researchers. Individual chapters offer support groups and other activities for families.

Publications: JDRF publishes the quarterly journal *Countdown* and a series of patient education brochures about insulin-dependent and non–insulin-dependent diabetes.

National Diabetes Education Initiative (NDEI)
125 Chubb Avenue
Lyndhurst, NJ 07071
800/471-7745
www.ndei.org

NDEI is a multicomponent educational program on type 2 diabetes that is designed for endocrinologists, diabetologists, primary care physicians, and other health care professionals. NDEI programs address issues such as epidemiology and pathophysiology, rationale for treatment and management guidelines, microvascular and macrovascular complications, therapeutic options and prevention.

National Diabetes Education Program (NDEP)
One Diabetes Way
Bethesda, MD 20814-9692
888/693-6337
www.ndep.nih.gov

NDEP is a federally sponsored initiative that involves public and private partners to improve the treatment and outcomes for people with diabetes, to promote early diagnosis, and ultimately to prevent the onset of diabetes. NDEP is sponsored by the National Institute of Diabetes and Digestive and Kidney Disease (NIDDK) of the National Institutes of Health (NIH) and the Division of Diabetes Translation of the Centers for Disease Control and Prevention (CDC).

Publications: NDEP offers a variety of publications and videos for use by the general public, people with diabetes, and health care providers. These materials are provided in both English and Spanish formats.

16

369

National Eye Institute (NEI)
National Eye Health Education Program (NEHEP)
31 Center Drive, MSC 2510
Bethesda, MD 20892-2510
301/496-5248
www.nei.nih.gov

NEI, one of the National Institutes of Health, supports basic and clinical research to develop effective treatments for diabetic eye disease. The institute's National Eye Health Education Program promotes public and professional awareness of the importance of early diagnosis and treatment of diabetic eye disease.

Publications: NEI produces patient and professional education materials related to diabetic eye disease and its treatment, including literature for patients, guides for health professionals, and education kits for community health workers and for pharmacists.

National Institute of Diabetes and Digestive and Kidney Diseases (NIDDK)
National Institutes of Health (NIH)
Bldg 31, Room 9A06
31 Center Drive, MSC 2560
Bethesda, MD 20892-2560
301/496-3583
www.niddk.nih.gov

NIDDK conducts and supports research on many of the most serious diseases affecting public health, including diabetes. The website has information about the NIDDK, news releases, event information, health information and education programs, patient recruitment, coordination of federal programs, and research funding and programs.

National Kidney Foundation
30 East 33rd St.
New York, NY 10016
212/889-2210 or 800/622-9010
www.kidney.org

The National Kidney Foundation is a major voluntary health organization, seeking to prevent kidney and urinary tract diseases, improve the health and well-being of individuals and families affected by these diseases, and increase the availability of all organs for transplantation. The web site has information for organ and tissue donors and recipients, health care professionals, patients, meetings and events.

Taking Control Of Your Diabetes

1110 Camino Del Mar, Suite B
Del Mar, CA 92014
800/99-TCOYD (800/998-2693)
or 858/755-5683 (main line)
858/755-6854 (fax)
www.tcoyd.org

Taking Control of Your Diabetes (TCOYD) is a nonprofit organization dedicated to promoting advocacy programs for people with diabetes. The two main goals of the organization are to (1) educate people with diabetes about how to live longer by learning about their condition, and (2) educate patients to be self-advocates and work within their health care program to get the help they need to maintain a high standard of care. TCOYD maintains their mission by producing large patient-oriented educational and motivational events nationwide, in addition to providing educational videos, audiotapes, and reading materials. TCOYD also conducts a series of medical education seminars for professionals. TCOYD has an 800 number help line and web site to assist people with diabetes and their families.

16

17

Abbreviations/Acronyms

A1C	glycosylated hemoglobin
AACE	American Association of Clinical Endocrinologists
AADE	American Association of Diabetes Educators
AAKP	American Association of Kidney Patients
ACCORD	Action to Control Cardiovascular Risk in Diabetes
ACE	angiotensin-converting enzyme
ACT-NOW	Actos Now for Prevention of Diabetes
ADA	American Diabetes Association
ADOPT	A Diabetes Outcome Progression Trial
AGI	alpha-glucosidase inhibitor
AHA	American Heart Association
ALLHAT	Antihypertensive and Lipid-Lowering Treatment to Prevent Heart Attack Trial
ALT	alanine aminotransferase
ARB	angiotensin II receptor blocker
AST	aspartate aminotransferase
AUC	area under the curve
BAS	bile acid sequestrant
bid	twice daily
BL	baseline
BMI	body mass index
BNP	B-type natriuretic peptide
BUN	blood urea nitrogen
CABG	coronary artery bypass grafting
CANA	canagliflozin
CAPPP	Captopril Prevention Project
CARDS	Collaborative Atorvastatin Diabetes Study
CARE	Cholesterol and Recurrent Events
CCB	calcium channel blocker
CDC	Centers for Disease Control
CGM	continuous glucose monitoring
CHD	coronary heart disease
CHF	congestive heart failure
CI	confidence interval
CPK	creatinine phosphokinase

17

CrCl	creatinine clearance
CRP	C-reactive protein
CV	cardiovascular
CVD	cardiovascular disease
DAIS	Diabetes Atherosclerosis Intervention Study
DCCT	Diabetes Control and Complications Trial
DPP-4	dipeptidyl peptidase-4
DESA	Diabetes Exercise and Sports Association
DKA	diabetic ketoacidosis
DPP	Diabetes Prevention Program
DREAM	Diabetes Reduction Assessment With Ramipril and Rosiglitazone Medication
EASD	European Association for the Study of Diabetes
ECG	electrocardiogram
ED	erectile dysfunction
ESRD	end-stage renal disease
EXEN	exenatide
FBG	fasting blood glucose
FDA	Food and Drug Administration
FDC	fixed-dose combination
FDPS	Finnish Diabetes Prevention Study
4S	Scandinavian Simvastatin Survival Study
FPG	fasting plasma glucose
GAD	glutamic acid decarboxylase
GDM	gestational diabetes mellitus
GI	gastrointestinal
GIP	glucose-dependent insulinotropic polypeptide
GLIM	glimepiride
GLP-1	glucogonlike peptide 1
GLUT2	glucose transporter 2
h	hour(s)
HCO3	concentration of bicarbonate
HDL	high-density lipoprotein
HGM	home glucose monitoring
HHNS	hyperosmolar hyperglycemic nonketotic syndrome
HIS	Indian Health Services
HMG-CoA	hydroxymethyl-glutaryl-coenzyme A
HOMA	homeostasis model assessment
HOMA-B	homeostatis model assessment–β-cell function

HOMA-IR	homeostatis model assessment–insulin resistance
HOPE	Heart Outcomes Prevention Evaluation
HPS	Heart Protection Study
HR	hazard ratio
ICA	islet cell antibody
IDF	International Diabetes Federation
IFG	impaired fasting glucose
IGT	impaired glucose tolerance
INSG	insulin glargine
ITT	intent-to-treat
IV	intravenous
JDRF	Juvenile Diabetes Research Foundation
K	concentration of potassium
K^+	potassium
LADA	latent autoimmune diabetes in adults
lb	pound
LDH	lactate dehydrogenase
LDL	low-density lipoprotein
LEAD	Liraglutide Effect and Action in Diabetes [trial]
LFT	liver function test
LIFE	Losartan Intervention for Endpoint Reduction in Hypertension [study]
LIRA	liraglutide
LOCF	last observation carried forward
LS	least square
MACE	major adverse cardiac events
MCP-1	monocyte chemoattractant protein-1
MDI	multiple daily injection
MET	metformin
MI	myocardial infarction
min	minute(s)
MTT	meal tolerance test
n, N	number [of subjects]
Na^+	sodium
NAVIGATOR	Nateglinide and Valsartan in Impaired Glucose Tolerance Outcomes Research
NCEP	National Cholesterol Education Program
NDCCB	nondihydropyridine calcium channel blocker
NDEI	National Diabetes Education Initiative
NDEP	National Diabetes Education Program
NEI	National Eye Institute

17

NFkappaB	nuclear factor kappa–binding
NIDDK	National Institute of Diabetes and Digestive and Kidney Diseases
NIDDM	non–insulin-dependent diabetes mellitus
NPH	neutral protamine Hagedorn [insulin]
NS	not significant
NSAID	nonsteroidal anti-inflammatory drug
NYHA	New York Heart Association
OAD	oral antidiabetic drug
OGTT	oral glucose tolerance test
ORIGIN	Outcome Reduction With an Initial Glargine Intervention
PAI-1	plasminogen activator inhibitor-1
PBO	placebo
PCI	percutaneous coronary intervention
PIO	pioglitazone
PPAR	peroxisome proliferator-activated receptor
PPG	postprandial glucose
PROactive	Prospective Pioglitazone Clinical Trial in Macrovascular Events
PVD	peripheral vascular disease
qd	every day
REMS	risk evaluation and mitigation strategy
RESULT	Rosiglitazone Early vs Sulphonylurea Titration [trial]
RSG	rosiglitazone
SAXA	saxagliptin
SC	subcutaneous
SD	standard deviation
SE	standard error
SEM	standard error of mean
SFU	sulfonylurea
SGLT2	sodium glucose cotransporter type 2
SMBG	self-monitoring of blood glucose
STOP-NIDDM	Study to Prevent Non–Insulin-Dependent Diabetes Mellitus
TCOYD	Taking Control of Your Diabetes
TENS	transcutaneous electrical nerve stimulation
tid	three times per day
TRIPOD	Troglitazone in the Prevention of Diabetes
TZD	thiazolidinediones
U	units
UKPDS	United Kingdom Prospective Diabetes Study

USDA	United States Department of Agriculture
UTI	urinary tract infection
VADT	Veterans Affairs Diabetes Trial
VA-HIT	Veterans Affairs High-Density Lipoprotein Intervention Trial
VALUE	Valsartan Antihypertensive Long-Term Use Evaluation [trial]
VLDL	very low-density lipoprotein
WBC	white blood cell (count)
WOSCOPS	West of Scotland Coronary Prevention Study
XENDOS	Xenical in the Prevention of Diabetes Mellitus in Obese Subjects
XR	extended release
y	year(s)

17

Note: Page numbers in *italics* indicate figures.
Page numbers followed by a "t" indicate tables.
Clinical trials are listed by their acronyms.

18

18

18

18

18

18

18

18

18

18

18

18

18

18

18

18

18

412

18

18

18

18